SECOND EDITION

Global Public Health
A new era

SECOND EDITION

Robert Beaglehole
Emeritus Professor,
University of Auckland,
New Zealand

Ruth Bonita
Emeritus Professor,
University of Auckland,
New Zealand

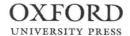

OXFORD
UNIVERSITY PRESS

OXFORD
UNIVERSITY PRESS

Great Clarendon Street, Oxford OX2 6DP
United Kingdom

Oxford University Press is a department of the University of Oxford.
It furthers the University's objective of excellence in research, scholarship,
and education by publishing worldwide.

Oxford is a registered trade mark of Oxford University Press in the UK
and in certain other countries

British Library Cataloguing in Publication Data
Data available

Library of Congress Cataloging in Publication Data
Data available

ISBN 978-0-19-923662-6

Contents

Preface to the second edition

There has been considerable progress in global public health since the first edition of this book was published in 2003. We are optimistic that public health is gradually moving closer to the centre of health affairs, both nationally and globally.

A key reason for our optimism is the availability of evidence on the effectiveness and cost-effectiveness of public health interventions for the improvement of overall levels of population health. However, we are not so certain that we have the tools, or the political will, for improving health equity, the other major goal of public health. Hopefully, the Report of the WHO Commission on the Social Determinants of Health will advance this critical public health challenge.

We recognize the major challenges ahead—both the unfinished agenda represented by the Millennium Development Goals, and the new agenda posed especially by global environmental changes and the pandemic of chronic noncommunicable diseases. There is a continuing need for increased advocacy for global public health, additional resources, and a strengthened public health workforce. An overarching challenge will be to maintain attention on health improvement and health equity in the face of the current global financial crisis.

The second edition of *Global Public Health* has been completely updated. The chapters on India, Canada, and the United Kingdom have been written by new contributors. The book addresses three major issues: the changing global context for public health, the state of public health theory and practice, and strategies for strengthening the practice of public health in the twenty-first century.

The aim of the second edition is to promote the practice of public health in all countries, with an emphasis on low- and middle-income countries. The prime audience for this book is public health practitioners and public health students. We hope to encourage this audience to be more fully engaged with the issues discussed in this book, especially the global aspects of public health. This engagement will go far in promoting global health improvement and health equity. The book will also be of interest to a more general audience with a concern for global health issues.

It has been a pleasure editing this book and we pay tribute to all the contributors.

Robert Beaglehole and Ruth Bonita
Auckland, New Zealand
January 2008

Preface to the first edition

The aim of *Global public health: A new era* is to promote the practice of public health in all countries, with an emphasis on developing countries. It stems from the evidence that public health as a discipline and set of activities has for too long been neglected. The reinvigoration of public health practice is long overdue; it is time for public health practitioners to prepare for the long delayed 'golden age.' This reinvigoration needs to be based on a realistic assessment of the challenges to be faced and the current state of public health practice globally. This is the justification for this book.

Public health is the organized global and local effort to promote and protect the health of populations and to reduce health inequalities. The scope of public health practice is broad and ranges from the control of communicable diseases to the leadership of intersectoral efforts to improve health. The key public health perspective is the population-wide approach to the prevention and control of health problems.

The public health workforce includes people who are involved in protecting and promoting the collective health of whole or specific populations (as distinct from activities directed to patient care). The public health workforce is characterised by its diversity and its complexity and includes people from a wide range of occupational backgrounds. An effective public health workforce is central to the improvement of health system performance in all countries; it contributes to the organization, delivery, and evaluation of health services directed towards both individuals and populations and leads efforts to ensure the health enhancing effects of other related sectors.

Despite impressive health gains in almost all countries over the last few decades, the challenges facing the public health workforce are great and even more difficult to address than in the past. The unfinished agenda of communicable disease control is now greatly complicated by the emergence of new pandemics, notably HIV/AIDS and noncommunicable diseases, the effects of violence in all its manifestations, and global health threats, such as environmental changes. The events of 11 September 2001 in New York, the anthrax attacks in the USA and the subsequent 'war on terrorism' have further widened the scope of public health.

Global public health: A new era grew out of a series of papers published in The Lancet in August and September 2000. The overarching theme of the series was the current state of public health theory and practice in the new and changing global context. The general theme of Global public health is similar to that of The Lancet series. Specifically, Global public health addresses three major issues: the changing global context for public health; the state of public health theory and practice in developed and developing countries; and strategies for strengthening the practice of public health in the twenty-first century.

This book is in three parts. The first part has two aims. Firstly, it surveys the complex old and new challenges facing public health practitioners. Secondly, it summarises the state of health globally using new data based on measures developed by the Word Health Organization and other groups to better describe population health status and trends.

Part two presents the first detailed review of the global state of public health. It analyses the public health situation in all regions of the world. Six chapters cover Europe, North and Latin America, and Australia and New Zealand. Three chapters cover China, Sub-Saharan Africa, and South Asia. The lessons from these chapters are surprisingly similar: the challenges are great; the public health workforce and infrastructure have long been neglected; and much needs to be done to reinvigorate the practice of public health.

The third section covers several cross cutting themes: the impact of the new public health threat from bioterrorism and its implications for the future of public health practice; the developing field of international public health ethics; and the central and neglected role of the public in strengthening the practice of public health. The final chapter summarises the major themes of the book and explores the opportunities for building the capacity of the public health workforce to respond to the major global health needs, Despite the enormity of the challenges facing public health practitioners, especially in developing countries, the tone adopted in the final section of this book is relatively optimistic. Perhaps this is a defensive reaction, but it is hard to imagine the global health situation improving, especially for the most disadvantaged populations, whether in poor or wealthy countries, without the efforts of a strong public health workforce.

This book is not a manual of public health practice; excellent handbooks already exist [1]. Nor is at an encyclopaedia of public health methods and issues; again the details can be found elsewhere [2].

The prime audience for Global public health is public health practitioners and public health students in developed and developing countries. After all, if this audience is not more fully engaged with the issues discussed in this book, the prospects for health of all populations will be bleaker than they should be. The book will also be of interest to a more general audience with a concern for global health issues.

It has been a pleasure editing this book and 1 pay tribute to all the contributors.

References

[1] Penchen D, Guest C, Melzer D, Muir Gray JA (eds.). Oxford Handbook of Public Health Practice, Oxford: Oxford University Press, 2001.

[2] Detels R, McEwen J, Beaglehole R, Tanaka H (eds.). Oxford Textbook of Public Health, 4th edn. Oxford: Oxford University Press, 2002.

Robert Beaglehole
November 2002

About the Editors

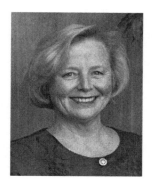

Ruth Bonita is an Emeritus Professor at the University of Auckland, New Zealand and, together with Robert Beaglehole, is a co director of International Public Health Consultants, a New Zealand based company addressing health policy in New Zealand, the Pacific, and globally. Between 1999 and 2005 Ruth was the director of Noncommunicable Disease Surveillance at the World Health Organization, Geneva, where she was involved with mapping the advancing epidemics of stroke and other chronic diseases and the major risk factors which predict them. She led the development a simplified surveillance system, the WHO STEPwise approach to Surveillance (WHO STEPS), suitable for collection of standardized data in low- and middle-income countries where the gaps in information for policy are the greatest.

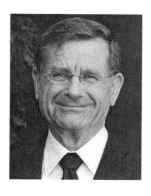

Robert Beaglehole is an Emeritus Professor at the University of Auckland, New Zealand, where he was Professor of Community Health. New Zealand. Between 2004 and 2007, he was the director of the WHO Department of Chronic Disease and Health Promotion, responsible for WHO's technical work in these areas. He developed an integrated and stepwise approach to the prevention and control of chronic diseases and led the development of the Bangkok Charter on Health Promotion in a Globalized World.

This professional couple bring a strong public health perspective to their work. They are authors of a large number of scientific papers, co-authors of several books on epidemiology and public health; Robert is also a co-editor of the Oxford Textbook of Public Health, Fifth Edition. They are now actively engaged in the theory and practice of public health with a focus on the prevention and control of chronic diseases, especially in low- and middle-income countries.

Contributors

Robert Beaglehole
Emeritus Professor, University of
Auckland, Auckland, New Zealand

Ruth Bonita
Emeritus Professor, University of
Auckland, Auckland, New Zealand

Richard Cash
Director, Program on Ethical Issues
in Global Health Research,
Department of Global Health and
Population, Harvard School of
Public Health, Boston, USA

Peter Davis
Professor of Sociology, School of
Population Health, University of
Auckland, Auckland, New Zealand

Delanyo Dovlo
Health Systems Adviser, World
Health Organization, Geneva,
Switzerland

Robin Gauld
Associate Professor of Health Policy,
Department of Preventive and Social
Medicine, University of Otago,
Dunedin, New Zealand

Robert Geneau
Research Scientist, WHO
Collaborating Centre on Chronic
Disease Policy, Public Health Agency
of Canada, Ottawa, Canada

Ehi Igumbor
Senior Lecturer, School of Public
Health, University of the Western
Cape, Bellville, South Africa

Alec Irwin
Associate Director, François-Xavier
Bagnoud Center for Health and
Human Rights, Harvard School of
Public Health, Boston, USA

Henri Jouval Jr
Adviser, International Cooperation
Oswaldo Cruz Foundation, Rio de
Janeiro, Brazil

Barbara Legowski
Senior Advisor International Programs,
WHO Collaborating Centre on
Chronic Disease Policy, Public Health
Agency of Canada, Ottawa, Canada

Liming Lee
Professor, School of Public Health,
Peking University, Vice President,
Chinese Academy of Medical
Sciences/Peking Union Medical
College, Beijing, China

Uta Lehmann
Associate Professor, School of Public
Health, University of the Western
Cape, South Africa

Vivian Lin
Professor of Public Health, School of
Public Health, La Trobe University,
Bundoora, Australia

Karen Lock
Senior Lecturer, Department of
Public Health and Policy, London
School of Hygiene and Tropical
Medicine, London, United Kingdom

Jun Lv
Associate Professor, School of
Public Health, Peking University
Health Science Center, Beijing,
China

Sarah Macfarlane
Senior Advisor, University of
California San Francisco Global
Health Sciences, USA

Martin McKee
Professor, European Centre on
Health of Societies in Transition,
London School of Hygiene and
Tropical Medicine, London,
United Kingdom

Anthony McMichael
Director, National Centre for
Epidemiology & Population Health,
Australian National University,
Canberra, Australia

Cristiani Vieira Machado
Researcher, Department of Health
Administration and Planning,
Sergio Arouca National School of
Public Health of the Oswaldo Cruz
Foundation, Rio de Janeiro,
Brazil

Colin Mathers
Co-ordinator, Mortality and Burden
of Disease, Department of Health
Statistics and Informatics, World
Health Organization, Geneva,
Switzerland

Wilma Meeus
Consultant, ETC Crystal, Leusden,
The Netherlands

José Carvalho de Noronha
Institute of Scientific and
Technological Communication
and Information, Oswaldo Cruz
Foundation, Rio de Janeiro, Brazil

Gudrun Persson
Senior researcher, Centre for
Epidemiology, National Board of
Health and Welfare, Stockholm,
Sweden

Mario Roberto Dal Poz
Coordinator, Human Resources
for Health Department, Health
Systems and Services, World Health
Organization, Geneva, Switzerland

K Srinath Reddy
President, Public Health Foundation
of India, New Delhi, India

David Sanders
Professor, School of Public Health,
University of the Western Cape,
South Africa

Fiona Sim
Senior Research Fellow, Health
Services Research Unit, London
School of Hygiene and Tropical
Medicine, London, United Kingdom

Sylvie Stachenko
Dean, School of Public Health,
University of Alberta, Edmonton,
Canada

Puja Thakker
Research Associate, Public Health
Foundation of India, New Delhi, India

Stig Wall
Professor, Epidemiology and Health Care Research, Director, Centre for Global Health Research, Umeå University, Sweden

Lars Weinehall
Professor in Epidemiology and Family Medicine, Umeå University, Sweden

Daniel Wikler
Mary B. Saltonstall Professor of Ethics and Population Health, Department of Population and International Health, Harvard School of Public Health, Boston, USA

Abbreviations

ANM	auxiliary nurse midwife		HDLC	high-density lipoprotein cholesterol
ART	anti-retroviral			
ASHA	accredited social health activist		HIPC	Highly Indebted Poor Countries
BMI	body mass index			
CHC	community health centre		HR	human resources
CHHI	Canadian Heart Health Initiative		HSR	health sector reform
			ICD-10	International Classification of Disease, 10th Revision
CIOMS	Council of International Organizations of Medical Sciences		ICF	International Classification of Functioning, Disability, and Health
CIS	Commonwealth of Independent States		ICIDH	International Classification of Impairments, Disabilities, and Handicaps
CMO	Chief Medical Officer			
CPHO	Chief Public Health Officer		IHR	International Health Regulations
CRG	Canadian Reference Group		IMF	International Monetary Fund
DALY	disability-adjusted life-year		IMR	infant mortality rate
DFLE	disability-free life expectancy		INCLEN	International Clinical Epidemiology Network
DHS	Demographic Health Survey			
DOTS	directly observed treatment, short course		IPCC	Intergovernmental Panel on Climate Change
ECLAC	Economic Commission for Latin America and the Caribbean		MCCD	Medical Certificate of Cause of Death
			MDG	Millennium Development Goal
EDR	extensively drug-resistant		MDR	multidrug-resistant
EPI	Expanded Programme on Immunization		MDR-TB	multidrug-resistant tuberculosis
ESI	Environmental Sustainability Index		MDS	Million Deaths Study
			MICS	Multiple Indicator Cluster Survey
FCTC	Framework Convention on Tobacco Control		MMR	maternal mortality rate, measles–mumps–rubella
GATS	General Agreement on Trade in Services		MTA	multilateral trade agreement
GBD	Global Burden of Disease		NCD	non-communicable disease
GDP	gross domestic product		NGO	non-government organization
GEC	global environmental change		OECD	Organization for Economic Cooperation and Development
GHI	Global Health Initiative			
GNI	gross national income		ORT	oral rehydration therapy
HALE	health-adjusted life expectancy		PCT	primary care trust
HDL	high-density lipoprotein			

PHAC	Public Health Agency of Canada	SIDS	sudden infant death syndrome
PHC	primary health care, primary health centre	SPP	specific-purpose payment
		SRS	Sample Registration System
		SSA	sub-Saharan Africa
PHM	People's Health Movement	STI	sexually transmitted infection
PHSWOW	Public Health Schools Without Walls	SWAps	Sector Wide Approaches
		TRIPS	Trade-Related Aspects of Intellectual Property Rights
R&D	research and development		
RMB	renminbi (Chinese unit of currency)	UHC	urban health centre
		UNCTAD	United Nations Conference on Trade and Development
SAP	Structural Adjustment Programme		
		UV	ultraviolet
SARS	severe acute respiratory syndrome	WTO	World Trade Organization
		YPLL	years of potential life lost
SHA	Strategic Health Authority		

Abbreviations which do not appear above are defined where they appear in the text.

Chapter 1

The global context for public health

Anthony McMichael and Robert Beaglehole

Introduction

A major transition in the health of human populations has been under way over the past half-century. In most populations there have been impressive gains in life expectancy. Fertility rates have been generally declining over the past several decades. The profile of major causes of death and disease is being transformed; in low- and middle-income countries, non-communicable diseases are replacing the previously dominant infectious diseases. In most countries there has been an uptrend in the prevalence of overweight and obesity, foreshadowing likely increases in the incidence of various major non-communicable diseases in future decades. Meanwhile, the pattern of infectious diseases, internationally, has become much more labile, along with an increased rate of emergence of new (mostly zoonotic viral) infectious diseases and a widespread increase in antimicrobial resistance [1].

The prospects for population health are coming under increasing influence from the diverse aspects of globalization, encompassing increases in economic, cultural, electronic, physical, and environmental connectedness. This growing influence of globalization applies particularly to the world's less wealthy populations. However, these relationships are complex, and their elucidation has been hampered by a lack of systematic research evidence [2,3]. Health prospects also depend increasingly on trends in global environmental conditions, changing in response to the increasingly vast and widespread pressures of economic activity. Climate change, the best known of these contemporary systemic environmental changes, is part of a larger syndrome of human-induced 'global environmental changes'. These relationships between social and environmental conditions and population health, present and future, are at the core of the 'sustainability transition' debate [4]. Overall, then, public health in the early twenty-first century remains at a substantive crossroads [5].

Improvements in the health status of Western populations during the past two centuries have resulted primarily from broad-based changes in the social, dietary, built, and material environments, due in large part to improved sanitation and other deliberate public health interventions. In less developed countries, health gains have occurred more recently in the wake of increased literacy, family spacing, improved nutrition, and vector control, assisted by the transfer of knowledge about sanitation, vaccination, and treatment of infectious diseases.

This brief review of the history of the fundamental influence on population health of social, environmental, economic, and technological changes is a reminder to public health researchers and practitioners, and those in the political and public realms with whom they interact, of the need to take a broad view of the determinants of population health. This essentially 'ecological' view recognizes that shifts in human ecology (encompassing community-wide patterns of social relations and ways of producing, consuming, and interacting with the natural environment) account for much of the ebb and flow of diseases over time [6,7].

In this chapter we describe this larger-scale context within which public health researchers and practitioners should address both traditional and new challenges to population health. These challenges are heightened by the even more fundamental contemporary challenge of helping our societies achieve a way of living, environmentally and socially, that will sustain good health in future.

The scope of public health

Broadly defined, public health is the art and science of preventing disease, promoting population health, and extending life through organized local and global efforts [8,9]. Two aspects of this public health task have been claiming increasing attention. First, because social and material inequalities within a society generate health inequalities, a central task is to identify, through research, the underlying political, social, and behavioural determinants of these health inequalities. That knowledge must then be applied, in part through professional practice, to the development and implementation of effective social policies. In its fullest sense, this includes the lessening of social inequalities. Secondly, longer-term changes in the structure and conditions of both the social and natural environments will affect the sustainability of good health within populations. A ready example is the rapid rise of obesity in urban populations everywhere, as ways of living become less physically active. Public health, as Virchow pointed out more than a century ago, is 'politics writ large'.

The goals of the contemporary public health effort must encompass these larger-scale dimensions: improvement of the health of whole populations and communities, reduction of health inequalities within and between populations, and striving for health-sustaining environments. In traditional, mostly self-contained, agrarian-based societies which produce, consume, and trade on a local basis and with low-impact technologies, the social and environmental determinants of health are predominantly local and relatively circumscribed. However, industrialization and modernization over the past century have altered the scale of contact, influence, and exchange between societies. Further, they have institutionalized hierarchical economic relations, reinforcing the modern world's 'structured unfairness' [10], and have exacerbated the rich–poor gap worldwide and increased the scale of human impact on the environment.

An important step towards addressing the goals of public health has been the widened recognition that the health of a population reflects more than the summation of the risk factor profile and health status of its individual members. It is also a collective characteristic reflecting the population's social history and its cultural, material, and ecological circumstances [11]. Epidemiological analyses that are confined to studying risk differences between individuals afford little insight into the causes of variations in population health indices, either between populations or in a particular population over time. For example, the effect of heat waves and cold spells on mortality differs between European populations at low and high latitudes, reflecting differences in culture, housing design, and environmental conditioning.

The inverse relationship seen in more developed countries between the within-population income gradient and average life expectancy cannot be satisfactorily explained at the individual level, even though mediating biomedical pathways relating to individual experiences of stress, status, or deprivation may be involved. Likewise, the apparent surge in excessive alcohol consumption that occurred in post-communist Russia (see Chapter 5) is essentially a population-level process which can only be partly understood by elucidating associated individual-level phenomena. The general point is that the individual-level perspective fails to conceptualize the population's health both as something that reflects prevailing ecological conditions and as a public good that affects social functioning, community morale, and collective economic performance [12]. Thus, analyses at the individual, community, and whole-population levels can address complementary, but qualitatively distinct, types of questions.

Thus, the public health endeavour is a broad and inclusive enterprise extending to political, social, and environmental leadership and management.

Clinical medicine is part of this overall public health effort to promote and protect population health, and to reduce the impact of illness and disease. In a rapidly changing world, with new and larger-scale influences on population health, implementing a broad-based multisectored public health effort becomes an increasingly important challenge. Currently, the public health workforce does not appear to be well equipped to meet these challenges.

Population health and sustainable development

The term 'sustainable development' is widely used and misused. Reflecting the dominance of economics in the policy arena, the phrase is often assumed to refer to achieving an economic system that can continue to grow over the foreseeable future. Thus, crucial issues are sidestepped—in particular the fact that we are already pressing up against, indeed exceeding, the capacity of the natural environment to supply our needs and absorb our waste. That, in turn, portends risks to human well-being, health, and survival—which points to the essence of 'sustainability'!

Our understanding of sustainability is becoming more enlightened as recognition grows that the human-made economic system is entirely dependent on the natural environment: thus 'sustainability' means that economic development must comply with maintaining the function and integrity of the ecosystems that support human societies and the things that they value [13].

In the popular view, human population health is often seen as an incidental beneficiary of the process of development, which has as its central goal economic growth. Further, population health is sometimes viewed from a utilitarian perspective, as an *input* to economic development—the healthier the population, the more efficient is that society's economic functioning. This view is evident in the work of WHO's Commission on Macroeconomics and Health which, while recognizing the importance of health in its own right, emphasizes the value of investing in health in order to promote economic growth [14]. Such approaches, by treating economic growth as society's primary desired endpoint, discount the fact that our reasons for seeking improvements in material and social conditions are to do with enhancing human experience—well-being, happiness, health, and survival.

Mainstream economic development thinking has not adequately internalized the role of population health as a central criterion of development strategy and of the measurement of success. To do so requires understanding that the population's health profile is an ecological characteristic which reflects the conditions of the social and natural environments. Instead, the conventional view of 'health' locates it mainly at the personal and family level. Thus, in wealthy countries, health is viewed primarily as an individual asset, a commodity even, to be managed by personal behavioural choices and personal access to the formal health-care system.

For the good health of any population to be sustained over generations, there is need for a stable and productive natural environment which yields assured supplies of food and fresh water, has a relatively constant climate in which climate-sensitive physical and biological systems do not change for the worse, and retains biodiversity (a fundamental source of both present and future value). For the human species, the stability, richness, and fairness of the social environment are also important to population health. In animal and plant populations, the size, vigour, and longevity of the population reflects the carrying capacity of the environment for that species. That is, the environment determines the maximum number that can be supported, and that number is the 'carrying capacity' of the local habitat [6]. However, human populations are not exclusively constrained by environmental conditions; through culture (including trade) and technology they can increase and supplement the carrying capacity of their local environments—at least temporarily. Eventually, the sustainability of this amplified carrying capacity becomes a critical issue.

Population health is more than a utilitarian input or an incidental consequence of economic development. It should be a *central focus of sustainable development*. The purpose of societal 'development', and specifically public health activity, is to improve the conditions, enjoyment, and healthiness of life for human societies and to do so in a way that entails sharing those benefits equitably. If the development process is not conducive to sustaining and improving health, then in a fundamental sense that process is not 'sustainable development'.

Human ecology as a prime determinant of population health

To add depth to our understanding of the determinants of population health, it is instructive to review how changes in ways of living and in human culture at large, over the ages, have affected patterns of health and disease [4].

A good example, extending over the past 10,000 years since some human societies first began farming, has been the nutritional impact of traditional staple-based, often monotonous, agrarian diets. Before the 'second agricultural revolution', which began in Europe in the nineteenth century, most agrarian societies experienced widespread malnutrition and recurring famine. The widening geographic spread of human populations has compounded this nutritional deficiency problem. For example, the extension of agrarian societies into highland and arid regions exposed many populations to dietary iodine deficiency, leading to iodine deficiency disorders [15]. Nevertheless, because of the great increase in environmental carrying capacity conferred by agricultural production and trade, farming populations have generally come to outnumber and replace smaller hunter–gatherer populations.

Many of the diseases that characterize modern wealthy societies, and increasingly poor societies, reflect a discordance between the evolved biological needs of the human animal and contemporary ways of living. For example, the radical industrial transformation of the food supply, entailing huge shifts in levels of consumption of saturated fats, simple sugars, salt, and dietary fibre, has contributed to the epidemics of non-communicable diseases (cardiovascular disease, diabetes, various cancers) which now characterize longer-living populations in wealthy countries and, increasingly, low- and middle-income countries. The local and long-distance spread of infectious diseases have been facilitated by urban crowding and migration, respectively. Physical inactivity in the modern mechanized environment predisposes to a rise in the prevalence of obesity, now becoming evident worldwide.

Nevertheless, various social and technical advances over the past two centuries have brought marked reductions in mortality, particularly in early life, with resultant gains in life expectancy and an ensuing reduction in birth rates. This composite process—the demographic and epidemiological transition—continues to transform life expectancies and patterns of disease in developing countries.

Explanations for recent trends in population health

There have been broad gains in life expectancy over the past half-century, and these gains are continuing in most regions [3]. However, substantial health inequalities between rich and poor nations and between rich and poor population subgroups persist. Further, setbacks have occurred in sub-Saharan Africa, primarily because of the ravages of HIV/AIDS, and in some of the former socialist countries of Central and Eastern Europe because of the turbulent social and economic disruptions that occurred in the early 1990s. Fertility rates are now declining on a wide front, and there have been widespread gains in maternal mortality and infant and child survival in developing countries. World population growth is, on current projections, expected to flatten out at around 8.5–9 billion by 2050, gaining up to another billion by 2100.

As noted earlier, as traditional infectious diseases recede in many lower-income countries, and as populations age, the incidence of the chronic non-communicable diseases of middle and later adulthood rises. Thus, health profiles are being transformed, with great implications for the health care system, public health strategies, and society at large.

The history of the decline in infectious disease epidemics in Western countries is instructive. It was long assumed that the decline was largely attributable to their 'conquest' by effective specific counter-measures, most recently by vaccines and antibiotics, and earlier by sanitation and improved water supplies. However, Thomas McKeown, using historical English data, showed that vaccines and antibiotics came too late to make major contributions [16]. For example, over 90 per cent of the recorded decline in tuberculosis mortality in England occurred before the advent of chemotherapy in the late 1940s. McKeown argued that improved nutrition, by enhancing host resistance, was the main determinant of the modern decline in fatal infection. The substantial historical increase in body size in wealthy countries attests to improved nutrition in infancy and childhood. The relationship between child nutrition and infection is generally reciprocal: better nourished children are more resistant to death from infection, and protection against infection reduces the nutrient losses caused by infection. Aspects of McKeown's thesis have been contested [5], and other aspects of social change and environmental regulation have been invoked as significant contributors. However, the central point stands: over the decades, major changes in population health have been primarily due to changes in social institutions, educational attainment, governmental policies, and ways of living.

Parents' understanding of how to care for their children appears to be very important, because child survival is enhanced if their parents have had school education. This effect of parental education is very powerful relative to other potential determinants of child mortality in low- and middle-income countries. Thus the social institutions of 'health care' and 'public health' should be understood to encompass various attributes of society, representing human and social capital (i.e. individuals, families, communities, and larger social groupings), and not just as narrow domains of professional practice [17].

The mortality decline in low- and middle-income countries is best explained by improvements in three domains: the material conditions of life (indicated, for example, by real incomes or child growth rates), institutional change, especially schooling for girls, and increased knowledge and knowledge application (Box 1.1). At any particular population income level, mortality reductions are mainly attributable to increases in the stock of scientific and practical knowledge and to institutional changes that apply this knowledge, especially via schooling for girls. One statistical analysis of increases in life expectancy in 115 low- and middle-income countries between 1960 and 1990 attributed 20 per cent to increased real incomes, 30 per cent to schooling for girls; and 50 per cent to the generation and use of new knowledge [12].

Box 1.1 Declining mortality in low-income countries

India provides a good example of how mortality can decline in a low-income country despite limited gain in the material conditions of living. During the twentieth century mortality in India declined markedly. By the century's end, the chance of dying before age 15 had been reduced from around one in two to one in eight, and the chance of dying between ages 15 and 65 had been reduced by about two-thirds to little more than one in four. Within India, region-specific declines in mortality have been associated much more strongly with indices of institutional modernization (such as high-school attendance rates for girls in rural areas) than with increases in income.

The mortality decline in the second half of the twentieth century occurred even more rapidly in East Asia (notwithstanding China's catastrophic famine in 1959–1961, which killed an estimated 30 million persons) and in Latin America. Death rates for adult males in Chinese cities are now amongst the lowest in the world, as are those in Caribbean states such as Jamaica and Cuba. However, the mortality decline has been much slower in sub-Saharan Africa. Indeed, in some countries severely effected by HIV (such as Zimbabwe, Malawi, and Zambia) and by civil war (such as Rwanda, Somalia, and Liberia), life expectancy fell in the last two decades of the twentieth century.

Each of these three 'factors' is a marker for a complex of social and economic processes. Thus, the first, economic development, brings not only increases in private incomes but also increases in important capital stocks, many of a public nature (roads and schools, teacher training, and electronic communications). Secondly, a marked degree of female autonomy is probably central to exceptional mortality declines, especially in poor but open societies. When girls are able to assume roles outside the house, even when adolescent and unmarried, and older women can appear in public on their own initiative, girls are more likely to remain at school and mothers are more likely to take themselves or sick children to health centres, wait in queues of mixed sex, and question male physicians.

The third factor, increases in knowledge, is also likely to be complex. For example, approximately 80 per cent of the world's children were estimated to have been immunized against measles in 2006, up from about 50 per cent in 1987. The knowledge contributing to this protection against early death encompasses the scientific knowledge embedded in the vaccine, the technical knowledge embedded in the 'cold chains' used to convey vaccines safely to remote areas, the 'organizational knowledge' about how best to conduct immunization programmes, and the knowledge embedded in communications technologies that almost certainly assisted the planning and implementation of these programmes.

Globalization: setting the scene

'Globalization', like 'sustainable development', is an elastic term. Here we use it to refer to the increasing interconnectedness of countries through cross-border flows of goods, services, money, people, information, and ideas, the increasing openness of countries to such flows, and the development of international rules and institutions dealing with cross-border flows. This is not a new phenomenon, although the current phase of globalization, dating from the 1980s, has seen an exceptionally rapid increase in interconnectedness and more radical changes in the international institutional framework than previous phases [2,3]. The core component of globalization is economic interconnectedness, including the associated ascendancy of deregulated markets in international trade and investment. Two other important domains are technological globalization, especially of information and communication technologies, and cultural globalization, where popular culture is increasingly dominated by the USA and the English language. There is also an emerging globalization of ethical and judicial standards which may render social and individual rights more secure (see Chapter 13).

Economic 'globalization' has been a long-evolving feature of a world dominated by Western society. The early twentieth century was a time of vigorous free trade, subsequently curtailed in the aftermath of the First World War. Contemporary globalization differs in both the scale and the comprehensiveness of change, and in the associated decline in the country's capacity to set social policy. The Western world's international development project following the First World War initially anticipated that countries everywhere would converge towards the Western model of national democratic capitalism. However, this project has evolved towards the building of an integrated and deregulated free-market global economy. These globalizing processes, in turn, have become a major determinant of national, social, and economic policies [18,19]. Thus, although responsibility for health care and the public health system remains with national governments, the fundamental social, economic, and environmental determinants of population health are increasingly supranational. This combination of liberal economic structures and domestic policy constraint promotes socio-economic inequalities and political instability, each of which adversely affects population health. Unless the moderating role of the state or international agencies is strengthened, increasing competition for the world's limited natural resources is likely to damage inter-country relations, local and global environments, and population health.

The principal promoters of a globalized market-based economic system are international agencies such as the World Bank, the International Monetary Fund (IMF), and transnational corporations. The main strategies have included the promotion of free trade through the rules of the World Trade Organization (WTO) and its multilateral trade agreements (MTAs), corporate taxation concessions and investment incentives allied to relaxation of wage controls and workplace standards, and support for the contraction of national public sector spending in the health, education, and welfare sectors.

Structural adjustment programmes imposed by the IMF on the economies of many poor countries, promoting particularly the wealth-creating role of the private sector, have often impaired population health. The curtailment of education under this imposed regime of economic rationalism has threatened advances in literacy in women, fertility reduction, and improved reproductive health [20]. The World Bank now recognizes the need for a strong state to carry out essential public functions, including public health, and to ensure well-functioning markets [21]. Meanwhile, tension persists between the philosophy of neoliberalism, emphasizing the self-interest of market-based economics, and the philosophy of social justice which sees collective responsibility and benefit as the prime social goal [22]. The practice of public health, with its underlying community and population perspective, sits more comfortably with the latter philosophy.

As economic liberalization has accelerated, there has been a polarization between richer and poorer countries. Income disparity has increased between high- and low-income countries and within many countries. Both trends have contributed to an increase in overall global inequality. There have been increases in inequality in Asia and Africa, and a massive increase in Eastern Europe, with smaller declines in the developed countries and Latin America [23]. With a combination of slowing growth and increasing inequality at the global level, it is not surprising that progress in reducing poverty has been disappointing.

Alongside this economic globalization has been the rapid development and international spread of information and communication technologies, facilitated by investments in infrastructure, improved technologies, and shrinking costs. However, the reach of the Internet is still limited within poor populations. Globally coordinated advertising, technological innovation, and marketing opportunities are increasingly driving modern consumer behaviours, as exemplified by the intensified global promotion of tobacco products [24].

Another feature of today's world is the increase in human mobility. Most movement is voluntary; some is involuntary and in response to conflict, civil disorder, and natural disaster. The number of environmental and political refugees has increased greatly over the past two decades. Increased mobility of labour can be of mutual economic benefit—many less-developed economies welcome cheap overseas labour, and international remittances from these workers assist their home economies. Meanwhile, human mobility is also important in the enhanced transmission of ideas, values, and microbiological agents.

Globalization and public health

From a public health perspective, globalization is having mixed effects [3]. On the one hand accelerated economic growth and technological advances have enhanced health and life expectancy in many populations. At least in the short to medium term, these material advances allied to social modernization and various health care and public health programmes yield gains in population health. On the other hand, aspects of globalization jeopardize population health via the erosion of social and environmental conditions, the global division of labour, the exacerbation of the rich–poor income gap between and within countries, and the accelerating spread of consumerism (Box 1.2).

One aspect of the growth in international trade with particularly deleterious public health consequences has been the escalation in the sales of weapons and associated equipment, much of it facilitated by Western governments. Sub-Saharan Africa provides many tragic examples of these effects, as does the continuing instability in the Middle East. The nature of modern conflict is such that most casualties are civilians, with women and children being particularly vulnerable [25].

Global environmental change and health

Over the past two centuries, three great changes in the human condition have occurred: industrialization, urbanization, and, latterly, increased control over human fertility. The fourth great change, which is ongoing, is globalization. The associated combination of receding infant and child mortality, followed by a downward trend in adult mortality, rapid population growth, and intensification of economic activities, has resulted in humans exerting enormous aggregate pressure on the natural environment. This pressure has begun to exceed the capacity of the environment to supply, replenish, restore, and absorb, causing a syndrome of 'overload' that is manifested as a range of global environmental changes (GECs) [26].

Box 1.2 Examples of health risks posed by globalization

The main health risks arising from the effects of globalization on social and natural environments include:

- Perpetuation and exacerbation of income differentials, both within and among countries, thereby creating and maintaining the basic poverty-associated conditions for poor health.
- The fragmentation and weakening of labour markets as internationally mobile capital acquires greater relative power and jeopardizes the health of workers by encouraging a lowering of occupational health and safety standards.
- The consequences of global environmental changes (includes changes in atmospheric composition, land degradation, depletion of biodiversity, spread of 'invasive' species, and dispersal of persistent organic pollutants).

Other, more specific, examples include:

- The spread of tobacco-caused diseases as the tobacco industry globalizes its markets.
- The diseases of dietary excesses as food production and food processing become intensified and as urban consumer preferences are shaped by globally promoted images and mass marketing.
- The diverse public health consequences of the proliferation of private car ownership, as car manufacturers extend their marketing.
- The continued widespread rise of obesity.
- Expansion of the international drug trade.
- Easier spread of infectious diseases because of increased worldwide travel.
- The apparent increasing prevalence of depression and mental health disorders in ageing and fragmented urban populations.

Humankind is now disrupting at global level some of the biosphere's life-support systems. These geophysical and ecological systems provide replenishment of soils, biological services (such as pollination), cleansing of water and air, recycling of nutrient elements, environmental stabilization, and natural constraints on infectious agents. These processes could be taken for granted in a less populated lower-impact world. However, today the global human population is changing the gaseous composition of the lower and middle atmospheres, there is a net loss of productive soils on all continents, depletion of most ocean fisheries, and many of the great aquifers upon which irrigated agriculture depends, and there is an unprecedented rate of loss of whole species and many local populations [6]. More than a third of the world's stocks of natural ecological resources have been lost since 1970. These changes to Earth's basic life-supporting processes pose long-term risks to human population health.

In 2007 the UN Environment Program released its *Global Environmental Outlook 2007* (GEO-4) containing a detailed assessment of the state and trajectories of Earth's main environmental and ecological systems [27] (Box 1.3). The report conveyed a heightened sense of urgency, including explicit recognition that social stability and human well-being, health, and survival are at increasing risk from these large-scale systemic environmental changes. It documented the adverse trends in the world's fertile soils (and in many regional agricultural yields), freshwater supplies, coastal and reef ecosystems, fish stocks, concentrations of human-activated nitrogen (mostly from nitrogenous

Box 1.3 Major environmental changes over past century

The GEO-4 report listed a range of environment-related indices that had undergone exponential growth since 1900, reflecting the surges in population size, energy use, material consumption, and waste generation. They include the following.

- Global population has grown from 1.6 billion to over 6.6 billion.
- Energy use has increased 16-fold.
- Industrial production has increased 40-fold, mainly due to growth in low- and middle-income countries.
- Water use has risen ninefold.
- Fish catch has soared 35-fold, with major stocks likely to crash by mid-century.
- Carbon dioxide emissions have increased 17-fold.
- Sulphur emissions have increased 13-fold, and other air pollutants have increased fivefold.
- Rates of both deforestation and desertification are accelerating.

fertilizers and fossil fuel combustion), acidity of the ocean, numbers and stocks of species, and the global climate.

Global climate change

Climate scientists forecast with very high confidence that the continued accumulation of heat-trapping greenhouse gases in the troposphere will change global patterns of temperature, precipitation, and climatic variability over the coming decades. The most recent five-yearly report of the UN's Intergovernmental Panel on Climate Change (IPCC) predicts a rise in average global surface temperature of 1.8–4.0°C by the end of the 21st century, with much of that uncertainty being due to inevitable uncertainties about the future pattern of global greenhouse gas emissions [28]. A rise of this order, greater at higher than at lower latitudes, would occur faster than any rise encountered by humankind since the inception of agriculture around 10,000 years ago.

The IPCC and various other national scientific panels have assessed the potential health consequences of climate change [29–31]. These risks to human health will arise from increased exposures to thermal extremes and from regionally variable increases in weather disasters. Other risks would arise from the disruption of complex ecological systems which determine the geography of vector-borne infections (such as malaria, dengue fever, and leishmaniasis) and the range, seasonality, and incidence of various food-borne and water-borne infections, the yields of agricultural crops, the range of plant and livestock pests and pathogens, the salination of coastal lands and freshwater supplies due to sea-level rise, and the climatically related production of photochemical air pollutants, spores, and pollens.

Public health scientists now face the task of estimating, via interdisciplinary collaborations, the future health impacts of these projected scenarios of climatic environmental conditions. For example, mathematical models have been used to estimate how climatic changes would affect the potential geographic range of vector-borne infectious diseases such as malaria and dengue. Some other health impacts, such as those resulting from displacement of coastal and degraded rural regions, will be harder to model or estimate, but may entail large burdens of poor health and premature death.

Stratospheric ozone depletion

Depletion of stratospheric ozone by human-made industrial and agricultural gases, such as chlorofluorocarbons and nitrous oxide, has occurred over recent decades. Stratospheric chlorine-equivalent levels (i.e. the suite of ozone-destructive chemicals) appear to have peaked in 2000 and are now decreasing; the ozone concentration has stabilized during the period 2002–2006.

Initial predictions were that there would be recovery of the ozone layer by 2050, but indications now are that human-induced climate change may delay this recovery by several decades [32]. There is strong evidence that ambient ground-level ultraviolet B (UVB) irradiation has increased over the period of ozone depletion, but since the late 1990s it has decreased at unpolluted sites in the southern hemisphere. However, in many locations, diminution of atmospheric aerosols and clearer skies during the 1990s has meant that ground-level UVB is now higher than previously.

The stratospheric ozone layer specifically filters out the UVB wavelengths of ambient UVR (with UVA wavelengths being unaltered). UVB is absorbed by cellular DNA and appears to be particularly important as a cause of adverse health effects, predominantly skin cancers and eye diseases [33]. Scenario-based modelling, integrating the processes of emissions accrual, ozone destruction, UVR flux, and cancer induction, indicates that European and US populations will experience a 5–10 per cent excess in skin cancer incidence during the middle decades of the coming century, assuming unchanged sun exposure behaviour [34]. Furthermore, it is estimated that by 2050 there will be 167,000–830,000 additional cases of cortical cataract of the eye attributable to ozone depletion, with substantial health costs [35].

However, these same UVB wavelengths are required for the initiation of vitamin D synthesis following UV irradiation of the skin. While vitamin D has well-known beneficial effects on bone health, the positive non-bone health effects of higher levels of vitamin D are increasingly being recognized [36]: lower incidence of various cancers (particularly colorectal cancer) and autoimmune diseases (including multiple sclerosis and type 1 diabetes) and improved cardiovascular health. Thus, increased UVB irradiation, under conditions of stratospheric ozone depletion, potentially has both beneficial and adverse effects on health [37], with the balance of effects not yet clearly defined.

Biodiversity loss and invasive species

As human demand for space, materials, and food increases, populations and species of plants and animals are rapidly being extinguished. An important consequence for humans is the disruption of those ecosystems that provide 'nature's goods and services'. Of particular concern, for example, is the actual and threatened loss of pollinating species—insects, birds, and small mammals [38]. An estimated 70 per cent of all food plant species require pollination by other organisms. Biodiversity loss also means the loss, before discovery, of many of nature's chemicals and genes of the kind that have already conferred enormous medical and health benefits. An estimated five-sixths of tropical vegetative nature's medicinal goods have yet to be recruited for human benefit [39].

Meanwhile, invasive species are spreading worldwide into new non-natural environments via intensified human food production, commerce, and mobility. The resultant changes in regional species composition have myriad consequences for human health. For example, the spread of water hyacinth, introduced from Brazil as a decorative plant, in Lake Victoria in eastern Africa has produced a breeding ground for the water snail that transmits schistosomiasis and for the proliferation of diarrhoeal disease organisms [40].

Impairment of food-producing ecosystems

Increasing pressures of agricultural and livestock production are stressing the world's arable lands and pastures. The twenty-first century began with an estimated one-third of the world's previously productive land seriously damaged by erosion, compaction, salination, waterlogging, and 'chemicalization' which destroys organic content [41]. Similar pressures on the world's ocean fisheries have left most of them severely depleted or stressed. Almost certainly we must find an environmentally benign, safe, and socially acceptable way of using genetic engineering to increase food yields if we are to produce sufficient food for another three billion persons (with higher expectations) over the coming half-century. If the choice is between re-engineering more land (e.g. irrigation, chemical supplementation, clearing more forest) or re-engineering crop plant genomes, we may have diminishing real choice anyway.

Modelling studies, allowing for future trends in trade and economic development, have estimated that climate change (entailing changes in temperature, rainfall, humidity, and extreme weather events) would cause a slight downturn globally of around 2–4 per cent in cereal grain yields (which represent two-thirds of world food energy). The estimated downturn in yield would be considerably greater in the food-insecure regions in South Asia, the Middle East, North Africa, and Central America [42]. By 2020, crop yields could increase by 20 per cent in East and Southeast Asia, but decrease by up to 30 per cent in Central and South Asia, and rain-fed agricultural output could drop by 50 per cent in some African countries [43].

Other global environmental changes

A number of additional items could be discussed here. They all illustrate the same general point—the sheer magnitude of human pressures on the natural environment is now beginning to cause systemic, often global, environmental changes of a kind not previously achievable by humans.

Freshwater aquifers in all continents are being depleted of their ancient 'fossil water' supplies. Agricultural and industrial demand, amplified by population growth, often greatly exceeds the rate of natural recharge. Water-related political and public health crises loom within decades. For example, Bangladesh faces the triple prospect of declining river flows from the Himalayas, as the headwater glaciers contract because of global warming, increased diversion, for irrigation, by India (Ganges) and China (Brahmaputra and Meghna), and a growth in downstream population pressures for food production in Bangladesh itself. Tensions, under-nutrition, and freshwater shortages could all affect aspects of population health.

The increasing concentration of carbon dioxide in the lower atmosphere is now causing acidification of the world's oceans. The absorbed carbon dioxide forms carbonic acid, and the pH (the logarithmic index of acidity) of seawater has measurably dropped over recent decades. The calcification processes (the formation of chalky structures) that are integral to the tiny creatures at the bottom of the marine food web—coral, zooplankton, copepods, crustaceans, and shellfish—are very sensitive to pH. Scientists estimate that, on current trends, acidification sufficient to seriously impair calcification will occur within three to four decades [28]. This GEC poses an additional threat to future food sources, nutrition, and health.

Various semi-volatile organic chemicals (such as polychlorinated biphenyls) are now disseminated worldwide via a sequential 'distillation process' in the cells of the lower atmosphere, thereby transferring chemicals from their usual origins in low to middle latitudes to high latitudes. Increasingly high levels are occurring in polar mammals and fish, and in the humans who eat them. Various chlorinated organic chemicals, butyl-tin, and other compounds adversely affect the immune and reproductive systems of mammals, including humans. Thus, chemical pollution is no longer just an issue of local toxicity.

Contribution of population increase to environmental change

The three main determinants of human disruption of the environment are population size, the level of material wealth and consumption, and technology. For several decades, and for largely political (not scientific) reasons, relatively little attention has been paid to the population factor. Interestingly, this has begun to change since the middle of the current decade, as it has become more widely recognized that, with critical limits being approached on several environmental fronts, there is a need to maximize the decline in fertility alongside the other major changes in technology choices and economic practices [44].

The ongoing climate change debate illustrates well the changing relativities between the environmental effects of increases in population and consumption. During the twentieth century, as population increased by just under four-fold, the annual fossil fuel emissions of carbon dioxide increased 12-fold [26].

Around the year 2000, the fifth of the world population living in high-emission countries accounted for almost two-thirds of carbon dioxide emissions, while the lowest-emitting fifth of the world's population contributed just a few per cent. Over the coming century the projected world population growth will contribute an estimated one-third of growth in carbon dioxide emissions, whereas economic growth (currently spearheaded by China and India) will account for the remaining two-thirds. Both are large figures.

Overall, the greater threat to environmental sustainability is not from increased human numbers *per se* but from the prospect of today's mildly environmentally disruptive humans becoming highly disruptive humans. This will happen if the prevailing development process generalizes the patterns of production and consumption typical of today's rich countries to a global population that is likely to expand to 9–10 billion before 2100, all of whom will come to expect a higher average standard of living. Today, the citizens of high-income countries each require approximately 4–9 hectares of Earth's surface to provide the materials for their lifestyle and to absorb their wastes, while India's population currently gets by on one hectare per person. Earth's surface area will not allow much more than one hectare of 'ecological footprint' per average person for a population of 9–10 billion [6].

The world needs substantial investment in the development and deployment of less environmentally disruptive technologies, and a much greater commitment to international equity, in order to achieve a smooth and timely transition to an ecologically sustainable world. For the moment, rich countries remain the main source of new knowledge and new technologies. Therefore they have the main responsibility for finding paths to sustainability. Meanwhile, the politically and culturally vexed issue of constraining population growth must come back onto the international policy agenda—again facilitated by concessionary and redistributive policies which must be part of a fairer cooperative world seeking, above all, sustainability. In all of this, minimizing the probabilities of long-term harm to health will be a major consideration and, hopefully, a spur to the achievement of global sustainable development.

Global environmental changes and health: challenges for scientists

These historically unprecedented global environmental changes pose a range of hazards to human health. Epidemiologists face some particular difficulties in assessing these environmentally induced risks [7]. First, most incipient environmental changes have not yet exerted detectable impacts on human health; such impacts are likely to emerge over several decades. Secondly, many of the causal pathways are of a complex and indirect kind, such as those likely to affect the transmission of vector-borne malaria and dengue fever, or the environmental impairment of agricultural yields and hence regional food insecurity. Thirdly, as usual, the causality of disease in human populations is multivariate and this difficulty is further amplified by there being coexisting impacts of various environmental changes.

Detecting the early health impacts of global environmental changes will be difficult. However, some clues have begun to emerge—as with the northerly spread of tick-borne encephalitis in Sweden in association with winter warming over the past two decades [45], and the similar northward movement of the water snails that transmit schistosomiasis in eastern China as the critical 'freezing zone' has drifted north in association with regional warming [46]. Some of the recent spread of malaria and dengue fever may have been due to the climate change that has occurred over the past quarter-century, although there are other competing explanations. Other evidence indicates that the tempo of extreme weather events and adverse human impacts has increased during the past decade. This may well reflect the climatic instability that characterizes global climate change [47].

The persistence of approximately 850 million persons suffering from malnutrition (marginally higher than the estimated 820 million at turn of century) may partly reflect the erosion of agro-ecosystem resources, along with the adverse impacts of various large-scale environmental changes on photosynthesis, plant physiology, and the occurrence of crop pests and diseases—and the persistence of unequal access to food supplies.

Conclusion

The combination of rapid socio-economic change, demographic change, and global environmental change, and their potential health impacts, requires a broad conception of the determinants of population health. A deficiency of social capital (social networks and civic institutions) adversely affects the prospects for health by predisposing to widened rich–poor gaps and weakened public health systems. The large-scale loss of natural environmental capital— manifested as climate change, stratospheric ozone depletion, degradation of food-producing systems, depleted freshwater supplies, biodiversity loss, and spread of invasive species—is impairing the biosphere's long-term capacity to sustain healthy human life.

Public health scientists and policy-makers face unfamiliar challenges in addressing these broader dimensions of population health, while at the same time continuing to identify, quantify, and reduce the risks to health that result from specific, often local, social, behavioural, and environmental factors.

This human ecology perspective will broaden the theory and practice of public health, and will help integrate the consideration of health outcomes into decision-making in all policy sectors. The sustained good health of populations requires enlightened management of our social resources, economic relations, and the natural world. There are win–win opportunities in this situation: many of today's public health issues, such as high population levels of obesity, have their roots in the same socio-economic inequalities and imprudent consumption patterns that jeopardize the future sustainability of health.

A major, and urgent, contemporary challenge for public health, and public policy at large, is to provide a satisfactory, healthy, and equitable standard of living for current and future generations. This must include adequate food yields, clean water and energy, safe shelter, and functional ecosystems. Human-induced global environmental changes jeopardize our ability to meet this challenge. Human population health should be a key criterion of 'sustainable development'. Population health in the medium to longer term is an indicator of how well we are managing our natural and social environments. History has shown that changes in human ecology and in humankind's relationship to the natural environment shape the patterns of population health and survival. Application of this ecological perspective will be critical if a sustainable future is to be achieved. These are great challenges for public health practitioners and researchers—challenges which most training programmes are not adequately addressing.

References

[1] Weiss RA, McMichael AJ. Social and environmental risk factors in the emergence of infectious diseases. *Nature Med* 2004; **10**: S70–6.

[2] Kawachi I, Wamala S. (eds). *Globalization and Health*. Oxford: Oxford University Press, 2007.

[3] Lee K. Globalization. In: Detels R, Beaglehole R, Lansang MA, Gulliford M (eds), *Oxford Textbook of Public Health* (5th edn). Oxford: Oxford University Press, 2009.

[4] McMichael AJ. Population, environment, disease, and survival: past patterns, uncertain futures. Lancet 2002; **359**: 1145–8.

[5] Beaglehole R, Bonita R. *Public Health at the Crossroads: Achievements and Prospects* (2nd edn). Cambridge: Cambridge University Press, 2004.

[6] McMichael AJ. *Human Frontiers, Environments and Disease: Past Patterns, Future Uncertainties*. Cambridge: Cambridge University Press, 2001.

[7] McMichael AJ. Population health as the 'bottom line' of sustainability: a contemporary challenge for public health researchers. *Eur J Public Health* 2006, **16**: 579–81.

[8] Acheson D. *Independent Inquiry into Inequalities in Health*. London: HM Stationery Office, 1998.

[9] Beaglehole R, Bonita R, Horton R, Adams O, McKee M. Public health for the new era: collaborative action for population-wide health improvement. *Lancet* 2004; **363**: 2084–6.

[10] Legge D. Challenges of globalization deserve better than simplistic polemics. *BMJ* 2002; **324**: 44.

[11] McMichael AJ. Prisoners of the proximate: epidemiology in an age of change. *Am J Epidemiol* 1999; **149**: 887–97.

[12] *The World Health Report 1999. Making a Difference.* Geneva: WHO, 1999.

[13] Rees W. A human ecological assessment of economic and population health In: Crabbé P, Westra L, Holland A (eds), *Implementing Ecological Integrity: Restoring Regional and Global Environmental and Human Health.* Dordrecht: Kluwer Academic, 2000.

[14] *Report of the Commission on Macroeconomics and Health. Macroeconomics and Health: Investing in Health for Economic Development.* Geneva: WHO, 2001.

[15] Hetzel BS. *The Story of Iodine Deficiency. An International Challenge in Nutrition.* Oxford: Oxford University Press, 1989.

[16] McKeown T. *The Modern Rise of Population.* London: Arnold, 1976.

[17] Powles JW, Cumio F. Public health infrastructures and associated knowledge as global public goods. In: Smith R, Beaglehole R, Woodward D, Drager N (eds), *Global Public Goods for Health.* Oxford: Oxford University Press, 2003.

[18] Gray J. *False Dawn: The Delusions of Global Capitalism.* London: Granta, 1998.

[19] Navarro V. Comment: whose globalization? *Am J Public Health* 1998; **88**: 742–3.

[20] Bassett M. Paper presented to Ecological Society of South Africa, Annual Scientific Conference, East London, 23–25 February 2000.

[21] World Bank. *The State in a Changing World: World Development Report 1997.* Oxford: Oxford University Press, 1997.

[22] Harvey D. *A Brief History of Neoliberalism.* Oxford: Oxford University Press, 2005.

[23] Milanovic B. True world income distribution, 1998 and 1993: First calculation based on household surveys alone. *Econ J* 2002; **112**: 51–92.

[24] *Report on the Global Tobacco Epidemic, 2008: The MPOWER Package.* Geneva: WHO, 2008.

[25] Levy BS, Sidel VW (eds). *War and Public Health.* New York: Oxford University Press, 1997.

[26] McMichael AJ, Powles JW. Human numbers, environment, sustainability and health. *BMJ* 1999; **319**: 977–80.

[27] UN Environment Program. *Global Environmental Outlook 2007.* Nairobi: UNEP, 2007.

[28] Intergovernmental Panel on Climate Change (WGI). *Climate Change, 2007—The Science of Climate Change: Contribution of Working Group I to the Second Assessment Report of the Intergovernmental Panel on Climate Change.* Cambridge: Cambridge University Press, 2007.

[29] McMichael AJ, Woodruff R, Whetton P, Hennessy K, Hales S. *Human Health and Climate Change in Oceania: A Risk Assessment 2002.* Canberra: Commonwealth Government, 2003.

[30] McMichael AJ, Campbell-Lendrum D, Ebi K, Githeko A, Scheraga J, Woodward A (eds). *Climate Change and Human Health: Risks and Responses.* Geneva: WHO, 2003.

[31] McMichael AJ, Woodruff RE, Hales S. Climate change and human health: present and future risks. *Lancet* 2006; **367**: 859–69.

[32] UN Environment Programme. *Scientific Assessment of Ozone Depletio, 2006: Executive Summary*. Geneva/Nairobi: WMO/UNEP, 2006.

[33] Norval M, Cullen AP, de Gruijl FR, et al. The effects on human health from stratospheric ozone depletion and its interactions with climate change. *Photochem Photobiol Sci* 2007; **6**: 232–51.

[34] Slaper H, Velders GJM, Daniel JS, de Gruijl FR, van der Leun JC. Estimates of ozone depletion and skin cancer incidence to examine the Vienna Convention achievements. *Nature* 1996; **384**: 256–8.

[35] West SK, Longstreth JD, Munoz BE, Pitcher HM, Duncan DD. Model of risk of cortical cataract in the US population with exposure to increased ultraviolet radiation due to stratospheric ozone depletion. *Am J Epidemiol* 2005; **162**: 1080–8.

[36] Lucas RM, Ponsonby AL. Considering the potential benefits as well as adverse effects of sun exposure. Can all the potential benefits be provided by oral vitamin D supplementation? *Prog Biophys Mol Biol* 2006; **92**: 140–9.

[37] Lucas RM, McMichael A, Smith W, Armstrong B. *Solar Ultraviolet Radiation. Global Burden of Disease from Solar Ultraviolet Radiation*. Geneva: WHO, 2006.

[38] Millennium Ecosystem Assessment. *Ecosystems and Human Well-being. Synthesis Report*. Washington, DC: Island Press, 2005.

[39] Myers N. Biodiversity's genetic library. In: Daily GC (ed), *Nature's Services: Societal Dependence on Natural Ecosystems*. Washington, DC: Island Press, 1997.

[40] Epstein PR. Weeds bring disease to the East African waterways. Lancet 1998; **351**: 577.

[41] World Resources Institute. *World Resources 1998–1999. Environment and Health*. Oxford: Oxford University Press, 1998.

[42] Intergovernmental Panel on Climate Change. *Climate Change 2007: Impacts, Adaptation and Vulnerability. Report of Working Group II*. Geneva: World Meteorological Organization, 2007.

[43] Intergovernmental Panel on Climate Change. *Climate change 2007: Impacts, Adaptation and Vulnerability. Contribution of Working Group II to the Fourth Assessment Report of the Intergovernmental Panel on Climate Change*. Cambridge: Cambridge University Press, 2007.

[44] Campbell M, Cleland J, Ezeh A, Prata N. Return of the population growth factor. Science 2007; **315**: 1501–2.

[45] Lindgren E, Gustafson R. Tick-borne encephalitis in Sweden and climate change. *Lancet* 2001; **358**: 16–18.

[46] Yang GJ, Vounatsou P, Zhou XN, Tanner M, Utzinger J. A potential impact of climate change and water resource development on the transmission of *Schistosoma japonicum* in China. Parasitologica 2005; **47**: 127–34.

[47] Intergovernmental Panel on Climate Change (WGI). *Climate Change, 2007. The Science of Climate Change: Contribution of Working Group I to the Second Assessment Report of the Intergovernmental Panel on Climate Change*. Cambridge: Cambridge University Press, 2007.

Chapter 2

Current global health status

Colin Mathers and Ruth Bonita

Introduction

The impressive improvements in health status worldwide over the last century are a cause for celebration. Public health professionals can feel proud of their contribution to these achievements, even as they appreciate the complexity of the underlying driving forces, many of which lie outside traditional public health work. However, satisfaction must be tempered by several concerns. First, the health improvements have not been shared equally and health inequalities among and within countries remain entrenched. Secondly, the fragility of health gains has repeatedly been demonstrated in response, for example, to economic and social changes and civil disruption. Thirdly, and as we have seen in Chapter 1, the global health situation is a complex and a challenging mixture of old and new health problems.

These factors suggest that, from a global perspective, sustainable and equitable health advancement is not yet secure, especially as the economic disparities between countries continue to grow. In this chapter we provide an overview of the global health status and highlight the importance of capturing, with a range of new measures, the health transformations that are taking place in the context of continuing global change.

Measures of health status

Mortality, risk of death, and life expectancy

The best known health status measure continues to be cause of death based on the death certificate. The system of classifying causes of death developed by William Farr 150 years ago still forms the basis of the International Classification of Deaths, now in its tenth version. This provides an invaluable source of information on patterns of death and trends over time. Unfortunately, complete cause specific death registration data are routinely available for only a minority of the world's countries. Approximately a third of the world's population are covered by national vital registration systems and there is a wide regional variation, ranging from over 95 per cent population coverage in the European region to less than 5 per cent population coverage in the African region of the WHO [1]. However, complete or incomplete vital registration data, together with sample registration systems now cover three-quarters of deaths. Survey data and indirect demographic techniques provide information on levels of child and adult mortality for the remaining quarter of global deaths. Data sources and methods are described in more detail elsewhere; these data are of variable quality and there are still a few countries for which no recent data on levels of adult or child mortality are available [2].

While much attention has been directed at obtaining data on children aged under 5 and maternal mortality (for example, from extensive child mortality surveys such as the Demographic Health Survey (DHS) or the Multiple Indicator Cluster Survey (MICS) programme of UNICEF), the most serious information gap now is for adult mortality. Fortunately, considerable effort has gone into developing alternatives to national routine death certification (Box 2.1).

In India, to compensate for a poor civil registration system, the Sample Registration System has successfully collected data on rural mortality and fertility since 1964–1965 through continuous recording by resident enumerators as well as retrospective half-yearly population surveys (Box 2.2). The data obtained through these operations are matched and discrepant events re-verified in the field. Data are collected on vital events in 4436 rural and 2235 urban sampling units with a population of about six million people covering almost all States and Territories. Comparison of these data with other survey and demographic estimates suggests that under-reporting of child deaths is minimal and of adult deaths is around 15 per cent. The Medical Certificate of Cause of Death (MCCD) provides information for deaths in urban India. A high coverage of all deaths (estimated at 95 per cent) has been achieved using these multiple approaches [5].

Two other developing countries which have dramatically improved their death registration systems in the last decade are Iran and South Africa. In 1999, the death registration system in Iran operated in four provinces, covering 5 per cent of all deaths in the country. This system was extended to 18 provinces in 2001, and by 2004 to 29 out of 30 provinces with an estimated coverage of around 65 per cent of all deaths in the country. Tehran province, the most populous province (population 12 million), was the only province not covered by the death registration system [9]. The 2004 data were coded to a condensed list of 318 cause categories, using the ICD-10 classification system. The completeness of death registration data for South Africa has increased from around 50 per cent in the early 1990s to around 90 per cent in 2004, although problems with miscoding of HIV deaths have increased in recent years [10].

Box 2.1 Improving vital statistics in China

In China provincial authorities have provided death data on a routine basis for the past decade from a nationally representative system of 145 disease surveillance centres (DSP) covering 1 per cent of the total Chinese population [3]. At each surveillance centre, a team which includes a physician, investigates each death using medical records and interviews with family members to assign a cause of death. Data on the age, sex, and cause of about 46,000 deaths are recorded each year for a sample population of a little over nine million. Periodic evaluations of the DSP data by resurveying households at random suggest a level of under-reporting of deaths of about 15 per cent[3].

In addition to the DSP, there has been substantial improvement in recent years in the Vital Registration System of the Ministry of Health in China, and this now provides additional useful information. Data on the age, sex, and cause of more than 300,000 deaths are collected annually from the Vital Registration System operated by the Ministry of Health, covering a population of 57 million (36 million in urban areas, 21 million in rural areas). While the data are not representative of mortality conditions throughout China, they are useful for suggesting trends in mortality, given the number of deaths covered, and also provide valuable information on cause-of-death patterns. A third source of data on mortality in China is the decennial population census which asks about deaths in the household in the past 12 months [4]. It has been possible to extrapolate from these three low-cost information sources to the national level, and to contribute to estimates of global patterns and causes of death.

These multiple sources have been used by WHO, together with information derived from specific epidemiological studies, to estimate life tables and cause-of-death patterns for all regions of the world [2,11]. WHO and the Health Metrics Network are also devoting considerable efforts to promoting the use of sample registration and survey and census methods, together with standardized and validated verbal autopsy methods, to address the information gaps for low- and middle-income countries [12]. These approaches should not be regarded as substitutes for complete civil registration, but rather as complementary to a surveillance system.

In particular, increased attention is being paid to the further development of standardized verbal autopsy instruments and improved validation and analysis

Box 2.2 The Million Deaths Study

During the early years of the twenty-first century, the methods used in the Sample Registration System (SRS) in India were substantially revised as part of the Million Deaths Study (MDS). As of 2002, causes of death have been ascertained using a verbal autopsy method, with re-sampling, double coding by physicians centrally, and other quality control efforts. The MDS is following the lives and deaths of 1.1 million households throughout India until 2014 [6]. This nationally representative survey will gather information about risk factors and causes of death for members of these households to yield a detailed picture of how and why people die [7]. The MDS provides a low-cost and large-scale means of tracking the health status of over a billion people. Preliminary data for a nationally representative sample of 62,553 deaths in 2001–2003 have been released, but validation studies of verbal-autopsy-assigned causes of death are still under way [8].

methods, to provide an economical and useful strategy for improving the quality of cause-of-death information where health workers have minimal training or where survey methods must be used (Box 2.3).

Disability and health status measures

While risk of death is the simplest comparable measure of health status for populations, there has been increasing interest in describing, measuring, and comparing health states of populations. These have been conceptualized in two main ways: in terms of disability and handicap [16], and in terms of multidimensional health profiles [17]. In the latter approach, a health state is a multidimensional attribute of an individual which reflects his/her level in the various domains of health. Thus, a health state differs from pathology, risk factors, or aetiology, and from health service encounters or interventions. Describing health states within and between populations is a central challenge in undertaking the measurement of health.

The WHO International Classification of Impairments, Disabilities, and Handicaps (ICIDH) defined *disability* as any restriction or lack of ability (resulting from an impairment) to perform an activity in the manner or within the range considered normal for a human being, and *handicap* as the social disadvantage resulting from an impairment or disability that limits or prevents the fulfilment of a normal role [18]. The second revision of the ICIDH, now called the International Classification of Functioning, Disability and Health

Box 2.3 Verbal autopsy

Verbal autopsy (VA) methods use a questionnaire administered to caregivers or family members of deceased persons to gather information on signs and symptoms and their duration, and other pertinent information about the decedent in the period before death. The validity of methods used for mapping this symptom information to underlying disease and injury causes of death is of central concern [13]. Most approaches have used panels of physicians to review the data collected and assign a probable cause of death. The precision of VA depends upon factors that vary across and even within countries, and can also change over time. Results of validation studies cannot usually be assumed to apply to other studies using different physicians. Categorical assignment of cause of death is inherently difficult for diseases without distinctive symptoms, such as malaria in children or some forms of cardiovascular disease in older adults. The use of Bayesian methods to develop probabilistic mappings of symptom patterns to underlying causes of death shows promise [14], and the WHO is working to standardize verbal autopsy instruments for use with children and adult deaths [15].

(or ICF) replaces the ICIDH concepts of disability and handicap by the concepts of *capacity* and *performance*, and applies these constructs to a single list of tasks and activities [16]. The term *disability* is now used broadly to refer to departures from good or ideal health in any of the important domains of health.

Within high-income countries, especially in the context of clinical trials, there has been substantial work on measuring functional health status, usually in terms of a set of 'core health domains' such as mobility, dexterity, pain, affect, cognition, vision, and hearing [17,19,20]. These instruments rely on self-report and none have solved the problem of comparability of responses across populations due to differences in expectations and norms for health. For example, the level of mobility described as 'moderate limitations' may differ across different cultures, across socio-economic groups within a society, across age groups, or between men and women. Despite innovative efforts to enhance comparability with methods such as anchoring vignettes, little progress has been made in the comparable measurement of functional health status [21–23] Development of instruments that can be used across cultural and linguistic groups will be crucial to improving population information on overall health states and disability in populations.

Recently, the WHO Global Burden of Disease (GBD) estimates for 2004 were used to estimate the prevalence of people with long-term disability for two severity thresholds of disability. Estimated regional distributions of disease and injury sequelae across seven disability classes were used, together with some specific assumptions about comorbidity, to estimate the prevalence of long-term disability (lasting for 6 months or more) for moderate and severe levels of disability [11,24].

Clinically and conceptually it is not usual practice to infer disability from diagnoses. In future revisions of the GBD study, increased effort will be devoted to direct estimation of the prevalences of impairments and disabilities, and to ensuring consistency with the disease- and injury-specific sequelae estimates. The GBD disability prevalence estimates have the virtue of comprehensiveness and at least some grounding in disease prevalence. However, they are only approximations, and are subject to very clear limitations in the way that they were compiled and the way in which comorbidity was addressed in adding across causes.

Summary measures combining mortality and morbidity

The epidemiological transition, characterized by a progressive rise in the average age of death in virtually all populations across the globe, has necessitated a serious reconsideration of how the health of populations is measured. Average life expectancy at birth is becoming increasingly uninformative in many populations where, because of the non-linear relationship between age-specific mortality and the life expectancy index, significant declines in death rates at older ages have produced only relatively modest increases in life expectancy at birth. Such considerations are critical for the planning and provision of health and social services, as resources are now devoted to reducing the incidence of conditions that cause ill health but not death.

Separate measures of survival and of health status among survivors, while useful inputs into the health policy debate, need to be combined in some fashion if the goal is to provide a single holistic measure of overall population health. Two classes of health status measures that combine mortality and morbidity into a single index have been developed: health gaps and health expectancies [25]. Both these types of summary measure use time as a common currency for years of life lived in various states of health and for time lost because of premature mortality.

Burden of disease and health gap measures

The GBD project developed a new summary measure which combines the impact of premature mortality with that of disability and captures the impact on populations of important non-fatal disabling conditions [26]. Disability-adjusted life-years (DALYs) combine time lost through premature death and time lived with disability. One DALY can be thought of as one lost year of 'healthy' life, and the measured disease burden is the gap between a population's health status and that of a normative reference population (with life expectancy at birth of 82.5 years for females and 80.0 years for males). The DALY is a generalization of the well-known mortality gap measure years of potential life lost (YPLL) to include lost good health. It also provides a way of linking information at the population level on disease causes and occurrence to information on both short- and long-term health outcomes, including impairments, disability, and death. This measure, like YPLL, weights causes of death that occur early in life more heavily than those that occur later in life and does not take into account competing risks but rather measures years lost against a normative standard.

The WHO has updated the assessment of the GBD for the years 2000–2004 based on an extensive analysis of mortality data for all regions of the world together with systematic reviews of epidemiological studies and population health surveys. These revisions draw on a wide range of data sources, and various methods have been developed to reconcile often fragmented and partial estimates of epidemiological parameters that are available from different studies [2,11].

The GBD study in general, and the DALY measure in particular, have stimulated considerable debate, in part because of the limitations of the basic data, the extrapolations from these data to entire regions, and the assumptions that are needed for these estimates. The greatest degree of uncertainty relates to the sub-Saharan estimates because of the scarcity of mortality data, particularly for adults. One of its major objectives of the GBD study is an assessment of all causes of disease and injury burden. Otherwise, limitations in the evidence base for certain causes or regions translate to 'no burden' rather than the best achievable uncertain estimates of burden, and health decision-makers would be presented with a misleading picture. Where the evidence is uncertain, incomplete, or even non-existent, the GBD study attempts to make the best possible inferences based on the knowledge base that is available, and to assess the uncertainty in the resulting estimates. This has generated controversy among epidemiologists who are more used to reporting only assessments with narrow uncertainty intervals primarily based on sampling error.

The social values and disability weights incorporated into the DALY have also attracted criticism. Some critics have argued against the use of age weights which give lower value to years of life lived in early childhood and older ages, and some recent burden of disease studies have used time discounting but not age weights [27,28]. These criticisms relate to concerns that priorities for health action might be set solely on the basis of the magnitude of the burden of disease (Box 2.4). Although other factors, such as effectiveness and cost-effectiveness of available interventions, equity, and other social and political considerations, also play an important and valid role in priority setting, the magnitude of disease burden at population level due to different causes and risks is also an important input to such policy debates.

Health expectancy measures

Another form of summary measure of population health—health expectancy—has been used to report on average levels of population health. Disability-free life expectancy (DFLE) was calculated and reported for many countries in the 1980s and 1990s [29,30]. Unfortunately, DFLE estimates based on self-reported health status information are not generally comparable across countries because of differences in survey instruments and cultural differences in reporting of health.

From 2000 to 2004, WHO reported annually on the average levels of population health for its member countries using health-adjusted life expectancy (HALE), which measures the equivalent number of years of life expected to be lived in full health [31]. Estimates for 2002 used improved methods and made use of survey data from 63 surveys in 55 countries from the WHO Multi-Country Survey Study [32], together with improved methods for taking account of

Box 2.4 'Health' and 'disability'

DALYs have received a great deal of criticism from disability advocates and some health analysts, who have seen the inclusion of disability in the DALY as implying that people with disability are less valued than people in full health. Some of this criticism relates to claims that cost-effectiveness analysis imposes an implicit utilitarianism on policy choices, but a more fundamental criticism is that the conceptualization of disability found in the DALY confounds the ideas of 'health' and 'disability', whereas in fact people with disabilities may be no less healthy than anyone else. In response to these critics, the conceptual basis for the measurement of health and the valuation of health states in the DALY has been further developed and clarified [2]. As used in the DALY, the term 'disability' is essentially a synonym for health states of less than full health and thus the disability weights reflect judgements about the 'healthfulness' of defined states, not judgements of quality of life or the worth of persons.

comorbidity in using inputs from the GBD study [24]. The authors have prepared updated estimates of healthy life expectancy for the year 2004 for this chapter using the GBD update for 2004 and the same methods as for previous WHO estimates [31].

Some commentators have argued that the data demands and complexity of the calculations make healthy life expectancy an impractical measure for use as a summary measure of population health [33]. Although the concept of healthy life expectancy is relatively simple to understand, health encompasses multiple domains and mortality risks, and with the additional requirement to ensure comparability of estimates across countries, current methods are inevitably complex and do not yet fully solve the problem of basing national-level estimates on national-level cross-population comparable data.

An overview of global health status

Life expectancy

Life expectancy at birth in 2004 ranged from 79 years in high-income countries down to below 50 years in Africa (Fig. 2.1). This is a 1.6-fold difference in total life expectancy across major regions of the globe. Female life expectancy in high-income countries reached an average of 82 years in 2006, and was 86 years in Japan. Overall, for the entire population of the world, average life expectancy at birth in 2004 was 65.6 years, an increase of almost 9 years over the last quarter century. As shown in Fig. 2.1, life expectancy increased during the 1990s for most regions of the world, with the notable exception of Africa and the low- and middle-income countries of Eastern Europe.

Mortality and causes of death

WHO estimates that almost 59 million people died in 2004, 10.4 million (or nearly 20 per cent) of whom were children less than 5 years of age. Of these child deaths, 99 per cent occurred in low- and middle-income countries. Just over 70 per cent of deaths in high-income countries occur beyond age 70, compared with 32 per cent in low- and middle-income countries. A key point is the comparatively high numbers of deaths in poor countries at young adult ages (15–59 years); just over 30 per cent of all deaths in these countries occur at these ages, compared with 15 per cent in wealthy regions.

The variations across regions of the world in the probability of premature death (for example, between birth and 5 years and between 15 and 60 years) give one indication of the potential for health improvement. The 25-fold variation in child mortality between different regions of the world is largely due to communicable diseases, malnutrition, and poverty (Fig. 2.2).

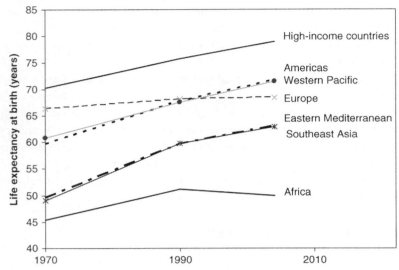

Fig. 2.1 Gains in average life expectancy at birth from 1970 to 2004, by region.
Note: Low- and middle-income countries are grouped by WHO region. High-income countries in all regions are grouped together as a single group. Countries were classified as high income if their 2004 GNI per capita was US$10,066 or more as estimated by the World Bank. The high-income countries were Andorra, Aruba, Australia, Austria, Bahamas, Bahrain, Belgium, Bermuda, Brunei Darussalam, Canada, Cayman Islands, Channel Islands, Cyprus, Denmark, Faeroe Islands, Finland, France, French Polynesia, Germany, Greece, Greenland, Guam, Iceland, Ireland, Isle of Man, Israel, Italy, Japan, Kuwait, Liechtenstein, Luxembourg, Malta, Monaco, Netherlands, Netherlands Antilles, New Caledonia, New Zealand, Norway, Portugal, Puerto Rico, Qatar, Republic of Korea, San Marino, Saudi Arabia, Singapore, Slovenia, Spain, Sweden, Switzerland, United Arab Emirates, UK, USA, and US Virgin Islands.

In contrast, the probability of death in adults aged between 15 and 60 years is due mostly to non-communicable diseases and injury, except in India and sub-Saharan Africa (Fig. 2.3). The probability of premature death varies widely between regions. For example, in the low- and middle-income countries of Europe, the death rate is similar to that in developing regions of Asia and the Middle East, and more than 2.5 times higher than in the high-income countries of Europe.

Low- and middle-income countries themselves are a very heterogeneous group in terms of mortality. A contrast between China (with more than one-sixth of the world's population) and Africa (with one-tenth of the global population) illustrates the extreme diversity in health conditions among developing regions. Less than 6 per cent of deaths in China occur below

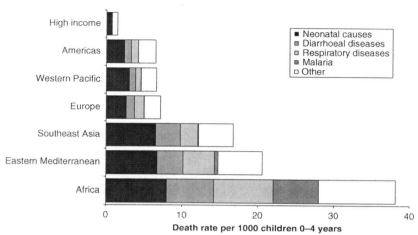

Fig. 2.2 Global variation in mortality rates of children under 5 years of age, 2004.
Note: High-income countries in all WHO regions are grouped together as a single group in this figure.
Source: WHO [11].

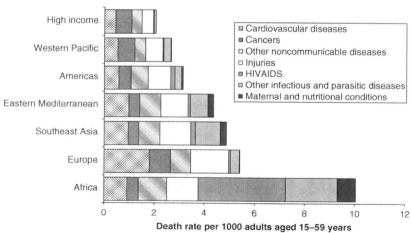

Fig. 2.3 Global variation in adult mortality rates for ages 15–59 years, 2004.
Note: High-income countries in all WHO regions are grouped together as a single group in this figure.
Source: WHO [11].

age 5 compared with 40 per cent in Africa. Conversely, 52 per cent of deaths in China occur beyond age 70 compared with only 12 per cent in Africa. Men in these two regions are three times more likely to die prematurely than men in Western industrialized populations. The variation in the proportion of women dying prematurely in these regions is much less dramatic, except for the differences between the wealthiest region and the poorest region.

There are major differences in adult mortality by sex and major cause group (Fig. 2.4). Overall, mortality is highest among men and women in sub-Saharan Africa, mainly because of high mortality due to communicable, perinatal, maternal, and nutritional causes, particularly HIV/AIDS. Men in Europe (excluding high-income countries) had the second highest mortality rates at ages 15–59 years, considerably higher than in Southeast Asia, the Eastern Mediterranean, and the Americas. In all regions, men had higher mortality rates than women. The largest differences were observed in Europe (male mortality 2.7 times higher than female mortality), the Americas (2.0), and high-income countries (1.9). In sub-Saharan Africa mortality among men is slightly higher than among women; this is entirely due to higher mortality as a result of injuries. At ages 15–59 years women have much higher mortality than men from HIV/AIDS, which causes more than half of all female deaths due to infectious and parasitic diseases, maternal, and nutritional causes and nearly 40 per cent of all female deaths. Maternal conditions were associated with 14 per cent of all deaths.

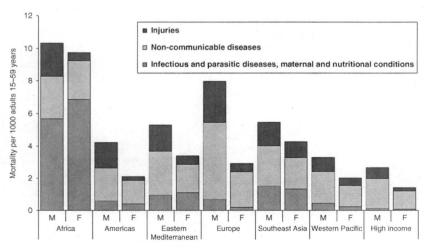

Fig. 2.4 Mortality rates for ages 15–59 years by sex, region, and cause of death, 2004.

Of the 59 million deaths in 2004, 35 million (60 per cent) were due to chronic (non-communicable) diseases, which killed twice as many people as communicable, maternal, perinatal, and nutritional causes combined (18.0 million, or 30 per cent of all causes). Injuries killed a further 5.8 million people in 2004— almost one in ten of the world's total deaths. The relative importance of these causes varies markedly across regions. Thus, in Africa, about one in four deaths are due to chronic diseases, compared with more than four out of five in high-income countries. Two-thirds of deaths in Latin America and close to 60 per cent in the low- and middle-income countries of Asia and the Western Pacific are due to non-communicable disease, reflecting the relatively advanced stage of the epidemiological transition achieved in these populations.

The top ten disease and injury causes of death in the year 2004 for high-, middle-, and low-income countries and the world are shown in Table 2.1. In high-income countries, ischaemic heart disease and cerebrovascular disease (stroke) were together responsible for 26 per cent of mortality, and death rates were higher for men than for women. Lung cancer was the third leading cause of death, again with a nearly threefold male excess. Another largely tobacco-related cause, chronic obstructive lung disease, was the fifth leading cause of death, accounting for 3.5 per cent of deaths in high-income countries. Road traffic accidents were no longer in the top ten causes of mortality, as there has been a decline in death rates due to road traffic accidents in high income countries since 1990.

The leading causes of mortality were very different in low- and middle-income countries (Table 2.1). While the five leading causes of death in middle-income countries are similar to those in high-income countries (with cerebrovascular disease leading ischaemic heart disease), road traffic accidents were the sixth leading cause of death and tuberculosis was also in the top ten causes. Chronic obstructive lung disease kills more people (1.5 million) in the Western Pacific region (primarily China) than anywhere else in the world, with over half of global mortality from the disease occurring there.

For low-income countries, in contrast, six of the top ten causes of death were infectious causes, and neonatal problems (prematurity and neonatal infections) were also in the top ten. Acute lower respiratory infection (primarily pneumonia) was the leading cause of death in low-income countries (more than half of these deaths were among children aged under 5). HIV/AIDS was the fourth leading cause of death for low-income countries in the year 2004, accounting for nearly 6 per cent of all deaths or 1.5 million deaths in total. Close to 85 per cent of these deaths occurred in Africa, making HIV the leading cause of death in this region, (approximately 15 per cent of total deaths). Malaria is the sixth leading cause of death in low-income countries, slightly

Table 2.1 The ten leading causes of death in low-, middle-, and high-income countries, 2004[1]

Disease or injury	Deaths (million)	Percentage total deaths
World		
1 Ischaemic heart disease	7.2	12.2
2 Cerebrovascular disease	5.7	9.7
3 Lower respiratory infections	4.1	7.0
4 COPD	3.0	5.1
5 Diarrhoeal diseases	2.1	3.6
6 HIV/AIDS	2.0	3.5
7 Tuberculosis	1.5	2.5
8 Trachea, bronchus, lung cancers	1.3	2.3
9 Road traffic accidents	1.3	2.2
10 Prematurity and low birth weight	1.2	2.0
Low-income countries		
1 Lower respiratory infections	2.9	11.0
2 Ischaemic heart disease	2.5	9.4
3 Diarrhoeal diseases	1.8	6.8
4 HIV/AIDS	1.5	5.7
5 Cerebrovascular disease	1.5	5.6
6 Malaria	1.0	3.7
7 COPD	0.9	3.6
8 Tuberculosis	0.9	3.5
9 Neonatal infections[2]	0.9	3.4
10 Prematurity and low birth weight	0.8	3.2
Middle-income countries		
1 Cerebrovascular disease	3.5	14.2
2 Ischaemic heart disease	3.4	13.9
3 COPD	1.8	7.4
4 Lower respiratory infections	0.9	3.8
5 Trachea, bronchus, lung cancers	0.7	2.9
6 Road traffic accidents	0.7	2.8
7 Hypertensive heart disease	0.6	2.5
8 Stomach cancer	0.5	2.2
9 Tuberculosis	0.5	2.2
10 Diabetes mellitus	0.5	2.1

Table 2.1 (continued) The ten leading causes of death in low-, middle-, and high-income countries, 2004[1]

Disease or injury	Deaths (million)	Percentage total deaths
High-income countries		
1 Ischaemic heart disease	1.3	16.3
2 Cerebrovascular disease	0.8	9.3
3 Trachea, bronchus, lung cancers	0.5	5.9
4 Lower respiratory infections	0.3	3.8
5 COPD	0.3	3.5
6 Alzheimer's and other dementias	0.3	3.4
7 Colon and rectum cancers	0.3	3.3
8 Diabetes mellitus	0.2	2.8
9 Breast cancer	0.2	2.0
10 Stomach cancer	0.1	1.8

COPD, chronic obstructive pulmonary disease.

[1] Income categories for 2004 as defined by the World Bank. Countries are divided among income groups according to 2004 gross national income (GNI) per capita. The groups are low income ($825 or less), middle income ($826–$10 065), and high income ($10 066 or more).

[2] This category also includes other non-infectious causes arising in the perinatal period, responsible for about 20 per cent of deaths shown in this category.

Source: WHO [11].

ahead of chronic obstructive lung disease and tuberculosis. Neonatal infections and prematurity are also in the top ten causes of death for low-income countries.

Globally, cancers of the trachea, bronchus, and lung are the most common cause of death among cancers among men, and this is also the case in all regions of the world apart from Africa. There were an estimated 1.32 million lung cancer deaths in 2004, an increase of 40 per cent in the 14 years from 1990. Of the 7.4 million cancer deaths estimated to have occurred in 2004, one in six (18 per cent) were due to lung cancer alone, and three-quarters of these occurred among men. Stomach cancer, which until recently was the leading site of cancer mortality worldwide, has been declining in all parts of the world where trends can be reliably assessed and caused 803,000 deaths in 2004, or about two-thirds as many as lung cancer.

For women, the most common cancer at the global level was breast cancer, followed by trachea, bronchus, and lung cancer and stomach cancer. Cervix cancer was the leading cause of cancer death for women in Southeast Asia and sub-Saharan Africa.

Morbidity and disability

The Global Burden of Disease study has estimated the incidence and prevalence of a comprehensive set of disease conditions and injuries for all regions of the world. Many of these estimates are based on a synthesis of data from relatively small numbers of epidemiological studies for each region, and in some cases estimates for regions with no data are based on neighbouring regions. The conditions which, at any given moment, affect the largest number of individuals are not very dramatic, and are easily overlooked and underestimated. Worldwide, at any given moment, more individuals have iron-deficiency anaemia than any other health problem. Even in high-income countries, iron-deficiency anaemia is common. Table 2.2 summarizes the estimated prevalences of selected conditions for the world and WHO regions in 2004. Recent data from the WHO World Health Surveys and the World Mental Health Survey are likely to lead to improved estimates of the prevalence of mental disorders. GBD prevalence estimates were also used to estimate the prevalence of moderate and severe disability by severity class in 2004 (Box 2.5)

Table 2.3 lists the major causes of disability according to the GBD estimates for 2004. Globally, adult onset hearing loss and refractive errors topped the list, with mental disorders such as depression, alcohol use disorders, and psychoses such as bipolar disorder and schizophrenia also appearing in the top 20 causes. The pattern differed between the high-income and middle- and low-income countries in that many more people were disabled due to preventable causes such as unintentional injuries and infertility arising from unsafe abortion and maternal sepsis in the lower-income countries. Also, the data reveal the lack of use of interventions for easily treated conditions such as hearing loss, refractive errors, and cataracts in low- and middle-income countries. Disability due to unintentional injuries among the younger population and cataracts among the older population was also far more common in low-income countries.

The GBD prevalence estimates are based on systematic assessments of the available data on incidence, prevalence, duration, and severity of a wide range of conditions, often based on inconsistent, fragmented, and partial data available from different studies. As a result, there are still very substantial data gaps and uncertainties, and improving the population-level information on the incidence, prevalence, and health states associated with major health conditions remains a major priority for national and international health and statistical agencies. Clinically and conceptually it is not usual practice to infer disability from diagnoses. In future revisions of the GBD study, increased effort will be devoted to the estimation of the prevalences of impairments and disabilities

Table 2.2 Prevalence of selected conditions by WHO region, 2004

	World (million)	Africa (million)	Americas (million)	Eastern Mediter-ranean (million)	Europe (million)	SE Asia (million)	Western Pacific (million)
Tuberculosis	13.9	3.0	0.5	1.1	0.6	5.0	3.8
HIV infection	31.7	21.8	2.9	0.5	2.1	3.3	1.1
Intestinal nematodes, high-intensity infection	150.9	57.7	5.8	8.5	0.0	37.7	41.2
Protein-energy malnutrition							
Wasting (children under 5)	53.2	11.8	1.3	6.3	1.3	24.9	7.5
Stunting (all ages)	182.6	47.8	8.0	17.3	4.0	77.5	28.0
Iron-deficiency anaemia	1159.6	194.0	66.8	89.1	77.8	462.6	269.3
Diabetes mellitus	220.5	9.8	46.6	18.0	45.4	44.7	56.0
Unipolar depressive disorders	151.2	13.4	22.9	12.5	22.2	40.9	39.3
Bipolar affective disorder	29.5	2.7	4.1	2.1	4.4	7.2	8.9
Schizophrenia	26.3	2.1	3.9	1.9	4.4	6.2	7.9
Alcohol use disorders	40.0	7.7	8.6	2.8	4.1	9.8	7.0
Epilepsy	125.0	3.8	24.4	1.1	26.9	21.5	47.3
Alzheimer's and other dementias	24.2	0.7	5.0	0.6	7.6	2.8	7.4
Parkinson's disease	5.4	0.2	1.2	0.2	2.1	0.7	1.1
Migraine[1]	324.1	12.6	60.0	16.3	77.4	70.3	87.5
Low vision[2]	277.1	25.6	26.3	19.4	27.6	82.9	95.3

Table 2.2 (continued) Prevalence of selected conditions by WHO region, 2004.

	World (million)	Africa (million)	Americas (million)	Eastern Mediterranean (million)	Europe (million)	SE Asia (million)	Western Pacific (million)
Blindness[3]	45.3	8.4	3.0	4.3	2.6	15.9	11.0
Hearing loss, moderate or greater[4]	275.5	37.6	31.2	19.6	44.5	89.7	52.9
Hearing loss, mild[5]	361.1	18.7	46.1	25.4	75.8	88.6	106.5
Angina pectoris	53.3	1.8	6.3	4.4	17.2	15.9	7.6
Stroke survivors	30.6	1.8	4.7	1.2	9.2	4.4	9.3
COPD, symptomatic cases	65.6	1.6	12.6	3.2	10.0	15.3	22.9
Asthma	234.8	30.0	53.6	15.5	28.8	45.7	61.2
Rheumatoid arthritis	23.7	1.2	4.7	1.3	6.2	4.4	6.0
Osteoarthritis	151.4	10.1	22.5	6.0	40.2	27.4	45.0

COPD, chronic obstructive pulmonary disease.
[1] Prevalence of migraine sufferers, not episodes.
[2] Low vision (<6/18 presenting visual acuity) due to glaucoma, cataracts, macular degeneration, or refractive errors.
[3] Blindness (<3/60 presenting visual acuity) due to glaucoma, cataracts, macular degeneration, or refractive errors.
[4] Hearing loss threshold in the better ear 41 dB or greater (measured average for 0.5, 1, 2, 4 kHz).
[5] Hearing loss threshold in the better ear 26–40 dB (measured average for 0.5, 1, 2, 4 kHz).
Source: WHO [11].

Box 2.5 Severity of disability

Severe disability includes conditions such as blindness, Down syndrome, quadriplegia, severe depression, and active psychosis. Moderate disability includes conditions such as angina pectoris, arthritis, low vision, or alcohol dependence. Of the nearly 6.5 billion of the world's population in 2004, 18.6 million (2.9 per cent) were severely disabled and another 79.7 (12.4 per cent) had moderate long-term disability, according to the definitions given above. The average global prevalence of moderate and severe disability ranged from 5 per cent in children aged 0–14 years, to 15 per cent in adults aged 15–59 years, and 46 per cent in older adults aged 60 years and over. Both moderate and severe levels of disability were higher in low- and middle-income countries than in high-income countries at all ages, and were higher in Africa than in other low- and middle-income countries. Although the proportion of older persons is much larger in high-income countries, they are relatively less disabled than their counterparts in low- and middle-income countries.

directly, and to ensuring consistency with the disease- and injury-specific sequelae estimates.

Population survey data on disability prevalence are limited in availability and comparability. The estimates derived from the GBD have the virtue of comprehensiveness, and at least some grounding in disease prevalence. Nevertheless, they are only approximations, and are subject to very clear limitations in the way they were compiled.

Global disease burden in 2004

The leading causes of DALYs worldwide, and for low-, middle- and high-income countries are shown in Table 2.4 for the year 2004. Lower respiratory infections, diarrhoeal diseases and unipolar depressive disorders were the three leading causes of DALYs globally. Reflecting the huge increase in HIV incidence between 1990 and 2000, HIV/AIDS has leapt from the 28th leading cause of DALYs (0.8 per cent) in 1990 to the fifth leading cause (3.9 per cent) in 2004. In Africa, HIV/AIDS was the leading cause of disease burden, responsible for 12.4 per cent of total DALYs.

Table 2.4 also highlights the marked contrast in epidemiological patterns between rich and poor regions of the world, even more so than comparisons based on deaths. Thus, in the high-income countries, the share of disease

Table 2.3 Estimated prevalence of moderate and severe disability[1] (in millions), by leading disease and injury causes and age, in high-, and low-, and middle-income countries, 2004

Disabling condition[2]	High-income countries[3]		Low- and middle-income countries		World
	0–59 years	60 years and over	0–59 years	60 years and over	All ages
1 Hearing loss[4]	7.4	18.5	54.3	43.9	124.2
2 Refractive errors[5]	7.7	6.4	68.1	39.8	121.9
3 Depression	15.8	0.5	77.6	4.8	98.7
4 Cataracts	0.5	1.1	20.8	31.4	53.8
5 Unintentional injuries	2.8	1.1	35.4	5.7	45.0
6 Osteoarthritis	1.9	8.1	14.1	19.4	43.4
7 Alcohol dependence and problem use	7.3	0.4	31.0	1.8	40.5
8 Infertility due to unsafe abortion and maternal sepsis	0.8	0.0	32.5	0.0	33.4
9 Macular degeneration[6]	1.8	6.0	9.0	15.1	31.9
10 COPD	3.2	4.5	10.9	8.0	26.6
11 Ischaemic heart disease	1.0	2.2	8.1	11.9	23.2
12 Bipolar disorder	3.3	0.4	17.6	0.8	22.2
13 Asthma	2.9	0.5	15.1	0.9	19.4
14 Schizophrenia	2.2	0.4	13.1	1.0	16.7
15 Glaucoma	0.4	1.5	5.7	7.9	15.5
16 Alzheimer's and other dementias	0.4	6.2	1.3	7.0	14.9

17 Panic disorder	1.9	0.1	11.4	0.3	13.8
18 Cerebrovascular disease	1.4	2.2	4.0	4.9	12.6
19 Rheumatoid arthritis	1.3	1.7	5.9	3.0	11.9
20 Drug dependence and problem use	3.7	0.1	8.0	0.1	11.8

COPD, chronic obstructive pulmonary disease.

[1] GBD disability classes III and above.

[2] Disease and injury causes of disability. Conditions are listed in descending order by global all-age prevalence.

[3] High-income countries are those with 2004 gross national income (GNI) per capita of $10,066 or more in 2004 as estimated by the World Bank.

[4] Includes adult-onset hearing loss, excluding that due to infectious causes, adjusted for availability of hearing aids.

[5] Includes presenting refractive errors, adjusted for availability of glasses and other devices for correction.

[6] Includes other age-related causes of vision loss apart from glaucoma, cataracts, and refractive errors.

Source: WHO [11].

Table 2.4 The ten leading causes of burden of disease (DALYs) for low-, middle-, and-high income countries[1] and the world, 2004

Disease or injury	DALYs (million years)	Percentage of total DALYs
World		
1 Lower respiratory infections	92.2	6.1
2 Diarrhoeal diseases	71.6	4.7
3 Unipolar depressive disorders	65.5	4.3
4 Ischaemic heart disease	62.6	4.1
5 HIV/AIDS	58.9	3.9
6 Cerebrovascular disease	46.6	3.1
7 Prematurity and low birth weight	44.3	2.9
8 Birth asphyxia and birth trauma	41.7	2.7
9 Road traffic accidents	41.2	2.7
10 Neonatal infections[2]	40.4	2.7
Low-income countries		
1 Lower respiratory infections	75.0	9.1
2 Diarrhoeal diseases	59.2	7.2
3 HIV/AIDS	42.9	5.2
4 Malaria	36.6	4.4
5 Prematurity and low birth weight	32.1	3.9
6 Neonatal infections[2]	31.4	3.8
7 Birth asphyxia and birth trauma	29.8	3.6
8 Unipolar depressive disorders	26.5	3.2
9 Ischaemic heart disease	26.0	3.1
10 Tuberculosis	22.4	2.7
Middle-income countries		
1 Unipolar depressive disorders	29.0	5.1
2 Ischaemic heart disease	28.9	5.0
3 Cerebrovascular disease	27.5	4.8
4 Road traffic accidents	21.4	3.7
5 COPD	16.1	2.8
6 Lower respiratory infections	15.9	2.8
7 HIV/AIDS	15.2	2.7
8 Alcohol use disorders	14.9	2.6
9 Refractive errors	13.7	2.4
10 Diarrhoeal diseases	12.9	2.2

Table 2.4 (continued) The ten leading causes of burden of disease (DALYs) for low-, middle-, and-high income countries[1] and the world, 2004

	Disease or injury	DALYs (million years)	Percentage of total DALYs
	High-income countries		
1	Unipolar depressive disorders	10.0	8.2
2	Ischaemic heart disease	7.7	6.3
3	Cerebrovascular disease	4.8	3.9
4	Alzheimer's and other dementias	4.4	3.6
5	Alcohol use disorders	4.2	3.4
6	Hearing loss, adult onset	4.2	3.4
7	COPD	3.7	3.0
8	Diabetes mellitus	3.6	3.0
9	Trachea, bronchus, lung cancers	3.6	3.0
10	Road traffic accidents	3.1	2.6

COPD, chronic obstructive pulmonary disease.

[1] Income categories for 2004 as defined by the World Bank. Countries are divided among income groups according to 2004 gross national income (GNI) per capita. The groups are low income ($825 or less), middle income ($826–$10,065), and high income ($10,066 or more).

[2] This category also includes other non-infectious causes arising in the perinatal period, responsible for about 20 per cent of deaths shown in this category.

Source: WHO [11].

burden due to communicable, maternal, perinatal, and nutritional conditions is typically around 5 per cent, compared with 70–75 per cent in Africa. Specifically, the leading causes of disease burden in low-income countries were acute lower respiratory infections (9.1 per cent), diarrhoeal diseases (7.2 per cent), HIV/ AIDS (5.2 per cent), and malaria (4.4 per cent), compared with depression, ischaemic heart disease, cerebrovascular disease, and senile dementias in the high-income countries. Road traffic accidents were the fourth leading cause of burden of disease in middle income countries, responsible for 3.7 per cent of all DALYs. Alcohol use disorders were also among the ten leading causes of DALYs in both middle- and high-income countries. The burden of alcohol use disorders was six times higher in men than in women. When DALYs rather than deaths are considered, the public health importance of injuries becomes more apparent. In the low- and middle-income countries of Europe and the Americas, more than 15 per cent of the entire disease and injury burden was due to injuries alone in 2004.

Measured in DALYs, 36 per cent of total disease and injury burden for the world in 2004 was in children aged less than 15 years, and almost 50 per cent

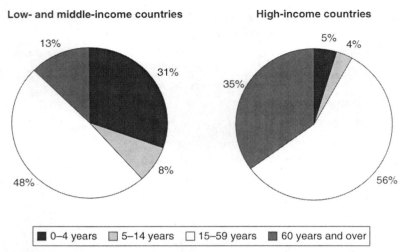

Fig. 2.5 Age distribution of burden of disease by income group, 2004.

in adults aged 15–59 years (Fig. 2.5). The disease burden for children fell almost entirely in low- and middle-income countries. While the proportion of total burden of disease borne by adults aged 15–59 was similar in both groups of countries, the remaining burden was predominantly among those aged 60 years and more in high-income countries. Note that DALYs are attributed to the age at which the disease, injury, or death occurred. Some of the YLD (lost years of health) associated with DALYs for children will be lived at older ages.

Healthy life expectancy

Overall, global HALE at birth in 2004 for males and females combined was 58.3 years, 7.3 years lower than total life expectancy at birth. In other words, poor health resulted in a loss of more than 7 years of healthy life per person, on average globally. Global HALE at birth for females was only 2.5 years greater than that for males. In comparison, female life expectancy at birth was 4.1 years higher than that for males. Global HALE at age 60 was 13.1 years and 15.0 years for males and females, respectively, 4.2 years lower than total life expectancy at age 60 for males and 5.1 years lower for females.

HALE at birth ranged from a low of 42.6 years for African males to 73.6 years for females in high-income countries (Table 2.5). This reflects an almost twofold difference in HALE between major regional populations of the world. The equivalent 'lost' healthy years (total life expectancy minus HALE) ranged from around 13 per cent of total life expectancy at birth in Africa to less than 10 per cent in high-income countries.

Table 2.5 Life expectancy (LE), healthy life expectancy (HALE), and lost healthy years as a percentage of total LE (LHE%), at birth and at age 60, by sex and WHO region, 2004. High-income countries from all regions are grouped separately as a single group

Region	Females			Males			Female–male difference		
	HALE (years)	LE (years)	LHE%	HALE (years)	LE (years)	LHE%	HALE (years)	LE (years)	LHE%
At birth									
High-income countries[1]	73.6	81.8	10.0	69.6	76.1	8.6	4.0	5.7	1.5
African Region	43.2	50.0	13.5	42.6	48.0	11.2	0.7	2.0	2.3
Region of the Americas	65.6	74.7	12.2	61.1	68.4	10.7	4.5	6.3	1.5
Eastern Mediterranean	55.1	63.7	13.5	52.7	59.6	11.6	2.4	4.0	1.8
European Region	64.0	72.5	11.8	56.7	62.8	9.7	7.2	9.7	2.1
Southeast Asia Region	54.9	63.5	13.7	54.5	61.3	11.2	0.4	2.2	2.5
Western Pacific Region	65.5	73.2	10.5	63.0	69.6	9.6	2.5	3.6	1.0
World	59.5	67.6	11.9	57.0	63.5	10.2	2.5	4.1	1.7
At age 60									
High- income countries	19.3	24.8	22.0	16.4	20.8	21.2	2.9	4.0	0.8
African Region	11.2	15.8	29.4	10.3	13.9	25.6	0.9	2.0	3.7
Region of the Americas	15.6	21.2	26.0	13.7	18.2	25.0	2.0	2.9	1.1
Eastern Mediterranean	12.3	17.4	29.3	11.1	15.4	27.7	1.2	2.0	1.6
European Region	14.6	19.3	24.4	11.9	15.6	23.8	2.7	3.7	0.6
South East Asia Region	11.8	17.1	31.0	11.1	15.4	27.9	0.6	1.6	3.1
Western Pacific Region	14.8	19.6	24.4	13.2	17.2	23.4	1.6	2.3	1.0
World	15.0	20.1	25.5	13.1	17.3	24.1	1.9	2.8	1.3

[1] See Fig. 2.1 for definitions of high-income category.

Regional healthy life expectancies at age 60 in 2004 ranged from a low of 8.3 years for men and women in Africa to a high of around 19 years for women in low mortality countries. The equivalent 'lost' healthy years at age 60 are a higher percentage of remaining life expectancy because of the higher prevalence of disability at older ages. These range from around 40–50 per cent in sub-Saharan Africa to around 20 per cent in low- and middle-income countries.

The female–male difference in healthy life expectancy is greatest for the low- and middle-income countries of Europe, at 7.2 years. In these countries, healthy life expectancy is 64.0 years for women, 9.6 years below the average for the high-income countries of Europe, but just 56.7 years for men, 12.9 years below the high-income European average. This is one of the widest sex gaps in the world, and reflects the sharp increase in adult male mortality since the early 1990s. The most common explanation is the high incidence of male alcohol abuse, which led to high rates of accidents, violence, and cardiovascular disease. From 1987 to 1994, the risk of premature death for Russian males increased by 70 per cent [34–36]. Life expectancy for males improved between 1994 and 1998, but has declined significantly again in the last 3 years. Similar rates exist for other countries of the former Soviet Union. This pattern is explored in greater detail in Chapter 5.

Figure 2.6 shows average healthy life expectancy at birth for 192 countries in 2004 plotted against income per capita (gross domestic product (GDP) measured in international dollars using purchasing power parity conversion rates). With some exceptions for countries with high HIV prevalence, average HALE at birth rises steeply with increasing income per capita to around $10,000 per capita, and then gradually flattens out showing no increase with increasing income per capita above around $30,000.

Projections of future trends in mortality

According to revised projections carried out by the WHO [37], the world will experience a substantial shift in the distribution of deaths from younger to older ages and from communicable diseases to non-communicable diseases during the next 25 years (Fig. 2.7). These revised projections take into account the latest projections by UNAIDS and WHO for HIV, and also updated World Bank forecasts for economic growth.

Large declines in mortality between 2002 and 2030 are projected for all the principal communicable, maternal, perinatal, and nutritional causes including HIV, tuberculosis, and malaria. Global HIV/AIDS deaths are projected to rise from 2.2 million in 2008 to a maximum of 2.4 million in 2012 and then to decline to 1.2 million in 2030 under a baseline scenario which assumes that coverage with anti-retroviral (ART) drugs continues to rise at rates currently being achieved.

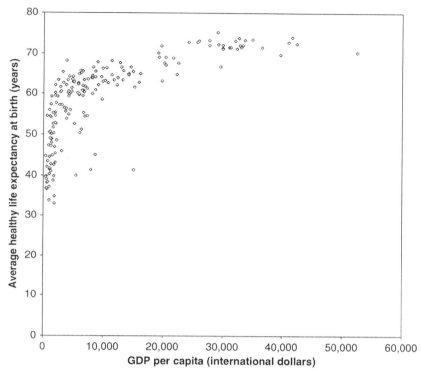

Fig. 2.6 Healthy life expectancy at birth versus GDP per capita in international dollars (purchasing power parity conversion) for 192 countries, 2004.
Source: Authors' calculations drawing on updated inputs from the Global Burden of Disease 2004 update [11].

Ageing of populations in middle- and low-income countries will result in significantly increasing total deaths due to non-communicable diseases over the next 25 years. Global cancer deaths are projected to increase from 7.4 million in 2004 to 11.8 million in 2030, and global cardiovascular deaths from 17.1 million in 2004 to 23.4 million in 2030. Overall, non-communicable diseases are projected to account for just over three-quarters of all deaths in 2030. For non-communicable diseases, demographic changes in all regions will tend to increase total deaths substantially, even though age-sex-specific death rates are projected to decline for most causes other than lung cancer. The impact of population ageing is generally much more important than population growth.

The projected 28 per cent increase in global deaths due to injury between 2004 and 2030 is predominantly due to the increasing numbers of road traffic deaths, together with increases in population numbers more than offsetting small declines in age-specific death rates for other causes of injury. Road traffic

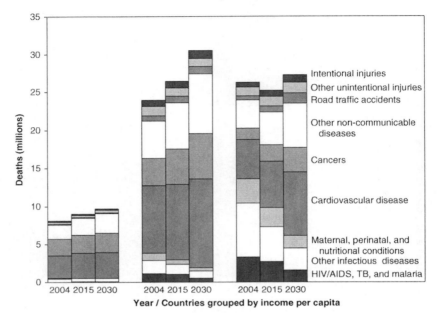

Fig. 2.7 Projected deaths by cause for high-, middle-, and low-income countries, 2004–2030. The group of bands on the Left side is High income, the middle group is Middle income and Right side group is Low income.

deaths are projected to rise from the ninth leading cause of death globally in 2004 to the fifth leading cause.

WHO's updated mortality projections were based on projections of economic and social development, and used the historically observed relationships of these with cause-specific mortality rates, including separate projections for HIV/AIDS, tuberculosis, lung cancer, and diabetes. Projected declining death rates reflect the observed declines in age-specific death rates for both infectious and chronic diseases with increasing levels of development in the available death registration data for 107 countries between 1950 and 2002. These projections do not specifically take account of trends in major risk factors, apart from tobacco smoking and, to a limited extent, overweight and obesity. If risk factor exposures do not generally decline with economic development and improving health systems in developing countries, the WHO projections may underestimate future non-communicable deaths in low- and middle-income countries.

Discussion

Advances in measuring population health

As the importance of health in the global agenda and the number of international partnerships and agencies targeting health problems grow, so does the responsibility to measure accurately the multiple dimensions of health and to assess the effects of increasing investments. Yet, too often, neither clinical care nor health policy formulation have an adequate evidence base.

While there have been noteworthy improvements in the coverage and quality of death registration data, with Iran and South Africa being two success stories in the last decade or so, only one-third of the world's population is covered by usable death registration data. China and India, the two most populous nations in the world, have both been redeveloping their verbal autopsy-based sample registration systems and new data are now becoming available. Apart from the as yet unsolved problems in obtaining valid cause-of-death information from verbal autopsy instruments, less than 5 per cent of the African population is covered by functioning death registration systems. Very little national-level information is available on the causes of child mortality or even on levels of adult mortality for most African countries [1].

Death rates do not tell the whole story about population health. For many conditions, such as blindness, mental disorders, or musculoskeletal diseases, the main effects are loss of health function. According to the GBD estimates, almost 40 per cent of global lost years of healthy life are attributable to loss of health function. Despite efforts to improve the cross-population comparability of self-reported functioning in health domains, little progress has been made in the comparable measurement of functional health status.

Over the last three decades there has been considerable advance in the coverage of household health surveys, and increasing use of these surveys to obtain physical measurements and biological samples for analysis. Advances in technology offer the opportunity to collect biomarkers—biological and clinical data—in existing large-scale national sample surveys. Such data on biomarkers could potentially result in significant improvement in the comparable and reliable measurement of prevalences for some diseases and risk factors. The substantial growth in representative population survey data for HIV prevalence has resulted in a major revision of the UNAIDS and WHO estimates of global prevalence and mortality for HIV [38].

There is now a very substantial database for data on levels of child mortality and coverage of key interventions for child health, with many countries having national surveys approximately every 5 years. A recent assessment of all the available survey evidence on trends in child mortality to age 5 concluded that child deaths worldwide have decreased from 13.5 million in 1980 to an estimated 9.7 million in 2005, and projected that global under-five mortality will decline by 27 per cent from 1990 to 2015, substantially less than the Millennium Development Goal 4 (MDG4) target of a 67 per cent decrease [39]. This rate of decline represents an annual decrease of 1.3 per cent, which is substantially slower than the 2.2 per cent rate of reduction recorded for the world between 1970 and 1985. Most regions of the world are undergoing declines that are considerably faster than 1.3 per cent, but areas with the slowest rates of reduction in fertility (sub-Saharan Africa) also have the slowest rates of decline in child mortality. The study concluded that, globally, we are not doing a better job of reducing child mortality now than we were three decades ago [39].

Worldwide interest in the monitoring of development, as exemplified in the Millennium Development Goals (MDGs), has generated pressure for high-quality and timely data for reporting on country progress [40,41]. Increased funding from donor organizations has also stimulated greater demand for accountability and data on effectiveness of interventions. This has exposed major gaps in the health statistics for developing countries, but has also provided major opportunities to address these gaps. However, within and outside the UN system, the emphasis on monitoring and evaluation is leading to proliferation of indicators and excessive reporting requirements, and needs to be refocused on systematic investments in data generation and analysis. The investment of $50 million by the Bill and Melinda Gates Foundation in the establishment of the Health Metrics Network is a step in this direction [42]. Its major objectives are to address gaps in country health information and to build capacity in health information systems at national and local levels. The Health Metrics Network is funding health information system capacity building projects in low-income countries, as well as providing technical advice and support (Box 2.6).

Health gains with widening health inequalities

While morbidity and disability assessment is of growing significance in all countries, mortality as a health status measure is still of great importance in the poorer countries. Of the estimated 59 million deaths worldwide each year, nine out of ten occur in low- and middle-income countries, reinforcing the fundamental importance of improving mortality statistics as a measure of health status in the developing world.

Overall, however, there have been impressive and unrivalled gains in health status worldwide in the past few decades. For example, life expectancy at birth has increased from a global average of 46 years in 1950 to 66 years in 2004; even since 1990, life expectancy has increased by 3 years. However, many populations in poor countries, and even a few in wealthy countries, still have life expectancies and disease profiles typical of European countries a century ago. Life expectancy at birth in high-income countries is almost double that of the most disadvantaged countries. However, life expectancies at birth may disguise smaller differences in the duration of later life; life expectancy for people in poor

Box 2.6 Improving measurement and use of data for policy

The Bill and Melinda Gates Foundation has provided substantial funding of $105 million over 10 years to establish an Institute for Health Metrics and Evaluation at the University of Washington, Seattle. This new research centre was established in 2007 and aims to conduct independent rigorous evaluations of health programmes worldwide. One of its first major projects, in collaboration with WHO and a number of other academic institutions, is to carry out a complete revision and update of the Global Burden of Disease over 3 years [43]. A large number of unresolved methodological and empirical challenges for better global and national estimates of disease burden remain. Academic research groups, such as the Institute for Health Metrics and Evaluation, will provide valuable partners for global health agencies, such as WHO, UNICEF, and the World Bank, in improving the measurement and policy use of information on population health, and on priorities for funding interventions to improve health.

countries who survive to reach middle age begins to approach that of people in wealthy countries, but with the potential of earlier functional ageing among survivors. Regional life expectancy data also hide important and sobering national and within-country differences and trends. For example, within the USA, the racial differences are large with African American men having a life expectancy at birth up to 20 years lower than that of white men [44]. Within the Eastern Mediterranean region of the WHO, life expectancy at birth for women in Djibouti is 23 years less than that for women in Cyprus.

The extent of the global inequalities in health is illustrated by the large variations in child (under 5 years of age) mortality rates. If all countries had the Japanese rates, the lowest in the world, there would only be one million child deaths each year, instead of the current 10 million deaths. Seven out of ten deaths in children under the age of 5 years still occur in low-income countries and can be attributed to just five preventable conditions—pneumonia, diarrhoeal diseases, malaria, measles, and malnutrition. These conditions overlap and are exacerbated by poverty. The eradication of polio may be achieved in the near future, and there have been impressive reductions in diarrhoeal disease and measles deaths. Malaria and malnutrition remain substantial challenges. A recent analysis estimated that 35 per cent (3.5 million) of child deaths under age 5 were attributable to malnutrition and sub-optimal breastfeeding [45].

Maternal mortality data are equally distressing, even though maternal deaths make up only about 1 per cent of all deaths. Although maternal deaths are often hard to measure and classify accurately, the maternal mortality rates vary enormously from as low as 4 per 100,000 in Australia to 2100 per 100,000 in Sierra Leone. Increasing the coverage of key maternal, newborn, and child health interventions is essential if MDG4 and MDG5 are to be reached.

In the absence of targeting, health interventions tend to be adopted initially by the wealthiest, and may later trickle down to the rest of the population who may emulate the behaviour of the elite groups. A recent analysis of the coverage of maternal, newborn, and child interventions in developing countries found that the coverage gap within countries ranged from an average of 29 per cent for the wealthiest quintile up to 54 per cent for the poorest quintile of the population [46]. Differences between the poorest and the wealthiest were largest for the maternal and newborn health intervention area and smallest for immunization.

The fragility of health gains

The fragility of recent health gains has become apparent in the face of social disruption as a result of economic and political disarray, as in the former Soviet Union (see Chapter 5), or war, as in the former Yugoslavia, Iraq, and Afghanistan. Less spectacular, but equally disturbing, is the recent increase in young adult male mortality in several northern and southern European countries. While the final pathway appears to be through alcohol in the north, HIV/AIDS (see Chapter 8) and road traffic crashes are responsible in the south [47].

Nearly 34 million people worldwide are currently living with HIV/AIDS, and 95 per cent of them are in low- and middle-income countries. In many countries, the development gains of the past 50 years, including the increase in child survival and life expectancy, are being wiped out by the HIV/AIDS epidemic. In sub-Saharan Africa, where nearly 25 million people are infected, HIV/AIDS is now the leading cause of death, with more women being infected than men. The HIV/AIDS crisis is a unique modern-day plague that threatens the political, economic, and social stability of sub-Saharan Africa and Asia [48].

Old and new public health challenges

The main item on the development agenda is the over one billion people whose life experiences have improved only slowly over the last half-century. Almost two-thirds of poor people live in Asia, with 17 per cent in Africa and 10 per cent in the rest of the world, and a substantial majority of the poor are women. The excluded billion need to be placed more firmly on the international development agenda, and increasingly this is being addressed through health programmes as well as more directly by economic means. A major goal of this agenda, as encapsulated in the MDGs, is the reduction by half of the number of people living in absolute poverty by the year 2015. Opinions differ as to whether this goal is achievable. Officially, the WHO is optimistic that, with a collaborative effort, this goal is attainable. However, progress is slow and, while the proportion of people living in extreme poverty fell in the last decade, the actual number of people living in poverty increased in South Asia and sub-Saharan Africa because of the failure of current policies of economic growth. Many national anti-poverty action plans remain vague and limited by poor governance, and do not consider the multidimensional nature of poverty [49]. The recent impact of rising fuel and food prices further threatens current policies for economic development as does the global financial crisis and climate change.

Tobacco use continues to increase in low- and middle-income countries, suggesting that the global impact on disease will also increase. Current estimates suggest that there are 3.9 million preventable tobacco-caused deaths each year; projections for the year 2030 suggest that this number will increase to 8.4 million [50]. More than three-quarters of these deaths are due to just three causes: cardiovascular disease, lung cancer, and chronic respiratory disease.

In wealthy countries, the ageing of the population is occurring in a relatively slow and predictable manner, and in some, such as Japan and Sweden, the rate of ageing is already slowing down. As a consequence of ageing, the global burden of disease is dominated by non-communicable diseases, with chronic diseases, such as heart disease, stroke, diabetes, cancers, and chronic respiratory diseases, now accounting for more than 60 per cent of deaths globally. Eighty per cent of these deaths occur in low- and middle-income countries. Projections by the WHO indicate that leading infectious diseases will become less important causes of death globally, and by 2030 three-quarters of all deaths in the world will be due to chronic non-communicable diseases [51]. Close to 50 per cent of the chronic disease deaths in low-and middle-income countries occur under the age of 70 years, compared with only 27 per cent in high-income countries. Over the next 25 years, the global distribution of deaths will shift from younger to older ages. Population ageing is driving a substantial increase in the numbers of chronic non-communicable disease deaths in low- and middle-income countries. While the proportion of the world's population aged over 65 years, currently 7 per cent, will more than double (to 16 per cent) in the next 50 years, the most explosive ageing will occur in some of the poorer regions of the world, particularly India, Indonesia, and China. Within the next half-century, the number of people aged 65 years or more will increase sixfold in the Southeast Asian region of the WHO [52].

The decline in chronic disease mortality observed in high-income countries in recent decades is probably due to improved control of risk factors such as high blood pressure, high blood cholesterol, and tobacco use and improved access to effective treatment interventions, even though levels of overweight/obesity and physical inactivity have worsened [53]. If economic development in low- and middle-income countries does not result in similar improvements, the burden of non-communicable diseases may increase even faster than projected by WHO.

WHO has estimated that over 70 per cent of cardiovascular disease deaths and around 50 per cent of all chronic disease deaths are attributable to a small number of known risk factors [54]. Four of the most important are unhealthy diet, physical inactivity, tobacco use, and high blood pressure. Globally, these risk factors are increasing as people's dietary habits change to foods high in fats, salt, and sugars, and people's work and living situations are much less physically active. The number of people who are overweight or obese will rise from one billion to more than 1.5 billion by 2015 if current trends continue.

Research published by *The Lancet* in its second series on chronic disease in December 2007 found that widespread efforts to curb salt intake and smoking and to ensure that those at risk of heart disease take the necessary drugs could prevent millions of deaths each year in 23 large low- and middle-income countries, and achieve in these countries the global goal set by WHO for reducing chronic disease deaths worldwide [55]. Reducing salt intake by 15 per cent and implementing tobacco control measures such as raising taxes, enforcing smoke-free workplaces, and public awareness efforts would prevent nearly 14 million deaths over 10 years at a cost of less than 40 cents per person in these 23 countries [56]. Identifying and treating people at high risk of heart disease in these 23 low- and middle-income countries could avert nearly 18 million deaths in 10 years through a daily regimen of aspirin, two common blood pressure pills, and a cholesterol-lowering drug [57].

The challenge will be to translate this knowledge into effective action in developing countries in order to avoid the predictable, but largely preventable, burden of chronic non-communicable diseases. It is difficult for poorer countries to focus on medium-term preventive strategies in the face of more immediate health problems, even though over 40 per cent of all deaths in the poorest 20 per cent of the world's population are already due to chronic diseases. The 'double burden' of disease is being superseded by the 'triple burden'. New health threats consequent on the new phase of globalization (see Chapter 1) are being added to the unfinished agendas of infectious and non-communicable disease prevention and control. These new challenges will potentially worsen regional and national health inequalities (see Chapter 1).

Conclusion

Improvements in global health status, as measured by gains in life expectancy and other measures, and the reductions in preventable deaths have been accompanied by widening health and poverty gaps between and within countries. People living in poor countries not only face lower life expectancies than those in richer countries but also live a higher proportion of their lives in poor health. Richer countries should be much more active in seeking ways to improve the health of the world's poor. The WHO has been a strong advocate for efforts to increase the resources available for this purpose.

Routine health status measures of health trends and inequalities are required to heighten awareness of their significance among policy makers, donors, and international agencies. The current international preoccupation with MDGs does not take into account the rapid health transition, which implies that health statistics should systematically include a much wider array of health issues from acute infectious diseases to chronic non-communicable diseases and injuries, disaggregated by socio-economic position. Better and more comprehensive data are a first step in the development of a stronger strategy to improve overall health and reduce inequalities in health status throughout the world. Insufficient emphasis is given to disease surveillance in most national health systems; this is a serious impediment to setting disease prevention and control priorities and measuring progress. Additionally, there is insufficient emphasis in national health data collections on the need for cross-population comparability. Despite the growing pressures of shrinking public sector resources, there is an urgent need for centralized organizations to collect data at both national and international level; there are some promising signs in this direction.

The global health scene has been characterized by major steps forward, but with some disturbing features. The measurement of health status is multifaceted and must take account of differences between and within nations that inevitably impinge on the comparability of data. As a first and essential step, there is need for better national and regional heath surveillance systems. Without such data, particularly in poorer regions of the world, it will be difficult to know if, and how much, progress is being made in improving global health status and reducing growing health inequalities.

Acknowledgments

The authors thank current and former WHO staff and others who have contributed to the measurement of global health status, in particular Robert Beaglehole, Ties Boerma, Somnath Chatterji, Majid Ezzati, Mie Inoue,

Alan Lopez, Doris Ma Fat, Chris Murray, Joshua Salomon, Claudia Stein, Kathleen Strong, and Bedirhan Ustun.

References

[1] Mathers CD, Ma Fat D, Inoue M, Rao C, Lopez AD. Counting the dead and what they died from: an assessment of the global status of cause of death data. *Bull WHO* 2005; **83**: 171–7.

[2] Mathers CD, Lopez AD, Murray CJL. The burden of disease and mortality by condition: data, methods and results for 2001. In: Lopez AD, Mathers CD, Ezzati M, Murray CJL, Jamison DT (eds), *Global Burden of Disease and Risk Factors*. New York: Oxford University Press, 2006; pp. 45–240.

[3] Yang GH, Hu J, Rao KQ, Ma J, Rao C, Lopez AD. Mortality registration and surveillance in China: History, current situation and challenges. *Popul Health Metr* 2005; **3**: 3.

[4] Bannister J, Hill K. Mortality in China, 1964–2000. *Popul Stud (Camb)* 2004; **58**: 55–75.

[5] Registrar General of India. *Medical Certification of Cause of Death Annual Report 1995*. New Delhi: Registrar General of India, Vital Statistics Division, 1996.

[6] Jha P, Gajalakshmi V, Gupta PC, *et al.* Prospective study of one million deaths in India: rationale, design, and validation results. *PLoS Med* 2006; **3**: e18.

[7] Jha P, Jacob B, Gajalakshmi V, *et al.* A nationally representative case–control study of smoking and death in India. *N Engl J Med* 2008; **358**: 1137–47.

[8] Registrar General of India. *Million Death Study, Preliminary Report on Causes of Death in India 2001–2003*. New Delhi: Registrar General of India, Centre for Global Health Research, 2008.

[9] Khosravi A, Taylor R, Naghavi N, Lopez AD. Mortality in the Islamic Republic of Iran, 1964–2004. *Bull WHO* 2007; **85**: 607–14.

[10] Rao C, Bradshaw D, Mathers CD. Improving death registration and statistics in developing countries: lessons from sub-Saharan Africa. *South Afr J Demogr* 2004; **9**: 81–99.

[11] WHO. *The Global Burden of Disease: 2004 Update*. Geneva: WHO, 2008.

[12] Hill K, Lopez AD, Shibuya K, Jha P. Interim measures for meeting needs for health sector data: births, deaths, and causes of death. *Lancet* 2007; **370**: 1726–35.

[13] Garenne M, Fauveau V. Potential and limits of verbal autopsies. *Bull WHO* 2006; **84**: 164.

[14] Murray CJ, Lopez AD, Feehan DM, Peter ST, Yang G. Validation of the symptom pattern method for analyzing verbal autopsy data. *PLoS Med* 2007; **4**: e327.

[15] Baiden F, Bawah A, Biai S, *et al.* Setting international standards for verbal autopsy. *Bull WHO* 2007; **85**: 570–1.

[16] WHO. *International Classification of Functioning, Disability and Health (ICF)*. Geneva: WHO, 2001.

[17] McDowell I, Newell C. *Measuring Health. A Guide to Rating Scales and Questionnaires* (2nd edn). Oxford: Oxford University Press, 1996.

[18] WHO. *International Classification of Functioning and Disability (ICIDH-2)* (beta-2 version). Geneva: WHO, 1999.

[19] Guyatt GH, Feeny DH, Patrick DL. Measuring health-related quality of life. *Ann Intern Med* 1993; **118**: 622–9.

[20] Salomon J, Mathers CD, Chatterji S, Sadana R, Ustun TB, Murray CJL. Quantifying individual levels of health: definitions, concepts and measurement issues. In: Murray CJL, Evans D (eds). *Health Systems Performance Assessment: Debate, Methods and Empiricism*. Geneva: WHO, 2003; pp. 301–18.

[21] Salomon JA, Tandon A, Murray CJL. Comparability of self rated health: cross sectional multi-country survey using anchoring vignettes. *BMJ* 2004; **328**: 258–61.

[22] King G, Murray CJL, Salomon JA, Tandon A. Enhancing the validity and cross-cultural comparability of measurement in survey research. *Am Polit Sci Rev* 2003; **93**: 567–83.

[23] Kapteyn A, van Soest A, Smith JP. Vignettes and self-reports of work disability in the United States and the Netherlands. *Am Econ Rev* 2007; **97**: 461–73.

[24] Mathers CD, Iburg KM, Begg S. Adjusting for dependent comorbidity in the calculation of healthy life expectancy. *Popul Health Metr* 2006; **4**: 4.

[25] Murray CJL, Salomon JA, Mathers CD. A critical examination of summary measures of population health. *Bull WHO* 2000; **78**: 981–94.

[26] Murray CJL, Lopez AD (eds). *The Global Burden of Disease: A Comprehensive Assessment of Mortality and Disability from Diseases, Injuries and Risk Factors in 1990 and Projected to 2020*. Cambridge, MA: Harvard School of Public Health for WHO and World Bank, 1996.

[27] Lopez AD, Mathers CD, Ezzati M, Murray CJL, Jamison DT. *Global Burden Of Disease and Risk Factors*. New York: Oxford University Press, 2006.

[28] Begg S, Vos T, Barker B, Stevenson C, Stanley L, Lopez A. *The Burden of Disease and Injury in Australia 2003*. Canberra: Australian Institute of Health and Welfare, 2007.

[29] Robine JM, Romieu I, Cambois E. Health expectancy indicators. *Bull WHO* 1999; **77**: 181–5.

[30] Robine JM, Jagger C, Mathers CD, Crimmins EM, Suzman RM. *Determining Health Expectancies*. Chichester: John Wiley, 2003.

[31] Mathers CD, Iburg K, Salomon J, *et al*. Global patterns of healthy life expectancy in the year 2002. *BMC Public Health* 2004; **4**: 66.

[32] Ustun TB, Chatterji S, Villanueva M, *et al*. The WHO Multicountry Household Survey Study on Health and Responsiveness 2000–2001. In: Murray CJL, Evans D (eds). *Health Systems Performance Assessment: Debates, Methods and Empiricism*. Geneva: WHO, 2003.

[33] Almeida C, Braveman P, Gold MR, *et al*. Methodological concerns and recommendations on policy consequences of the World Health Report 2000. *Lancet* 2001; **357**: 1692–7.

[34] McKee M, Shkolnikov V. Understanding the toll of premature death among men in Eastern Europe. *BMJ* 2001; **323**: 1051–5.

[35] Shkolnikov V, McKee M, Leon D. Changes in life expectancy in Russia in the mid-1990s. *Lancet* 2001; **357**: 917–21.

[36] Gavrilova NS, Semyonova VG, Evdokushkina GN, Gavrilov LA. The response of violent mortality to economic crisis in Russia. *Popul Res Policy Rev* 2000; **19**: 397–419.

[37] WHO. *World Health Statistics 2008*. Geneva: WHO, 2008.

[38] UNAIDS and WHO. *AIDS Epidemic Update: December 2007*. Geneva: UNAIDS, 2007.

[39] Murray CJL, Laakso T, Shibuya K, Hill K, Lopez AD. Can we achieve Millennium Development Goal 4? New analysis of country trends and forecasts of under-5 mortality to 2015. *Lancet* 2007; **370**: 1040–54.

[40] Murray CJL. Towards good practice for health statistics: lessons from the Millennium Development Goal health indicators. *Lancet* 2007; **369**: 862–73.

[41] Murray CJ, Frenk J. Health metrics and evaluation: strengthening the science. *Lancet* 2008; **371**: 1191–9.

[42] AbouZahr C, Boerma T. Health information systems: the foundations of public health. *Bull WHO* 2005; **83**: 578–83.

[43] Murray CJL, Lopez AD, Black RE, *et al*. Global Burden of Disease 2005: call for collaborators. *Lancet* 2007; **370**: 109–10.

[44] Murray CJL, Michaud,CM, McKenna MT, Marks JS. *US Patterns of Mortality by County and Race: 1965–1994*. Cambridge, MA: Harvard Center for Population and Development Studies and Centres for Disease Control, 1998.

[45] Black RE, Allen LH, Bhutta Z, *et al*. Maternal and child undernutrition: global and regional exposures and health consequences. *Lancet* 2008; **371**: 243–60.

[46] Boerma JT, Jennifer B, Yohannes K, *et al*. Mind the gap: equity and trends in coverage of maternal, newborn, and child health services in 54 Countdown countries. *Lancet* 2008; **37**: 1259–67.

[47] Leon DA, Chenet L, Shkolnikov VM, *et al*. Huge variation in Russian mortality rates 1984–94: artefact, alcohol, or what? *Lancet* 1997; **350**: 383–8.

[48] http://www.unitaid.eu (accessed 4 April 2009).

[49] UN Development Programme. *Poverty Report 2000: Overcoming Human Poverty*. New York: UN, 2000.

[50] Mathers CD, Loncar D. Projections of global mortality and burden of disease from 2002 to 2030. *PLoS Med* 2006; **3**: e442.

[51] Strong KL, Mathers CD, Leeder S, Beaglehole R. Preventing chronic diseases: how many lives can we save? *Lancet* 2005; **366**: 1578–82.

[52] UN Population Division. *World Population Prospects: The 2006 Revision*. New York: UN, 2007.

[53] Ford ES, Ajani UA, Croft JB, *et al*. Explaining the decrease in US deaths from coronary disease, 1980–2000. *N Engl J Med* 2007; **356**: 2388–98.

[54] Ezzati M, Vander Hoorn S, Lopez AD, *et al*. Comparative quantification of mortality and burden of disease attributable to selected major risk factors. In: Lopez AD, Mathers CD, Ezzati M, Murray CJL, Jamison DT (eds). *Global Burden of Disease and Risk Factors*. New York: Oxford University Press, 2006; pp. 241–396.

[55] Abegunde DO, Mathers CD, Adam T, Ortegon M, Strong K. The burden and costs of chronic diseases in low-income and middle-income countries. *Lancet* 2007; **370**: 1929–38.

[56] Asaria P, Chisholm D, Mathers C, Ezzati M, Beaglehole R. Chronic disease prevention: health effects and financial costs of strategies to reduce salt intake and control tobacco use. *Lancet* 2007; **370**: 2044–53.

[57] Lim SS, Gaziano TA, Gakidou E, *et al.* Prevention of cardiovascular disease in high-risk individuals in low-income and middle-income countries: health effects and costs. *Lancet* 2007; **370**: 2054–62.

Chapter 3

Public health in the United Kingdom

Karen Lock and Fiona Sim

Introduction

Population health in the United Kingdom (UK) has continued to improve over the last 50 years. However, while overall life expectancy and mortality rates improve, health inequalities between socio-economic groups and between geographical areas have continued to widen. These inequalities in risk factors and health outcomes are influenced by a range of environmental and socio-economic factors, and present the greatest challenge to UK public health in the early twenty-first century.

The UK has a 60 year history of universal health care provision, free at the point of use, through the National Health Service (NHS). In recent years, this model has been under increasing strain as demands on the service have continued to rise because of the ageing of the population and technological developments. As a result of concerns about the future sustainability and affordability of the NHS, public health has tended to be marginalized, particularly because of the lack of explicit resource allocation. The capacity to deliver public health initiatives has also been weakened by reductions in the specialist public health workforce.

Since the Labour government came to power in 1997 there has been a welcome change towards long-term proactive health policies. Public health strategies have tackled a wide range of issues from inequalities to alcohol, teenage pregnancy, smoking, obesity, and communicable disease control. However, the government has lacked a coherent approach to public health, with greater emphasis being placed on individual rather than societal change. This has led to tensions and some contradictions between policies, with some, such as obesity strategies, focusing on individual behaviour change, and others, such as smoking policy, using legislation to protect the public from strong industry pressures.

Changing patterns of health

Life expectancy

Over the last 20 years, strong economic growth, higher standards of living, and improved health care across the UK have contributed to the population living longer, but the extra years of life have not necessarily been lived in good health. Life expectancy reached 77 for men and 81 for women in 2006. Both life expectancy and healthy life expectancy have increased, although life expectancy has increased at a faster rate than healthy life expectancy (Fig. 3.1); women live for longer in poor health than do men. Of concern, there has been no reduction in inequalities in life expectancy between social class groups in the past three decades. Striking geographical variations in life expectancy across the UK are largely explained by deprivation [1]. Between 2004 and 2006 older men and women in the most affluent areas of London could expect to live 12.6 years and 10.2 years longer, respectively, than people living in deprived areas of Glasgow in Scotland [2]. There has also been no change in healthy life expectancy by level of deprivation across the country [3].

These demographic and health trends have received attention in the UK during the past decade, mainly focusing on the rising costs of medical and long-term social care of the increasing elderly population. The compression of morbidity theory predicted that there are limits to human life expectancy and that changes in lifestyle which modify risk factors for mortality will also delay the age of onset and progression of non-fatal disabling conditions [4]. There is evidence of an increase in rates of healthy life expectancy in the USA and in some European Union (EU) countries such as Sweden [4,5]. This reflects reductions in exposure to major risk factors, such as smoking, and improvement of modern health care in tackling avoidable mortality in the EU [6]. However, it is not clear why this compression of morbidity has not yet been seen in the UK.

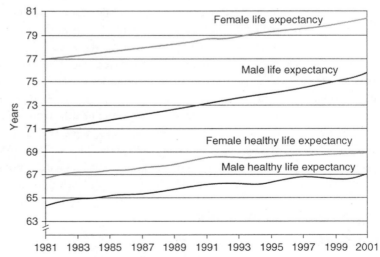

Fig. 3.1 Life expectancy and healthy life expectancy at birth by sex, United Kingdom. (Source: Office for National Statistics.)

Mortality trends

Overall mortality rates have been decreasing for both men and women. Between 1950 and 2005, age-standardized cancer mortality in England and Wales changed very little. However, mortality from the other main causes (heart disease, stroke, diabetes, accidents, and infectious diseases) has declined (Fig. 3.2). There are clear social class differences in mortality for ischaemic heart disease, cerebrovascular disease, respiratory diseases, lung cancer, and accidents. Between 1980 and 2002, despite reductions in mortality from major diseases, relative inequalities in mortality increased. In Scotland mortality for men under 65 years fell by 49 per cent in the least deprived areas compared with a decrease of only 2 per cent in the most deprived [7].

Changing patterns of disease risk factors

There are clear links between the reductions in mortality and some risk factor changes. However, the population health picture reveals complex changes in health behaviours and emerging public health priorities. Policies designed to tackle these major risk factors will be covered later in this chapter.

Tobacco use

Smoking rates in the UK have decreased dramatically over the last 30 years. In 2004–2005, 26 per cent of men and 23 per cent of women were regular

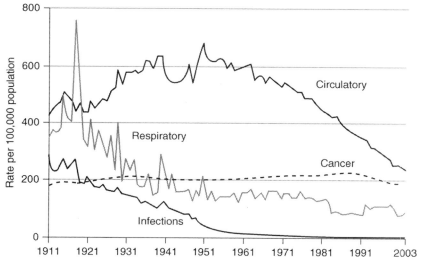

Fig. 3.2 Age-standardized mortality rates for selected disease groups, 1911–2003, England and Wales.
(Source: Office for National Statistics.)

cigarette smokers, compared with 50 per cent of men and 40 per cent of women in the early 1970s. Since the early 1990s the prevalence of cigarette smoking has been highest among 20–24 year olds [8]. While less than 1 per cent of 11–12 year old children smoke, 20 per cent of children in England are regular smokers by the age of 15, despite the fact that it is illegal to sell any tobacco product to those aged under 18 years in England and Wales. Since 1986, girls have consistently had higher smoking rates than boys. In 2006, among 15 year olds, 24 per cent of girls regularly smoked compared with 16 per cent of boys [8]. There are clear inequalities in smoking because of the differential decline in smoking by higher social classes that occurred in the 1970s and 1980s. By 2005, 29 per cent of adults in manual occupations smoked compared with 19 per cent of those in non-manual occupations [8]. There are also huge differences in smoking rates between different ethnic groups in the UK. In UK men, smoking rates range from 20 per cent (Indian) to 40 per cent (Bangladeshi) compared with the national average of 24 per cent. In UK women, the rates range from 2 per cent (Bangladeshi) to 26 per cent (Irish) compared with the national average of 23 per cent [9].

Alcohol use

Harmful alcohol use is the third leading cause of premature death and illness in the EU, behind tobacco and high blood pressure [10]. In the UK, total recorded alcohol consumption doubled between 1960 and 2002. Cirrhosis mortality rates, an important indicator of population levels of alcohol harm, have also increased steeply. Between the periods 1987–1991 and 1997–2001, cirrhosis mortality in men in Scotland more than doubled (104 per cent increase), and in England and Wales it rose by over two-thirds (69 per cent). Mortality in women increased by almost half (46 per cent in Scotland and 44 per cent in England and Wales) [11]. These relative increases are the steepest in Western Europe, and contrast with the declines apparent in other countries, particularly those of Southern Europe. Cirrhosis mortality rates in Scotland are among the highest in Europe; in 2002 they were 45.2 per 100,000 in men and 19.9 per 100,000 in women. Alcohol consumption is also frequently implicated in accidental injury, the major cause of mortality in men under 44 years of age. Both the amount and pattern of alcohol consumption are important. Twenty-four per cent of male drinkers in the United Kingdom describe themselves as weekly binge drinkers, with rates higher than in most of Western Europe. Binge drinking has been clearly associated with an increase risk of death, particularly from injury and myocardial infarction [12].

Obesity

The UK is the most overweight country in Europe with 24 per cent of the population obese (BMI >30 kg/m^2). Between 1995 and 2005 the rates of overweight and obesity (BMI >25 kg/m^2) in English adults increased from

58 to 67 per cent in men and from 49 to 58 per cent in women. Between 1984 and 2003, the prevalence of obesity (>95th centile for age) in children aged 5–10 years increased from 1.2 to 6.0 per cent in boys and from 1.8 to 6.6 per cent in girls, with rates accelerating in the most recent years. These increases are most marked among children from lower socio-economic households [13]. If current trends continue unchanged, it has been forecast that by 2010 childhood obesity prevalence will increase by 7 per cent for those in the lowest socio-economic households, compared with 2 per cent for the highest socio-economic backgrounds [14]. Government modelling estimates that, by 2050, 60 per cent of adult men, 50 per cent of adult women, and about 25 per cent of all children under 16 could be obese [15].

Diet

Although there has been a marked change in the British diet since the early 1970s, it does not appear to explain the rise in overweight and obesity. The Health Survey for England found no evidence that the average calorific intake or consumption of foods rich in fat and added sugar has increased in the past few decades. Reductions in the contribution of total fat to total energy intake and saturated fat have been observed over the same period. Data from the National Food Survey between 1971 and 2000 suggest that household consumption of some foods is increasingly in line with dietary recommendations, although this is not true for all food types and population groups. For example, consumption of both butter and margarine is now only about a quarter of the level of 1971. This is linked to a sharp rise in consumption of low- and reduced-fat spreads. Consumption of fruit and vegetables has increased from approximately 200 to 300 grams per person per day. Red meat intake has fallen by up to 80 per cent from 1970–2000. In contrast, consumption of poultry increased from 134 to 253 grams per person per week over the same time [16].

Physical activity

Population levels of physical activity have reduced in both adults and children over the last 20–30 years but do not fully explain the increased obesity rates [17]. Since the early 1990s there has been a steady increase in the use of cars and a 26 per cent decrease in walking and cycling to school or work. The Health Survey for England found that the proportion of children aged 5–10 years who walked to school fell from 61 per cent in 1992–1994 to 52 per cent in 2002–2003, mirroring the equivalent 10 per cent rise in the proportion of school journeys by car (from 30 to 40 per cent).

Infectious diseases and sexual health

Patterns of communicable diseases have also been changing. The UK has one of the highest rates of HIV infection in Europe, and newly diagnosed cases of

HIV have been increasing since the mid-1990s. In 2006 there were an estimated 73,000 persons of all ages living with HIV in the UK, and 21,600 of these were estimated to be unaware of their infection [18]. Homosexual men accounted for up to three-quarters of UK-acquired HIV infections, and remain the behavioural group at greatest risk of acquiring HIV. An estimated 24,800 people born in sub-Saharan Africa were living with HIV in the UK in 2006. An increasing number of black Africans are now being infected heterosexually in the UK, accounting for almost half of all new HIV diagnoses in 2006. Eleven per cent of all new HIV diagnoses in 2006 were in young adults.

The incidence of sexually transmitted infections (STIs) has also been rising in the UK. The Health Protection Agency noted that young adults (aged 16–24) account for more than half of all STI diagnoses. Chlamydia is the most common sexually transmitted infection, and the number of cases has more than tripled from 30,794 cases diagnosed in 1995 to 109,958 in 2005. Between 2006 and 2007, 10 per cent of the 14,939 young adults screened in the English National Chlamydia Screening Programme outside the specialist clinic setting were infected with chlamydia [19].

The poor sexual health of adolescents is coupled with the UK having the second highest teenage birth rate in the developed world after the USA [20]. Birth rates among 15–19 year olds were seven times those in the Netherlands where, although rates of adolescent sexual activity are comparable, contraceptive use is much more common. The number of teenage conceptions and births in the UK peaked in 1998, and then declined after the implementation of the teenage pregnancy strategy in 1999 [21]. However, UK rates are still much higher than in comparable EU countries, and there is significant geographical and socio-economic variation with half of under-18 conceptions occurring in the 20 per cent of most disadvantaged areas [22].

The poor sexual health and high rates of tobacco, alcohol, and drug use among UK teenagers compared with other European countries has raised concern that there is fundamental problem with public health policies aimed at young people [23].

In summary, while overall life expectancy and mortality rates in the UK continue to improve, health inequalities in risk factors and health outcomes between socio-economic groups and between geographical areas remain unchanged or have widened.

Delivery of the public health function

Public health has appeared to have a more prominent role in government policy in the UK since the election of a Labour government in 1997, initially led by Tony Blair as Prime Minister and, since 2007, by Gordon Brown. Since 1998 the responsibility for health care and public health has been devolved to the national governments of Scotland, England, Wales, and Northern Ireland. Key differences in health service and public heath are summarized in Box 3.1. It is difficult to say whether any differences in population health in the separate countries of the UK can be attributed to the different delivery systems as this has been a largely unplanned, and unevaluated, natural experiment (Box 3.1). In this chapter we will concentrate on the development of major public health policies in England.

Responsibility for public health

In the English Department of Health a Minister of State for Public Health, first appointed in 1997, is responsible for policies relating to prevention and health promotion, health inequalities, communicable diseases, and sexual health in England. The ministerial position has been variably successful, depending largely upon the competence and personal commitment of the incumbent. The post is at a relatively junior level in government, solely based within the Ministry of Health and not across government, and usually with several additional, and frequently unconnected, policy briefs. Its impact has not been helped by the rapid turnover of ministers—there have been six incumbents between 1997 and 2008, with the post-holders mostly promoted to larger ministerial roles in other government departments.

The implementation of public health policy has been a function of the NHS since 1974. Before that, public health was a function of local government. Since 1984 there have been widespread and constant changes to the structure and organization of the NHS, largely intended to improve the efficiency of the service, which have influenced both how public health specialists work and the focus of public health policy and practice. In 2001, a Department of Health paper, entitled *Shifting the Balance of Power*, outlined a further restructuring of the NHS delivery system including arrangements to strengthen the public health function at a local level [24]. Most public health strategy is now delivered via local primary care trusts (PCTs) which have the responsibility to improve population well-being and tackle inequalities by identifying a local population's health and health-care needs, and then working with other local organizations, including hospital trusts, general practitioners, and local authorities, to commission health and social services. Reorganization has continued, with the number of PCTs in England reduced from 303 to 152 on 1 October 2006. About 70 per cent of PCTs now mirror the geographical boundaries of local authorities with social services responsibilities [25].

Box 3.1 Health in the four devolved administrations of the UK

Differences in service provision

England, Wales, and Northern Ireland have a purchaser–provider organization where local health organizations commission services from local hospital and community providers for a defined community. England is unusual in having introduced a 'payment by results' system that rewards providers of care for volumes of work undertaken, and an independent health care sector as a provider of mainstream health services to NHS patients.

Scotland has re-integrated health services and abandoned any purchaser–provider split.

Northern Ireland is unique amongst the four countries in its longstanding integration of health and social care services in a single Ministry.

Differences in public health policy

Public health policy is now developed in each country, with differences in priorities. For example, bans on smoking in public places were introduced in Scotland in 2006, Wales and Northern Ireland in early 2007, and England on 1 July 2007. Similarly, plans for pandemic influenza are specific to each country, with coordination at national level.

Compared with England, the public health function has a more central role in the three devolved governments.

In Northern Ireland, the public health work of the Ministry is supported by two agencies: the Health Promotion Agency and the Communicable Disease Surveillance Centre.

In Wales, the office of the Chief Medical Officer reports directly to the Welsh Assembly and oversees the National Public Health Service which provides public health support to the local health boards, which are responsible for the local public health function.

Health improvement is also a central part of Scotland's health policy. All local Scottish health boards have directors of public health, and Health Scotland is a national agency for health promotion and public health.

In England, the Secretary of State for Health is supported by regional Directors of Public Health based in strategic health authorities (SHA). SHAs are responsible for performance management of PCTs in their delivery of public health policy.

Public health policy: recent progress

The development of public health policy since 1997 has seen a shift from short-term reactive policies focused on ill health to a more long-term proactive public health agenda.

Initially the Labour government seemed to make public health a priority with a commitment to tackle inequalities. Its first public health strategy *Saving Lives: Our Healthier Nation* in 1999 [26] acknowledged the roles of communities and government as well as individuals in reducing the wider determinants of ill health. However, the implementation of many of the proposals was shelved because of the overwhelming focus on reforming the NHS and improving acute patient care. Some of the initiatives which emphasized this 'new' public health agenda targeted deprived communities, using community development and regeneration approaches. Initiatives included Health Action Zones, Sure Start, and Healthy Living Centres, with the last of these funded from the National Lottery. Most of these faded or disappeared because of their short-term funding and the inability of local NHS commissioning (in PCTs) to identify the resources required to sustain them as part of local services.

In 2002, a former banker, Derek Wanless, was asked by the Treasury to report on ways of ensuring the long-term affordability of a publicly funded NHS. He estimated the amount of money that health care would require up to 2023. It led to the Chancellor's decision to increase annual NHS funding by 7.4 per cent in real terms from 2002–2003 up to 2007–2008. One of his key concepts, from a public health perspective, was the introduction of what he called the 'fully engaged' scenario, through which people would understand how to make informed decisions which have implications for their own and their family's health [27].

In 2004, the government published Wanless's second report, *Securing Good Health for the Whole Population*, which analysed the record of the government's public health initiatives. This made a clear case for investing in the health of the population, emphasizing the importance of policy engagement with the determinants of health. One major outcome of the report was the recommendation that the Department of Health change its focus from treating to preventing illness. It highlighted the government's responsibility for making people aware of health risks and gaining the benefits of healthy lifestyles. It advised that more funding was needed to address the UK's largest population health problems, which it proposed were smoking, alcohol-related harm, obesity, and STIs.

The 2004 Public Health White Paper *Choosing Health: Making Healthier Choices Easier* followed rapidly and represented the Department of Health's view of how to achieve Wanless's vision. It set out broad proposals for government regulation and policy targeting determinants of the major disease risk factors. These included:

* Smoking to be banned in some public places (later changed to all public places after public consultation).
* Restrictions on 'junk food' advertising to children.
* Food labelling using the 'traffic light' coding approach.
* Improved access to sexual health clinics.
* Clearer labelling on alcohol.
* Access to 'personal health trainers' on the NHS (short-term-funded initiative)

An extra £211 million was allocated to be invested into public health projects in England through PCTs. Despite claims that public health was a top priority, the Department of Health would not ring-fence this money specifically for public health initiatives, arguing that it was up to individual PCTs to determine health priorities in different areas. However, at the same time PCTs were under immense pressure to reduce NHS budget deficits to achieve financial balance, a top priority for health service managers. This resulted in budget cuts across all departments, including public health, to balance the NHS budget at the expense of investment in disease prevention and health improvement.

Public health regulation: tobacco control

Despite these local financial pressures, several important national public health polices have been implemented. In July 2004 the government set a new target to reduce the overall proportion of cigarette smokers in England from 28 per cent in 1996 to 21 per cent or less by 2010, with a reduction from 32 to 26 per cent or less among manual occupation groups. Several policies have been introduced to achieve this. In 1999 the government introduced the banning of tobacco advertising on billboards and in newspapers and magazines. On 1 July 2007 the English smoke-free regulation came into effect, resulting in smoking being banned in all enclosed public spaces. This followed public smoking bans in Scotland in March 2006, and in Wales and Northern Ireland in April 2007. The smoking bans have been an exceptionally high-profile public health intervention, and have been accompanied by nationwide campaigns encouraging people to stop smoking and increased investment in local smoking cessation services. In England, PCTs have been financially incentivized through local smoking reduction targets. Twelve months after the introduction of smoke-free legislation in England, evaluations have shown that compliance with the law has been extremely high (98 per cent of all locations inspected) [28] and that 76 per cent of people support the ban [29]. Research also suggests that the smoking ban is encouraging people to quit. A survey of 32,000 people in England showed that that smoking rates fell by 5.5 per cent in the 9 months after the ban compared with only 1.6 per cent before, with the effect seen in all social groups [30]. Based on these figures, it is estimated that 400,000 people in England quit smoking in the 12 months since the ban was introduced. Local NHS stop smoking services have experienced over 23 per cent increased demand [28]. A report by industry analysts AC Nielsen in January 2008 recorded a drop of 3.9 per cent in cigarette sales for the 12 months from January 2007 to January 2008 (compared with a 2 per cent decline in 2006). Air quality in bars has improved dramatically, with concentrations of particulate matter (PM2.5) dropping by 91 per cent to levels comparable to outdoor air levels. The exposure of bar workers to secondhand smoke has also been reduced, with mean salivary cotinine levels in non-smoking bar workers falling by 76 per cent 2 months after the ban [31]. There have been similar research findings on the impact of the smoking ban in Scotland.

Alcohol: harm reduction

In contrast, alcohol has mainly been seen by government as a criminal justice and not a health issue. Rates of alcohol consumption and binge drinking have been increasing, keeping alcohol on the political and media agenda because of its links to violence and antisocial behaviour. The Department of Health estimated that the annual cost of alcohol-related harm to the NHS in 2005–2006 was £2.7 billion [32]. While public smoking has been reduced through the smoking bans, drinking hours in public bars in England and Wales have been extended following a reform of the licensing laws. Public health evidence, which showed that increased opening hours are associated with increased alcohol consumption and alcohol-related problems, was ignored [33]. The Licensing Act 2003 now permits 24-hour bar opening in England and Wales. Government ministers claimed that a Continental 'café culture' would be encouraged by extending bar opening hours, but according to a range of statistics there has been little evidence of this cultural shift and no reduction in bingeing, particularly among young women.

In 2004, the government published the *Alcohol Harm Reduction Strategy for England* [34]. This was the first cross-government statement on the harm caused by alcohol. It focused on better education through health promotion campaigns on binge drinking and drink driving, combating alcohol-related crime and disorder through the use of new enforcement powers in the Licensing Act 2003 (and more recently the Violent Crime Reduction Act 2006), and working with the alcohol industry on a voluntary scheme that would lead to alcoholic drinks carrying health information and warning labels. By 2007, there had been very little progress, and the government launched an updated strategy, *Safe. Sensible. Social*, which included a commitment to review alcohol promotion and pricing activities such as happy hours and marketing [35]. This also focused on developing local multisectoral strategies to cut problem drinking, but little extra funding was provided.

A 2008 study to determine the extent to which the government's alcohol-labelling agreement with industry was being followed showed that many retailers were not following the voluntary codes on displaying the number of units of alcohol contained and only 2.4 per cent of products had sensible drinking guidelines in the agreed format [36]. There has been much criticism from a range of medical and public health organizations, including the British Medical Association and the Royal College of Physicians, that the government has worked too closely with the alcohol industry and pursued policies of deregulation and liberalization regarding alcohol control, while ignoring effective interventions such as price interventions, strict advertising restrictions, and reducing availability. Current alcohol policies in the UK need to be assessed by the extent to which they can successfully halt the adverse trends in liver cirrhosis mortality; to date they appear to be increasing consumption levels and alcohol-related problems.

Tackling obesity

Most recently, obesity has been seen as the greatest public health priority, with various estimates that the health impact of increasing incidence in both adults and children will soon cost the NHS £3.3–£3.7 billion per year. By 2006, the government had allocated more than £1 billion for a range of preventive programmes, particularly around children's nutrition and physical activity, including improving school meals, through which it aimed to address childhood obesity [37]. A public service agreement target for child obesity was set in July 2004 to '… halt the increase in obesity among children under the age of 11 by 2010'. However, in 2006 a joint report published by the Audit Commission, the Healthcare Commission, and the National Audit Office concluded that without better leadership across government departments, this target would not be met [37]. Although the policy lead for obesity rests with the Department of Health in England, many of the programmes supporting the target were led by the Department for Education and Schools, the Department of Culture, Media and Sports, local authorities, schools, and sports bodies, over which the Department of Health has no direct control. The report found that a lack of timely guidance has meant that the various organizations which will need to work together to deliver reduction in obesity prevalence have been unclear about their roles, resulting in those further down the delivery chain potentially wasting resources on ineffective or inappropriate interventions that fail to target those children most at risk.

The Office of Science Foresight Programme *Tackling Obesities: Future Choices* was launched in October 2007 to produce a long-term vision of how the government could deliver a sustainable response to obesity in the UK over the next 40 years. Its findings draw parallels with the complexity of tackling climate change [15]. The government had a year to draw up a policy response. Just 3 months later, in January 2008, the Government launched a £372 million cross-government strategy to combat obesity—*Healthy Weight, Healthy Lives* [38]. This is part of a new approach to targeting childhood obesity which is now the joint responsibility of the newly created Department of Children, Schools and Families and the Department of Health.

In reality this new strategy repackages several initiatives already proposed and implemented. For example, it includes within 'healthy schools' approaches such as school fruit and vegetable schemes (rolled out nationally in 2004, initially with National Lottery funding), the new school meal standards (led by the School Food Trust and launched in 2005), and increasing the amount of sport in the school curriculum. It also announced the importance of banning junk food advertising to children, and pledged to 'review' advertising restrictions for food and drinks high in fat, salt, or sugar during or between TV shows aimed at 4–9 year olds which had been introduced in April 2007 by Ofcom (the independent regulator and competition authority for the UK communications industries).

Another strand of the policy comprised voluntary agreements with the food and drink industry around healthy food codes of practice. This includes the 'traffic light' colour-coded front-of-pack food-labelling scheme launched by the Food Standards Agency in 2006. The scheme has failed to achieve its aim of standardizing and simplifying food labelling for consumers. Despite being adopted voluntarily by a large number of retailers and manufacturers in the United Kingdom, five of the top food manufacturers (PepsiCo, Danone, Kraft, Nestlé, and Kellogg's) and the largest UK supermarket chain (Tesco) refused to accept traffic light labelling and have introduced their own more complicated scheme based on guideline daily amounts.

The final focus of the recent obesity strategy is on personalized advice and support, including the proposal of personal financial incentives to maintain a healthy weight. This includes a new three year £75 million social marketing campaign launched in January 2009 to promote healthy lifestyles called *Change 4 Life*. This initiative involves partnerships with voluntary and commercial sectors including large multinational food companies such as PepsiCo, Unilever, and Tesco. There is criticism that the terms of engagement for industry are not sufficiently transparent or robust to protect the new brand because Change 4 life partners have not had to comply with any standards requiring meaningful commitments to public health, such as, for example, adopting traffic light food labelling. While the evidence is that a multifaceted approach to obesity is likely to be the most effective, there is little evidence as yet to determine whether the government's current range of policies, programmes, and initiatives is sufficient to achieve a reduction in rates of obesity.

Lack of policy coordination

Despite the wide range of public health strategies introduced since 1997, the UK public health agenda is not coherent or coordinated. The government has tended to respond to population health concerns by tackling individual problems separately. This is most clearly highlighted when looking at the public health issues of adolescents [23]. For example, the appointment of a 'Drug Tsar' to tackle street drug use in 1997, the 1998 Teenage Pregnancy Strategy, and the 2004 Alcohol Harm Reduction Strategy all focus on the behaviour of adolescents and young people, yet the obvious upstream links and synergies between the public health issues have been ignored. More recently, cross-governmental strategies, for example for childhood obesity, have attempted to attain 'joined-up' government working. However, as the National Audit Office report on childhood obesity showed, these intersectoral initiatives have had limited impact because of the lack of leadership and lack of clarity regarding the roles of the various organizations involved [37].

Inequalities—a cross-cutting theme

In 2008 the NHS was 60 years old. Since 1948, in accordance with its core principle of equity, access to health care has been free at the point of use for all, with a few exceptions, such as charges for prescriptions in England and for ophthalmic and dental services. Where charges have been introduced, there is commonly a means-tested exemption, so that people who cannot afford to pay are entitled to free access to the service they need.

Despite greatly improved access to comprehensive health care, as described earlier in this chapter the UK has witnessed growing inequalities in health, whether measured through life expectancy at birth, infant mortality or premature mortality from a range of common diseases, or increasingly through differences in morbidity from chronic conditions such as type 2 diabetes. Although health inequalities are associated with many factors, including age, gender, ethnicity, geography, and social class, the strongest association is with poverty. Whilst the NHS ensures some degree of equity of access to health care, evidence has been available for several years that differences in the social and economic determinants of health are more influential than access to health care.

By 1981 the Black Report, published by the then Chief Medical Officer in England, clearly demonstrated England's health inequalities. Perhaps the most important source of evidence was the Whitehall Study, a longitudinal study which demonstrated that it was less affluent workers, with little control over their working lives, who were most likely to suffer premature death. The Conservative government led by Margaret Thatcher (1979–1990) did not recognize inequalities in health as relevant to their political vision and renamed them 'variations' in health, so removing any government responsibility for their occurrence.

By 1997, the inequalities gap had widened substantially, with differences in life expectancy between the most and least affluent more marked, and it became less easy for an incoming Labour administration to ignore. Indeed, one of the first decisions of the new government was to commission an independent inquiry on health inequalities, to be led by another former Chief Medical Officer, Sir Donald Acheson. This report [39] highlighted actions necessary to reduce inequalities, and stressed that long-term vision was needed, with an emphasis on preconceptual and early years, if health inequalities were to be addressed effectively. Another important development was clarifying that a range of sectors were central to tackling health inequalities, for if early years were crucial, education, social care, housing, and employment were all factors that would ensure a change in health experience for future generations.

The Acheson Report was greeted by a government commitment to tackling health inequalities. After this, the government commissioned its first cross-cutting review of health inequalities to determine the role and responsibilities of each government department in addressing them [40]. This was followed by the publication, in 2003, of the government's *Health Inequalities Programme for Action*, which was supported by 12 government departments, and the Treasury review of NHS funding and progress in tackling health inequalities [27].

In the UK, the National Institute for Health and Clinical Excellence is responsible for providing national evidence-based guidance on both treatment and health improvement. In 2004, it concluded that the evidence base for tackling health inequalities is, at best, patchy. There is no shortage of evidence demonstrating the magnitude and nature of the challenge, but far less evidence on what community-wide changes would make a real difference. Short-term government initiatives which aimed at tackling deprivation, such as Sure Start and Health Action Zones, have had limited impact on inequalities at a local level.

In June 2008, the Department of Health produced a new strategy for tackling health inequalities [41]. This acknowledged that health inequalities in the UK have not only persisted, but in some cases widened. The strategy reiterated the government target to reduce inequalities in health outcomes (infant mortality and life expectancy) by 10 per cent by 2010. The report launches action on three main levels: first, acting on wider social determinants of health, including investments in early childhood development, using work to improve well-being and reducing discrimination; secondly, promoting health lifestyles through reducing smoking, alcohol use, and obesity (through the existing polices discussed earlier in the chapter); finally, improving access to health services in most deprived areas. Despite pledging an extra £34 million for inequalities in 2008–2009, many of the initiatives put forward in the strategy, such as the new cross-government Child Health Strategy and the Obesity Strategy, have already been developed and/or introduced for other objectives and appear to have been repackaged with a focus on tackling inequalities for this report.

Although health inequalities have remained on the national political agenda, there has been little progress in reducing them despite a range of policy initiatives since 1997. Alongside its commitment to reducing inequalities, the Labour government has also shown an increasing desire to develop an agenda of personal 'choice', particularly around health care and public health. This approach appears to work in opposition to tackling inequalities as a societal issue. At its simplest, only those people who possess the capacity to exercise choice do so; others fall further behind, widening the gap.

Changing public trust in government and its impact on health

An emerging debate, which has started to influence public health, has been the perceived lack of public trust in the Department of Health and NHS. This is most apparent in the recent debates over childhood immunization. Over the past 50 years a key factor in the reduction of infectious diseases and associated morbidity and mortality in the UK has been the childhood vaccination programme. Nearly all children are now immunized against tetanus, diphtheria, polio, whooping cough, *Haemophilus influenzae b*, meningitis C, and measles, mumps, and rubella. Current government immunization targets are for 95 per cent of children to be immunized against these diseases by the age of 2 years. The measles–mumps–rubella (MMR) vaccine was introduced in 1988. However, in recent years, concerns by parents and the media over the safety of the MMR combined vaccine (after publication of now discredited research claiming links to autism) have led to a fall in the proportion of children immunized to below 80 per cent in 2003–2004, rising again to 85 per cent in 2006–2007. In the worst hit areas of London the immunization rate was below 64 per cent. This has led to a re-emergence of measles and mumps outbreaks across the UK, with associated avoidable child mortality and morbidity.

Although there have been claims that there is not evidence for a crisis of trust, there is evidence of a culture of public suspicion [42]. This has resulted in a new ethos of accountability throughout the NHS. Performance is monitored and subjected to quality control and quality assurance. The idea of audit has been exported from its original financial context to cover ever more detailed scrutiny of non-financial processes and systems. Performance indicators are used to measure adequate and inadequate performance with supposed precision and have been increasingly applied to public health policy initiatives locally, for example the public service agreement targets for obesity and smoking cessation, and indicators used by the Healthcare Commission in its inspectorial role over PCTs.

The capacity of the public health workforce to implement change

The ability to implement changes in public health policy has been hit by funding and reorganizations, but also by the reduction of the UK specialist public health workforce in real terms in recent years. Without the infrastructure or workforce to deliver public health initiatives themselves, public health specialists have had to adapt modes of working so that they are now seen as a 'catalyst', working with others in both health and local government to effect changes at the local level that are conducive to health improvement. Faced with multiple competing priorities in local government and the NHS, it is no surprise that this model has produced only modest achievements.

This multisectoral approach has been facilitated by significant changes in public health training. Until the 1990s specialist status in public health could only be obtained by spending time in designated training posts and passing postgraduate medical examinations. This professional route was closed to non-physicians. By the late 1990s it became clear that this situation was becoming untenable, given the evolving public health agenda, and it became necessary to redefine the specialist workforce to include those people from other disciplines who were making a major contribution to public health practice. In 2000, the Faculty of Public Health dropped its suffix 'Medicine' and permitted membership by examination for non-medically qualified graduates in a move which most public health specialists support in terms of the new and much-needed skills brought to the workforce by people from backgrounds in the social sciences, geography, politics, economics, health intelligence, and others beyond medicine.

The development of a revised curriculum, finally agreed in 2007, created common training requirements for medical and non-medical public health specialists. At the same time, training posts within the NHS in England became multidisciplinary, and most senior posts in public health became open to both medically and non-medically qualified public health specialists. Despite this coordination of training and employment, an important issue remained. Only one part of the specialist workforce (those who were medically trained) was now regulated, leaving populations potentially vulnerable to unsound professional practice. In 2003 a new official regulating organization, the United Kingdom Voluntary Register for Public Health Specialists, was established with government support. Non-medical specialists are now expected to register prior to taking up senior posts in the NHS in England.

These reforms addressed specialist training but also highlighted the recurrent problem of how to define the boundaries of the public health workforce. This issue was addressed by the UK government's senior medical adviser, the Chief Medical Officer (CMO) for England. In a 2001 report on strengthening Public Health he identified three major categories in the public health workforce: 'specialist', 'practitioner' and 'wider workforce'. The public health practitioner workforce comprises a diverse mix of core disciplines – from health visitors and community nurses to health promotion practitioners and environmental health officers. Their common denominator is their day-to-day responsibility for influencing population health, through front-line, operational interventions, often with individuals or families. Public health practitioners may have obtained their core education in areas such as teaching or clinical practice, although some, such as environmental health officers, may have trained primarily in a core public health discipline.

The most diverse of the CMO's three categories is the 'wider' public health workforce, which includes people from all sectors and at all levels of organizations, from chief executives to front-line service providers. Potentially, they include journalists, pharmacists, social care staff, teachers, and workers in the retail, leisure, and hospitality sectors. This is a largely undefined and substantially under-utilized workforce in public health terms. In 2002, the size of the 'wider' public health workforce in London (population 7.5 million in 2005) was estimated to be of the order of a quarter of a million people. The policy implication is that future prevention initiatives and public health gains will require involvement of this wider workforce, who are often not trained in public health but may now be expected to deliver public health improvements for little or no targeted funding [43].

Conclusion

The wide and uncoordinated range of public health initiatives over the last 10 years clearly shows that the UK government has not developed a coherent approach to public health policy. Despite a welcome change in emphasis away from illness to health, there is a fundamental policy tension caused by a lack of any explicit statement of values on the balance between the state and the individual underpinning its health strategy. Government policy has emphasized individual behaviour change and lifestyles, which have been at the centre of its agenda to promote choice in all areas, including health-care provision. The individual focus prevails despite the Department of Health acknowledging that people face constraints, including structural, organizational, psychological, and informational barriers, in making choices, and this influences health inequalities. This has resulted in contradictions in health policy between allowing people to decide on their own, the need to recognize the limitations in their ability to do this effectively [44], and the responsibility of the state in protecting population health. This is clearly illustrated in the contrast between the willingness of government to legislate against tobacco advertising and for smoke-free public places, and food, obesity, and alcohol policy where the government has mainly focused on health education and voluntary agreements with industry. Together with a culture of accountability in the health system, driven by public health targets and performance monitoring at local levels, the ability to tackle health inequalities, and the broader structural determinants of public health in the UK, has so far been severely constrained.

References

[1] Woods L, Rachet B, Riga M, Stone N, Shah A, Coleman M. Geographical variation in life expectancy at birth in England and Wales is largely explained by deprivation. *J Epidemiol Community Health* 2005; **59**: 115–20.

[2] Office for National Statistics. *Inequalities in Life Expectancy at 65 in the UK*. London: UK Statistics Authority, 2007.

[3] Bajekai M. Healthy life expectancy by area deprivation and trends in England 1994–1999. *Health Stat Q* 2005; **25**: 18.

[4] Fries J. Measuring and monitoring success in compressing morbidity. *Ann Intern Med* 2003; **139**: 455–9.

[5] Parker M, Thorslund M. Health trends in the elderly population: getting better and getting worse. *Gerontologist* 2007; **47**: 150–8.

[6] Newey C, Nolte E, McKee M. *Avoidable Mortality in the Enlarged European Union*. Report, Institut des Sciences de la Santé, Paris, 2004.

[7] Leyland A, Dundas R, McLoone P, Boddy F. Cause-specific inequalities in mortality in Scotland: two decades of change. A population-based study. *BMC Public Health* 2007; **7**:172.

[8] Goddard E. *General Household Survey: Smoking and Drinking Among Adults 2005*. London: Office for National Statistics, 2006.

[9] Office for National Statistics. *The Health of Minority Ethnic Groups. Health Survey for England 2004*. London: Office for National Statistics, 2006.

[10] Rehm J, Taylor B, Patra J. Volume of alcohol consumption, patterns of drinking and burden of disease in the European region 2002. *Addiction* 2006; **101**: 1086–95.

[11] Leon D, McCambridge J. Liver cirrhosis mortality rates in Britain from 1950 to 2002: an analysis of routine data. *Lancet* 2006; **367**: 52–6.

[12] Kauhanen J, Kaplan G, Goldberg D, Salonen J. Beer binging and mortality: results from the Kuopio ischaemic heart disease risk factor study, a prospective population based study *BMJ* 1997; **315**: 846–51.

[13] Stamatakis E, Primatesta P, Chinn S, Rona R, Falascheti E. Overweight and obesity trends from 1974 to 2003 in English children: what is the role of socioeconomic factors?. *Arch Dis Childhood* 2005; **90**: 999–1004.

[14] Zaninotto P, Wardle H, Stamatakis E, Mindell J, Head J. *Forecasting Obesity to 2010*. London: NatCen, University College London, for the Department of Health, 2006.

[15] Government Office for Science. Foresight. *Tackling Obesities: Future Choices*. London: Government Office for Science, Department for Innovation, Universities and Skills, 2007.

[16] Office for National Statistics. Changing patterns in the consumption of foods at home 1971–2000. *Social Trends 32*. London: Office for National Statistics, 2002.

[17] Chief Medical Officer. *At Least Five a Week: Evidence on the Impact of Physical Activity and its Relationship to Health. A Report from the Chief Medical Officer*. London: Department of Health, 2004.

[18] Health Protection Agency. *Unlinked Anonymous HIV Surveillance*. London: Centre for Infections, Health Protection Agency, 2007.

[19] National Heath Service. *Maintaining Momentum. Annual Report of the National Chlamydia Screening Programme in England 2006/7*. London: NHS, 2007.

[20] UNICEF. *A League of Teenage Births in Rich Nations. Innocenti Report Card 3*. Florence, Italy: UNICEF Innocenti Research Centre, 2001.

[21] Wilkinson P, French R, Kane R, *et al*. Teenage conceptions, abortions, and births in England, 1994–2003, and the national teenage pregnancy strategy. *Lancet* 2006; **368**: 1879–86.

[22] Department for Education and Skills, Department of Health, Department of Communities and Local Government. *Local Strategic Partnerships and Teenage Pregnancy*. London: Department for Education and Skills, 2007.

[23] McKee M. Sex and drugs and rock and roll. Britain can learn lessons from Europe on the health of adolescents. *BMJ* 1999; **318**: 1300–1.

[24] Department of Health. *Shifting the Balance of Power*. London: Department of Health, 2001.

[25] Talbot-Smith A, Pollock AM. *The New NHS: A Guide*. Abingdon, Oxon: Routledge, 2006.

[26] Secretary of State for Health. *Saving Lives: Our Healthier Nation*. London: Department of Health, 1999.

[27] Wanless D. *Securing Our Future Health: Taking a Long-Term View. Final Report*. London: HM Treasury, 2002.

[28] Department of Health. *Smokefree England: One Year On*. London: Department of Health and NHS, 2008.

[29] Office for National Statistics. *Smoking Related Behaviour and Attitudes 2007*. London: Office for National Statistics, 2008.

[30] West R. *Key Performance Indicators on Smoking Cessation in England: Findings from the Smoking Toolkit Study*. London: Cancer Research UK, McNeil, Pfizer, and GlaxoSmithKline, 2008.

[31] Semple S, van Tongeren M, Gee I, Ayres J. *Smokefree Bars 07. Changes in Bar Workers' and Customers' Exposure to Second-Hand Smoke, Health and Attitudes*. University of Aberdeen, Institute of Occupational Medicine, John Moores University, 2008.

[32] Department of Health, Health Improvement Analytical Team. *The Cost of Alcohol Harm To the NHS in England. An Update to the Cabinet Office (2003) Study*. London: Department of Health, 2008.

[33] Academy of Medical Sciences. *Calling Time: The Nation's Drinking as a Major Health Issue*. London: Academy of Medical Sciences, 2004.

[34] Prime Minister's Strategy Unit. Alcohol Harm Reduction Strategy for England. London: Prime Minister's Strategy Unit, 2004.

[35] HM Government. *Safe. Sensible. Social. The Next Steps in the National Alcohol Strategy*. London: Department of Health, Home Office, Department for Education and Skills, Department for Culture, Media and Sport, 2007.

[36] Campden and Chorleywood Food Research Association Group. *Monitoring the Implementation of the Alcohol Labelling Regime*. London: Department of Health, 2008.

[37] National Audit Office. *Tackling Child Obesity: First Steps*. London: National Audit Office Value for Money Report by the Comptroller and Auditor-General prepared jointly by the Audit Commission, The Healthcare Commission, and the National Audit Office 2006.

[38] Department of Health. *Healthy Weight, Healthy Lives. A Cross Government Strategy for England*. London: Department of Health, 2008.

[39] Acheson D. *Independent Inquiry into Inequalities in Health*. London: HMSO, 1998.

[40] Department of Health. *Tackling Health Inequalities: A Cross-Cutting Review*. London: Department of Health, 2002.

[41] Department of Health. *Health Inequalities: Progress and Next Steps*. London: Department of Health, 2008.

[42] O'Neill O. *A Question of Trust: The BBC Reith Lectures 2002*. Cambridge: Cambridge University Press, 2002.

[43] Sim F, Lock K, McKee M. Maximizing the contribution of the public health workforce: the English experience. *Bull WHO* 2007; **85**: 935–940.

[44] McKee M, Raine R. Choosing health? First choose your philosophy. *Lancet* 2005; **365**: 369–371.

Chapter 4

Public health in Sweden: facts, visions, and lessons

Stig Wall, Gudrun Persson, and Lars Weinehall

Introduction

Sweden has a long tradition of public health information. Vital statistics and death cause registration were initiated in Sweden earlier than in any other European country by the Commission of Tables, founded in 1749. The Commission became the Central Bureau of Statistics in 1858 and is now Statistics Sweden [1]. From 1854 provincial medical officers were required to submit annual reports on the health of their populations. Doctors were responsible for death certification in urban areas by 1860 and in rural areas by 1911 when a standardized cause of death list was established [2]. Even though the systematic preventive maternity and child health services have been county council responsibilities for more than 60 years, the broad population perspective on health gradually fell into abeyance as a consequence of progress in medicine and continuing specialization.

According to the Medical Services Act, the major emphasis of the government with respect to health until the early 1980s was to supply medical care. A renewed interest in public health from Swedish health authorities occurred during the 1970s with a changing perspective from medical care policy to health policy [3]. The Health and Medical Services Act, adopted in 1982, included provisions that covered all health services, i.e. services provided by both county councils and municipalities. The aim of this legislation was to provide a good health service on equal terms for the entire population. The Swedish Parliament [Riksdag] emphasized that health services were responsible both for treating disease and injury that had already occurred and for active efforts to prevent disease and injury from occurring. In 1984, in conjunction with the WHO *Health for All by the Year 2000* strategy [4], a national Health Care Commission presented a model for systematic description of the population and its health risks, health problems, and care facilities. As a consequence, the government proposed that a review and analysis of the health of the population should be published every third year. The task was undertaken by the National Board of Health and Welfare. Sweden's first national *Public Health Report* was published in 1987 [5].

In this chapter we examine the Swedish public health scene from three perspectives, each of which involves different actors: public health *policy*, public health *reporting*, and public health *research*. By combining the three we emphasize their interdependence and provide some examples of successes and failures in Swedish health and welfare programmes.

We now summarize the public health situation in Sweden as mirrored by its national *Public Health Reports* (1987–2005) and identify major themes in Swedish public health research and policy. We also describe the lessons learnt from trying to promote and evaluate public health changes at the local community level.

Demographic and health trends

Health information

Sweden is known for the availability of good-quality central disease and population registers [6–8]. Public health reporting is the responsibility of the Centre for Epidemiology within the National Board of Health and Welfare. Since 1994 Public Health and Social Reports have been published in parallel. The sixth *Public Health Report* was published in 2005 [9] and the fourth Social Report in 2006 [10]. These reports provide a basis for health and social policy and give a broad description and analysis of health and socio-economic trends. They are used by national and local politicians and their organizations, health professionals, journalists, and public health training programmes. Data from national registers, surveys of living conditions and work environments, and labour force surveys provide the empirical basis for public health reporting. The Swedish personal identification number makes it possible to link health registers to census data, income registers, and education registers. National legislation (The Personal Data Act) sets the rules for ethical conduct and the use of these data [11].

Life expectancy continues to increase

Between 1900 and 2006 life expectancy at birth increased by roughly 25 years for both men and women to 78.8 years and 82.9 years, respectively. Only men in Iceland and Japan live longer. During the past few decades, men's life expectancy has grown more quickly than that of women and, indeed, life expectancy in women is greater in some other European countries, such as Spain, France, and Switzerland, than in Sweden.

The recent increases in life expectancy are due mainly to increased survival among middle-aged and elderly people, which in turn is largely due to reduced mortality from cardiovascular diseases, with men benefiting more than women (Fig. 4.1). As well as the trend for women to give birth to fewer children (1.5–2 children per woman during the last decade), population growth is tapering off as the population ages. The trend towards an increasing proportion of old people is similar in many European countries as a consequence of very low fertility and high average length of life. This development will be partially balanced by increased immigration from countries outside Europe.

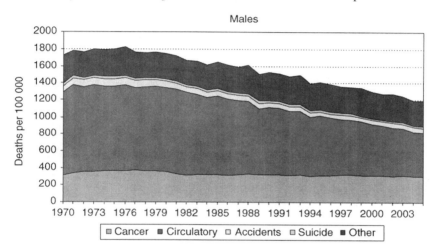

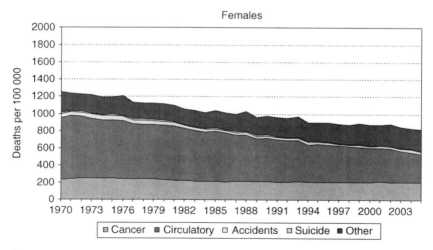

Fig. 4.1 Age-standardized deaths per 100,000 from different causes 1970–2005. Source: Cause of Death Register, EpC/National Board of Health and Welfare.

Infant mortality continues to decline

During the past 20 years infant mortality has more than halved to a low of 2.8 deaths during the first year of life per 1000 live births in 2006. The decline in infant mortality during the past few decades has been more pronounced during the first month of life, whereas the opposite occurred during earlier periods. This shift is explained largely by improved neonatal care and the fact that more very premature babies survive their first year of life. During the 1970s and 1980s the number of cases of sudden infant death syndrome (SIDS) increased in Sweden as in many other countries. The situation improved when increasing numbers of children were sleeping in a safe position on their backs—a successful non-medical intervention [12]. Another significant risk factor for SIDS is maternal smoking during pregnancy which has considerably declined. During the 1990s the rate of SIDS deaths in Sweden declined rapidly and has continued to decrease, falling to 0.2 per 1000 live births in 2004.

Longer life—better health?

What then is the quality of the years added to life? According to calculations in earlier *Public Health Reports*, it is chiefly years with slight ill health that have been added [13]. Health development during the last 25 year period has favoured those aged 45 or older rather than younger adults. Self-reported good health has improved most for men older than 55 years and women aged 55–74; women over 75 years reported a worsening of health. At the same time, there has been an improvement in mobility and fewer with daily living difficulties, partly an effect of knee and hip arthroplasty. Vision has improved because of the large number of cataract operations. Dental health has also improved considerably. Mild mental problems, such as anxiety and sleep problems, are being reported less than formerly in this age group. However, there are signs that there was an increased prevalence of many chronic illnesses among the population aged 65–84 years between the periods 1988–1994 and 2001–2005, especially among those having at least three chronic illnesses: diabetes, hypertension, and heart disease. Since disease is strongly related to age, this is partly a consequence of increased survival in general and indicates a greater need for care of the elderly population in the future.

During the 1990s mental ill health problems, such as anxiety, worry, and sleep problems, became more common in younger age groups (16–44 years), and particularly among women. This coincided with the economic depression during the first half of the 1990s when there was high unemployment in Sweden; at the same time decreasing sickness absence was noted. Many studies have shown that the level of sick leave is associated with the current economic situation [14]. In times of prosperity the number of unemployed people decreases while sick leave increases. During a recession, the opposite is the case.

Recent data from the 2009 *Public Health Report* [15] suggest that mental well-being appears to have improved except for adolescents since the beginning of 2000. Work-related problems have also declined, and the increase in overweight and obesity has levelled off in adults. A few small studies from Stockholm and Gothenburg point in the same direction in children. Alcohol consumption, which had been increasing since the mid-1980s, is no longer increasing. Smoking has long shown a downward trend and this is continuing. Dental health is continuing to improve among both adults and children. During this period Sweden has had a prosperous economy.

Cardiovascular disease—fewer new cases and more survivors

Mortality from cardiovascular diseases in the age group 15–74 years more than halved in Sweden between the mid-1980s and 2004 because of reductions in incidence and case fatality [16]. Cardiovascular diseases still accounted for approximately 45 per cent of the total mortality in 2005 (Fig. 4.1), and one in five deaths occur under the age of 75 years. The decreased risks of cardiovascular disease are due to improvements in the major risk factors, predominantly reduced smoking and improved dietary habits, while the reduced case fatality is largely due to medical care efforts [9]. The proportion of daily smokers has been declining since about 1960 among men and since 1980 among women. In 2006, 12 per cent of men and 17 per cent of women were daily smokers, one of the lowest rates in Europe. The proportion of daily snuff-taking has increased among women since the 1990s (now 3 per cent) and among men over a period of about 30 years (24 per cent) (Table 4.1).

The number of cancer survivors is increasing

Cancer is the second most common cause of death after cardiovascular disease (Fig. 4.1). Life expectancy for people diagnosed with cancer today is an average of 7 years more than for those who were diagnosed with cancer in the middle of the 1960s [17]. Early detection and better treatment are behind the improved survival. Cancers of the breast and prostate are most common, and together they account for one-third of all new cases. Lung cancer accounted for 7 per cent of all new cancers in men and women in 2006.

Table 4.1 Proportion of daily smokers and of daily snuff users among women and men in various age groups, 2006

Age	Daily smokers		Daily snuff users	
	Women	Men	Women	Men
16–24	16	8	4	23
25–34	14	12	3	32
35–44	19	12	3	29
45–54	24	15	6	28
55–64	22	14	1	19
65–74	10	14	1	18
75–84	5	7	0	8
16–84	17	12	3	24

Source: Survey of Living Conditions, Statistics Sweden (2008).

Inequalities in health

Widening gap in inequalities

A major obligation for public health practitioners is to increase the visibility of social and gender differentials in health. The first *Public Health Report* [5] noted that:

> ... although, during the 70's material conditions equalized between people, class differences increased with regard to exposure for such living conditions that had health impacts, e.g. smoking, unemployment, stress and monotonous work.

Subsequent *Public Health Report*s have found persistent social differences in health [9]. They are greatest among men; male upper white-collar workers at age 35 are expected to live 2 years longer than unskilled male blue-collar workers, and female upper white-collar workers are expected to live 0.7 years longer than female unskilled blue-collar workers. The *Public Health Report*s have also shown that, in many respects, health in several immigrant groups is poorer than in native-born Swedes. However, mortality among non-Nordic people is comparable with that of those born in Sweden, although people from the other Nordic countries, especially those born in Finland, have significantly raised death risks.

A probable explanation of social differences in morbidity and mortality is that health risks cluster among individuals in certain social groups, beginning early in life and in response to social conditions. Unhealthy living habits (including high energy intake that can lead to excess weight, smoking, and high alcohol consumption), which are now more common among blue-collar workers, were previously more common among white-collar workers. A tenth of the Swedish population has an accumulation of welfare problems such as low income, economic problems, difficulties in obtaining employment, and problems on the housing market or low housing standards. They also report more health problems and unhealthy living habits which tend to accumulate among those who are socially exposed and vulnerable [9,10]. The same pattern of social differences is observed for different educational levels. The importance of education is further supported by the fact that educational advantage *within* all socio-economic strata seems to be beneficial [18].

Comparing the first half of the 1990s with a decade earlier, relative inequalities in total mortality increased in Scandinavia while absolute social differences were fairly stable. The increasing relative social gap was mainly attributable to cardiovascular mortality in view of its steeper decline in the upper socio-economic groups [19]. From a social equality perspective, absolute mortality or morbidity in the socially or economically worst-off groups may be more relevant as a comparative measure of how well countries are looking after their population's health [20].

Social differences in health risks, ill-health, and death are conspicuous and have increased in some areas. Blue-collar workers, those with a lower level of education, single men, single mothers, and those born in other countries generally have poorer health. Particular attention should be paid to health developments in the group of people born abroad; for instance, their mental health is much poorer than that of the remainder of the population. There are still major differences between blue-collar and white-collar workers with regard to dental health.

The social differences have often increased when a positive trend has been observed; for example, the percentage of non-smokers has increased more rapidly among white-collar workers than among blue-collar workers. The systematic differences in health that prevail between different groups in the population are largely related to people's different living conditions and habits. The health level enjoyed by well-to-do groups can give an indication of what it is possible to achieve. Many of today's health problems can be reduced through preventive work. To be effective, this requires measures at national, community (Box 4.1) and individual levels. Preventive work requires long-term thinking and should be regarded as an investment.

Public health policy in Sweden

Background

Public health policy in Sweden traditionally addressed preventive health by emphasizing specific areas such as alcohol and tobacco, the environment,

Box 4.1 Community commitment to intervention

Epidemiological studies from the late 1970s showed that the county of Västerbotten had the highest cardiovascular mortality in Sweden [3], and as a result a long-term prevention programme, the Västerbotten Intervention Programme, was initiated in 1985. The community intervention in Norsjö—the municipality with the highest mortality—combined individual and population-oriented efforts. Popular movement activities in the community brought ideas out into the public arena. A unique feature of the programme is that the health sector and its primary health-care providers took an active role in the work [21,22]. All individuals at ages 30, 40, 50, and 60 were invited to participate in educational screening including health counselling (Fig. 4.2). In the 10 year evaluation the intervention area had a significantly larger decline in cholesterol, systolic blood pressure, and predicted coronary heart disease mortality [23]. People with lower education levels seemed to benefit the most from the prevention programme (Fig. 4.2), suggesting that reduction of health inequity is possible through this type of approach, as was recognized by the WHO Commission on Social Determinants of Health [24].

traffic, and chronic disease prevention. However, until recently there were no overall national objectives for public health. For this reason, in 1997 the Swedish government appointed a committee to produce national objectives for health development. In 2003 the Riksdag adopted *Objectives for Public Health* (Government bill 2002/03:35). The national public health strategy was based on the overall aim of creating social conditions that would ensure good health on equal terms for the entire population [25]. This overriding goal remains after the recent change in government.

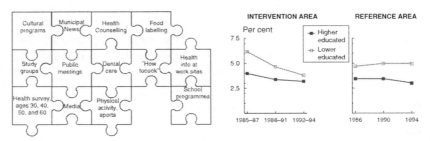

Fig. 4.2 Components in the Norsjö intervention and the estimated risk of dying of cardiac infarction compared with Northern Sweden (reference area) stratified by educational level.

The process

The Swedish Parliament decided on a comprehensive national public health policy in 2003. The new policy aims to strengthen health promotion and disease prevention initiatives, contribute to a reduction of health inequalities between groups, and make health consequences an important consideration in all decision-making at every level of society. The proposal was developed by a National Committee for Public Health, appointed in 1997. A number of experts and researchers within various areas collaborated on the development of the proposal and 19 different expert-produced reports were published (Fig. 4.3). During the three years of its work the Committee fostered a broad discussion with the public and with politicians and civil servants at state and municipal level, with research workers, and with representatives of different organizations and trades. Furthermore, the Committee invited representatives of different organizations and popular movements to provide active input.

Focusing on the determinants of health

Three public health issues were identified by the National Committee as important to address: the steadily increasing life expectancy; the pattern of declining self-estimated good health among young people; and the remaining health gap between different social strata. In its final proposal the Committee defined 18 health objectives. Some of these objectives included initiatives to develop the social capital, to counteract wider disparities in income and reduce relative poverty, to give all children the opportunity to grow up on fair and safe

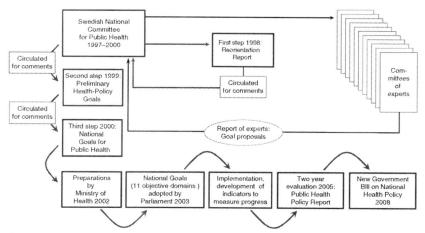

Fig. 4.3 The process of developing the Swedish National Public Health Policy from committee work to formulation, adaptation, and evaluation of national objectives.

terms, to support high employment, to create accessible areas for recreation, and to promote safe environments and products. Other objectives dealt with preconditions for public health research and public health information, or aimed at stronger collaborations at the local level, based on a proposed new Public Health Law. The focus on lifestyle factors (food, activities, drugs) should not 'blame the individual', but support and facilitate healthier living. The importance of partnerships with health-care providers was recognized, and these are challenged to focus more on disease prevention and health promotion and to foster intersectoral work. The proposals aimed to prevent ill health that restricts the freedom of the individual and urged for changes to take place in the labour market, in welfare policy, and in consumption patterns, as well as with regard to health-care policy.

Setting objectives

The Ministry of Health circulated the Committee proposals among national and regional authorities, universities, research bodies, county councils, municipalities, unions, and community groups in order to obtain comments and reactions. Finally, the Minister of Health summarized the Committee proposals and the comments from different bodies in Swedish society in a governmental bill and presented it to Parliament, which adopted the bill in 2003 (Fig. 4.3). Eleven general objectives and a large number of policy areas in which efforts should be made to affect public health were specified [25]. The 11 general objectives cover the most important determinants of health (Box 4.2), and it was expected that, by directing measures to these areas, better and more equal public health would be achieved. The first six objectives concern factors in society, termed structural circumstances, while the remaining five focus on living habits which individuals themselves can affect.

In contrast with many other national health policies, Swedish health objectives mainly address determinants of health [25]. The objectives are directed to the level of society and culture and attempt to put health issues on the political as well as the social agenda [26].

Coordination

National public health policy is coordinated by the government. A number of actions and challenges are defined for national, regional, and local authorities, as well as for the private and voluntary sectors. Monitoring and evaluation of the national public health objectives are reported to the government every four years in a public health policy report from the National Institute of Public Health [27]. In 2008 the government presented a Green Paper on *A Renewed*

Box 4.2 General health objectives for the Swedish population

- Participation and influence in society
- Economic and social security
- Secure and favourable conditions during childhood and adolescence
- Healthier working life
- Healthy and safe environments and products
- Health and medical care that more actively promote good health
- Effective protection against communicable diseases
- Safe sex and good reproductive health
- Increased physical activity
- Good eating habits and safe food
- Reduced use of tobacco and alcohol, a society free from illicit drugs and drug-taking, and a reduction in the harmful effects of excessive gambling

Public Health Policy (2007/08:110). This proposal preceded a bill presented to Parliament confirming the objectives outlined above.

Future scenarios in public health

A governmental task force presented a *Balance Sheet for Welfare of the 1990s* in terms of health, education, work, economy, social security and relations, and political resources [28]. Major negative changes were seen during the decade, as had been documented in the previous public health and social reports. These changes occurred even though death rates continued to drop, infant mortality halved, and education levels improved even further. Particularly vulnerable groups were lone mothers with meagre economical resources, immigrants with declining social positions, and young people increasingly experiencing perceived ill health and social insecurity.

People in Sweden will continue to be healthier than earlier generations, and future disease patterns will be dominated by problems associated with ageing. Mortality rates will continue to decrease for many reasons. Paradoxically, however, reduced risks together with successes in medical care are creating new problems. If tobacco and alcohol consumption decline and eating and activity patterns continue to improve, disease risks will be reduced. However, despite general improvements in both food and exercise habits, the proportion of overweight people has increased. Lower European Union-adjusted alcohol prices may lead to increased alcohol consumption and more alcohol-related injuries. In general, there is no indication that serious mental disease is on the increase, rather the reverse; however, many people experience increased worry and anxiety, partly because of increased stress in working life [9]. The number of people living with cancer in Sweden has increased substantially [29]. The decline in cardiovascular diseases may continue if current risk factor trends prevail, unless disease trends are counteracted by the increasing overweight problem.

Children and young people in Sweden have had a very favourable health development for many years, although there are some disturbing trends, such as the increase in juvenile diabetes. Signs of increasing psychosocial problems among Swedish schoolchildren may relate to the individualization of the modern society with less security. This has generated an initiative from the Royal Academy of Sciences to undertake a systematic review of school health in Sweden and a subsequent state of the art conference.

Lessons for public health

Swedish research supports the view that work and other living conditions interact with other early risk factors to produce and reproduce health inequalities. How then do we respond to the challenge of the social differences within a modern society? Since social inequality is manifested through the accumulation of risk factors among vulnerable groups, prevention should focus primarily on the social situation rather than on the individual risk factors. We still lack a basic understanding of how people in different social positions take advantage of and adopt society's well-meant health messages, for example on lifestyle changes, many of which are more suited to well-educated people. Should the widening social gap be interpreted as a result of the general and nonspecific structure of public health policy? Does equity in health call for targeted prevention approaches? What lessons for health policy can be learnt from the inequalities in health between and within countries and from the observations that an unequal society in itself is a risk factor over and above that of the individual's social position?

The point of departure for several studies comparing Sweden with other countries has been the hypothesis that our social policy and relative social homogeneity should yield less health inequity. However, the mechanism underlying social inequality in health is probably more related to fundamental issues than to short-term health and social policy. More decisive changes require a sustainable policy [30]. Others suggest that equality has become politically outdated [31]; it has been suggested that the ethical principle of autonomy is a hindrance in that it prevents targeting of vulnerable groups [32]. Public health work should not add to risks and needs to establish its ethical platform. We need an evidence-based public health policy; this implies that we must also be prepared to analyse the health consequences of the many structural interventions imposed by current welfare politics [33].

It is time to act in accordance with what we know about the social circumstances beyond individual control—the evidence on social inequalities is overwhelming and needs no further documentation [34]. What is needed is a committed public health policy and local interventions for social and behavioural change involving the community. Evaluations of such actions must focus on structure and process as well as on outcome and discuss measures and criteria of success not only in disease terms but also in areas such as cultural and democratic development, and psychological and emotional well-being. We need to move beyond analysing the impact of social factors on health to documenting the contribution of health and health care to society and economic development. We also need to move the perspective from disease orientation to health promotion [35,36].

Although public health research in Sweden is multidisciplinary, it is mainly the reponsibility of medical faculties and its scope has been widened to include the functioning and quality of the health care as well as its role as a partner in preventive work. The research agenda on social inequalities in health has, to a large extent, been set by medical sociologists and epidemiologists. The recognized importance of the field is shown by a governmental commission to develop a national research programme to counteract social inequalities in health [37] and by the establishment of a centre for research on health equity. In parallel with the increasing demands for health interventions, there is a need for research on the benefits from such interventions. There is a considerable gap between the epidemiological identification of risk factors and the documentation of the effects of intervention and a potential in prevention. The challenge lies in bringing the development of epidemiological theory closer to public health efforts [38]. This calls for conceptual and methodological development of evaluations of public health interventions in terms not only of their efficacy but also of cost-effectiveness, social acceptance, and ethical consequences. Medical practice also needs a clearer public health perspective in everyday work [9].

Globalization implies greater interdependence between people and countries, bringing positive as well as negative local effects, calling for global thinking and local action. This analysis of public health in Sweden has attempted to illustrate the close links between public health policy, reporting, and research. Globalization creates new imperatives for public health research [39] both outside health care, highlighting governance in health policy, gender issues, and working patterns, and within health systems, addressing ongoing health transitions and the role of health care for public health.

References

[1] Documents of Death Cause Statistics. *Hygeia* 1856; **18**: 798–817.

[2] Luther G. The birth of official statistics in 18th century Sweden. In: *Bulletin of the International Statistical Institute, 52nd Session, Finland,* 1999. Available online at: http://www.stat.fi/isi99

[3] Rosén M. Epidemiology in planning for health—with special reference to regional epidemiology and the use of health registers. *Umeå University Medical Dissertations, New Series* 1987; **188**: 1–158.

[4] World Health Organization. Global Strategy for Health by the Year 2000. Geneva: WHO, 1981.

[5] *Public Health Report 1987.* Stockholm: National Board of Health and Welfare. 1987.

[6] Wall S, Källestål C. *Epidemiology Research in Sweden—Structure, Conditions and Need. A Task Force Report.* Stockholm: Swedish Medical and Social Research Councils, 1996.

[7] *Evaluation of Swedish Epidemiological Research.* Stockholm: Swedish Council for Social Research, 1997.

[8] Rosén M. National Health Data Registers: a Nordic heritage to public health. *Scand J Public Health* 2002; **30**: 81–5.

[9] Persson G, Danielsson M, Rosén M, *et al.* (eds). Health in Sweden: The National Public Health Report 2005. *Scand J Public Health* 2006: **34** (Suppl 67).

[10] Biterman D (ed). Social Report 2006. The National Report on Social Conditions in Sweden. *International Journal of Social Welfare* 2007; **16** (Suppl 3): 1–240.

[11] Allebeck P. The Helsinki Declaration. Good for patients? Good for public health? *Scand J Public Health* 2002; **30**: 1–4.

[12] Högberg U, Bergström E. Suffocated prone: the iatrogenic tragedy of SIDS. *Am J Public Health* 2000; **90**: 527–31.

[13] Rosén M, Haglund B. From healthy survivors to sick survivors: implications for the twenty-first century. *Scand J Public Health* 2005; **33**: 151–5.

[14] Alexanderson K, Norlund A (eds). Sickness absence: causes, consequences and physicians' sickness certification practice. A systematic literature review by the Swedish Council on Technology Assessment in Health Care. *Scand J Public Health* 2004; **32** (Suppl 63): 1–263.

[15] Danielsson M (ed). The National Public Health Report 2009 in Sweden (in press)

[16] Lundblad D, Holmgren L, Jansson J-H, Naslund U, Eliasson M. Gender differences in trends of acute myocardial infarction events: the Northern Sweden MONICA study 1985–2004. *BMC Cardiovasc Disord* 2008; **8**: 17.

[17] Talbäck M, Stenbeck M, Rosén M, *et al.* Cancer survival in Sweden 1960–98: developments across four decades. *Acta Oncol* 2003; **42**: 637–59.

[18] Erikson R. Social class assignment and mortality in Sweden. *Soc Sci Med* 2006; **62**: 2151–60.

[19] Mackenbach JP, Bos V, Andersen O, *et al.* Widening socioeconomic inequalities in mortality in six Western European countries. *Int J Epidemiol* 2003; **32**: 830–7.

[20] Vågerö D, Eriksson R. Socioeconomic inequalities in morbidity and mortality in western Europe. *Lancet* 1997; **350**: 516–17

[21] Weinehall L, Westman G, Hellsten G, *et al.* Shifting the distribution of risk: results of a community intervention in a Swedish programme for the prevention of cardiovascular disease. *J Epidemiol Community Health* 1999; **53**: 243–50.

[22] Weinehall L. Partnership for health. On the role of primary health care in a community intervention programme. *Umeå University Medical Dissertations, New Series* 1997; **531**: 1–161.

[23] Weinehall L, Hellsten G, Boman K, *et al.* Can a sustainable community intervention reduce the health gap? 10-year evaluation of a Swedish community intervention program for the prevention of cardiovascular disease. *Scand J Public Health* 2001; **29** (Suppl 56): 59–68.

[24] Marmot M. Achieving health equity: from root causes to fair outcomes. *Lancet* 2007; **370**: 1153–63.

[25] Pearson TA. Scandinavia's lessons to the world of public health. *Scand J Public Health* 2000; **28**: 161–3.

[26] Health on equal terms: national goals for public health. Final report by the Swedish National Committee for Public Health. *Scand J Public Health* 2001; **29** (Suppl 57): 1–68.

[27] Hogstedt C, Lundgren B, Moberg H, *et al.* (eds). The Swedish Public Health Policy and the National Institute of Public Health. *Scand J Public Health* 2004:**32** (Suppl 64): 1–64.

[28] *Välfärdsbokslut för 1990-talet (Balance Sheet for Welfare of the 1990s).* Stockholm: Statens Offentliga Utredningar, 2001; 1–299.

[29] Stenbeck M, Rosén M, Sparén P. Causes of increasing cancer prevalence in Sweden. *Lancet* 1999; **354**: 1093–4

[30] Vågerö D. Health inequalities: searching for causal explanations. In: *Inequality in Health: A Swedish perspective.* Stockholm: Socialvetenskapliga Forskningsrådet, 1998.

[31] Lindbladh E, Lyttkens CH, Hanson BS, Östergren PO. Equity is out of fashion? An essay on autonomy and health policy in the individualized society. *Soc Sci Med* 1998; **46**: 1017–25.

[32] Lindbladh E, Lyttkens CH, Hanson BS, *et al.* An economic and sociological interpretation of social differences in health-related behaviour: an encounter to guide social epidemiology. *Soc Sci Med* 1996; **43**: 1817–25.

[33] Wall S. Epidemiology in transition. *Int J Epidemiol* 1999; **28**: S1000–4.

[34] Krasnik A, Rasmussen NK (eds). Reducing social inequalities in health: evidence, policy and practice. *Scand J Public Health* 2002; **30** (Suppl 59): 1–79.

[35] Yach D. Economics and public health: reflections from the past, challenges for the future. *Scand J Public Health* 2001; **29**: 241–4.

[36] *Towards a More Health-Promoting Health Service. Summary of Study Material, Government Bills, Parliamentary Decisions, Draft Indicators, and Examples of Application.*

Stockholm: Swedish National Institute of Public Health, 2006. (available online at: www.fhi.se/upload/ar2006/Rapporter/R200630_health_promoting_0702.pdf).

[37] Carsjö K, Erikson R, Hogstedt C, *et al.* (eds). A status report on Swedish public health research: history, inventory and international evaluation. *Scand J Public Health* 2005; **33** (Suppl 65): 1–84.

[38] Wall S. Epidemiology for prevention. *Int J Epidemiol* 1995; **24**: 655–64.

[39] Wall S. Globalization makes new demands on public health research (editorial). *Scand J Public Health* 2007; **35**: 449–53.

Chapter 5

Public health in Central and Eastern Europe and the former Soviet Union

Martin McKee

Introduction

In the period after the Second World War many aspects of life in Western Europe changed beyond recognition while progress in Eastern Europe was much slower. Between 1945 and 1990 the countries in the communist bloc shared an experience that continues to have profound implications for the health of their populations, as well as their ability to respond to them, almost 20 years after the Soviet Union ceased to exist. The Soviet regime was isolated from the West by physical barriers, most obviously the Berlin Wall, but there was an equally important cultural divide. Yet this region is also very diverse, politically, geographically, and culturally. Geopolitically, the region divides into three parts:

- ten countries in Central and Eastern Europe that were Soviet satellites (or, in the case of the Baltic States Estonia, Latvia, and Lithuania, part of the Soviet Union) but are now members of the European Union (hereafter referred to as countries of Central and Eastern Europe (CCEE));

- the remaining ex-Soviet republics (hereafter referred to as the Commonwealth of Independent States (CIS));

- the countries of the western Balkans, comprising Albania and most of what was Yugoslavia. Within each grouping, there is also considerable diversity among and, especially in the case of the larger ones, within countries.

Patterns of health: the single same, but different

Life expectancy

At the risk of generalization, it is possible to ascertain differences in health relating to the broad political groupings of countries. Figure 5.1 shows trends

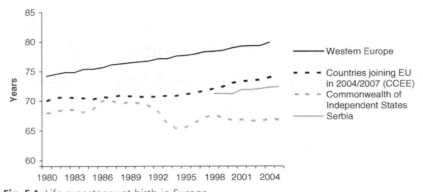

Fig. 5.1 Life expectancy at birth in Europe.
Source: WHO, Health for All database, Copenhagen: WHO, 2008.

in life expectancy at birth in Western Europe, the countries of Central and Eastern Europe joining the European Union in 2004 and 2007, the CIS, and Serbia as an example of a country in the western Balkans.

While noting all its limitations as a broad summary measure of health, the whole region had attained a relatively high level of life expectancy at birth by the mid-1960s. Soon after, however, things began to go wrong. While life expectancy in Western Europe steadily increased, in the CCEE it stagnated so that, by 1990, it was 6 years behind that in the West [1]. In the Soviet Union, in contrast, life expectancy actually deteriorated, falling by 2 years between 1970 and 1980. It then began a series of unexpected fluctuations in which it improved dramatically in 1985 before falling back after 1987 and then accelerating downwards [2]. This pattern was relatively consistent across the 15 republics which then made up the Soviet Union.

Since 1990, the individual countries have followed different health trajectories, although some sub-regional patterns can be ascertained. Rapid gains in life expectancy were seen in the German Democratic Republic, which was rapidly absorbed into the German Federal Republic [3], Czechoslovakia (and its successor states, the Czech Republic and Slovakia following their split in 1993) [4], and Poland [5]. Hungary followed soon after, followed in the mid-1990s by Romania [6] and Bulgaria. The three Baltic States followed almost exactly the same trajectory as the rest of the ex-Soviet Union until 1998, since when they have experienced considerable gains. The countries emerging from the Soviet Union suffered greatly in the aftermath of its break-up. The downward trend in life expectancy accelerated, reversing briefly in 1994, to be followed by a further decline after 1998 coinciding with an economic crisis in Russia [7]. Since 2000, life expectancy in most of the CIS has stagnated, although there was a brief, apparently short-lived, recovery in Russia in 2006. The 1990s were largely a lost decade for the countries of the western Balkans [8]. All of them were afflicted, to some degree, by conflict, leading to tens of thousands of deaths and massive destruction of infrastructure.

Vital statistics systems

Despite its many drawbacks, communism bequeathed to epidemiologists a high-quality system of vital statistics [9]. Some countries did conceal data at various times, either withholding data completely, as the Soviet Union did in the early 1980s, or 'losing' certain sensitive causes such as homicide, suicide, and cirrhosis in non-specific categories, as occurred in the German Democratic Republic in the 1970s and 1980s. However, in all cases comprehensive mortality data sets have now been reconstructed [10] and provide a unique resource for understanding adult mortality in middle-income countries that is not available in other parts of the world, such as Latin America [11]. However, there are some problems. Data collection has suffered in areas experiencing conflict, such as the western Balkans and the countries of the Caucasus [12].

Infant mortality rates

The greatest problems have been in recording events at the beginning of life. Some countries introduced fees for registering births, with the result that births were only recorded when children entered school. Thus, in many parts of Central Asia and the Caucasus official infant mortality rates are significant underestimates [13] (Table 5.1). In some countries there are difficulties in calculating denominators because of unrecorded migration. Nonetheless, a high proportion of deaths are still subject to autopsy, albeit often somewhat

Table 5.1 Infant mortality according to official data and surveys in Central Asia

	Official infant mortality	Infant mortality according to survey data
Armenia	15.4 (1996–2000)	36 (1996–2000)
Azerbaijan	17.2 (1996–2000)	74 (1996–2000)
Georgia	15.2 (1995–1999)	43 (1995–1999)
Kazakhstan	24.8 (1994–1999)	62 (1994–1999)
Kyrgyzstan	29.1 (1993–1997)	61 (1993–1997)
Tajikistan	24.1 (1996–2000)	89 (1996–2000)
Turkmenistan	38.9 (1995–2000)	74 (1995–2000)
Uzbekistan	30.2 (1992–1996)	49 (1992–1996)
Sub-regional average	25.8	59.4

Source: Rechel et al. [13].

basic, and, at least for adults, the available data are believed to be generally accurate in most places.

A conceptual framework: explaining patterns of mortality

Nearly all the Soviet republics experienced a dramatic increase in life expectancy in 1985 and, perhaps more surprisingly as they were by then all independent, a steep fall between 1991 and 1994, followed by a short-lived improvement and then another decline after 1998. This pattern was relatively consistent across the 15 republics that made up the Soviet Union. Several distinct and apparently unrelated causes of death, such as injuries and heart disease, contributed to these changes, indicating a phenomenon that must have its origins at a societal level, acting through multiple biological and social pathways. Importantly, cancer rates did not change substantially, indicating that the fluctuations were real and not due to artefacts caused by problems with numerators or denominators. Although cancer is clearly affected by societal forces, there are long lag periods between exposure and death. Thus, deaths today from stomach cancer reflect conditions several decades ago when those affected were young children [14], and deaths from breast cancer have been linked to historical trends in birth rates [15].

Patterns of mortality

In this section the pragmatic separation of the different parts of this region will be maintained, reflecting their quite different experience of mortality, although, as will be seen later, there are also certain common factors, in particular in relation to mechanisms of disease (Box 5.1).

The most significant impact of mortality patterns in the region relates to deaths in early middle age. In the CCEE, deaths in this age group increased

Box 5.1 Gender differences in mortality

Mortality can be disaggregated in many ways. Looking first at gender, it is apparent that men have been particularly vulnerable [16]. In all industrialized countries men have a lower life expectancy than women, but the gap is particularly large in this region. In 2005, life expectancy at birth for men was almost 13 years less than that for women, indicating that factors such as environmental pollution, to which both sexes are equally exposed, cannot explain the poor health in this region. Unmarried men [17,18] and those with low levels of education have been particularly vulnerable [19].

steadily throughout the 1980s. Subsequently, each country has experienced an improvement, but beginning at different times. In Poland and the Czech Republic it began almost at once, while in Hungary and Bulgaria it only started in the mid-1990s. In Romania it was delayed until 1997. This age group was also affected most in the CIS, with their deaths driving the large fluctuations in overall mortality [2].

The causes of death underlying these changes are extremely complex, and the following description is, of necessity, a simplification. Most countries in the CCEE experienced a short-lived increase in deaths at the time of transition, largely due to deaths from external causes, especially traffic accidents, which have continued to decline. Later, sustained improvements in life expectancy, beginning at different times in the 1990s, have been largely due to falls in cardiovascular disease. In some cases, such as Poland, life expectancy has risen quite steeply [5]. In some parts of Southern Europe, where rates were previously extremely high, a decline in deaths from cirrhosis has also contributed.

To understand the very different trends in the Soviet Union it is necessary to go back to events in 1985, when Mikhail Gorbachev, the Secretary General of the Communist Party of the Soviet Union, implemented an initially highly effective and wide-ranging anti-alcohol campaign [20]. This led to an immediate improvement in life expectancy, due largely to a decline in cardiovascular diseases and injuries. Smaller contributions were made by a range of causes known to be associated with alcohol, including acute alcohol poisoning and pneumonia. Importantly, other major causes of death, such as cancer, were unaffected. In the subsequent large fluctuations in mortality the same causes have been implicated [2]. Thus, it is apparent that it is impossible to interpret the changing pattern of mortality in the former Soviet Union without understanding the role played by alcohol. This, in turn, requires some knowledge of the nature of drinking.

Alcohol consumption: a critical factor

Although the products drunk throughout this region are changing, in part as a result of aggressive marketing by Western alcohol manufacturers, there are some important regional patterns which ultimately reflect climate and thus traditional patterns of agriculture. In a band of countries in the southern part of this region, from Slovenia through Hungary and Romania to Moldova, and extending across the Black Sea to the Caucasus the main source of spirits is fruit, distilled into brandy. Much was traditionally home-made and, as a result, contains high levels of toxic long-chain alcohols [21]. These countries have high levels of cirrhosis [22], although there is still some debate about whether this reflects the presence of toxins or simply the high level of consumption.

The remaining countries in the CIS are characterized by high levels of consumption of vodka, produced from grain [23,24]. This has been produced widely from the seventeenth century onwards; before then the main source of alcohol was mead, fermented from honey, or kvass, fermented from bread [25]. Drinking in this region is frequently characterized by episodes of extremely high levels of consumption. The Russian word *zapoi* describes a drinking episode in which the individual concerned is incapacitated for several days at a time. Deaths from acute alcohol poisoning are common. However, recent work has identified the very important role played by other sources of alcohol, in particular a range of substances that are not sold officially for consumption but which are easily available in several countries (including Russia, Ukraine and the Baltic States) [26–28] (Box 5.2). Historically, there are many accounts of these being drunk during the Soviet era but circumstantial evidence suggests that they are now much more widely available.

It was estimated that a combination of *zapoi* and drinking non-beverage alcohols accounted for almost 40 per cent of deaths in Russian working-age men. Importantly, in part as a consequence of this research, the Russian government introduced restrictions on the sale of these substances in January 2006. While these restrictions have been only partly effective, they have been associated with a marked drop in deaths from alcohol poisoning and an

Box 5.2 Ethanol 'aftershaves'

The most important source of non-beverage alcohol is to be found in 'aftershaves', known in Russian as *odekolon*. Until recently these were sold in 250 ml bottles, bearing brightly coloured labels. Although marked as not for consumption, most include no scents (a few contain lemon, although this is labelled as a flavour) and they consist of 95 per cent ethanol. They are untaxed and thus, in terms of volume of pure alcohol, are about one-sixth the price of vodka. Other sources include medicinal tinctures, sold in pharmacies, and a wide range of technical liquids, including industrial cleaners and fire-lighting liquid. A study in a typical Russian city found that these substances were being drunk regularly by about one in 12 men of working age, with substantially higher rates among those with least education and in unskilled jobs [29] while a subsequent survey found them to be widely available across Russia [28]. A case–control study found a very strong and specific relationship between consumption of these substances and deaths form alcoholic psychosis, cirrhosis, and cardiomyopathy (odds ratio, 25.5) [30].

increase in male life expectancy at birth of 1.5 years, a marked departure from the previous stagnating trend, although it now seems this gain may have only been temporary.

Other causes of death

A few specific conditions emerge as major causes of the health gap with Western Europe: injuries and violence, cardiovascular disease, cancer, and some alcohol-related diseases such as cirrhosis.

Injuries and violence (external causes)

In 2004 the death rate from external causes was about five times higher in the CIS than in Western Europe; in the CCEE it was about double that in the West. While all causes of injury are more common in this region, the gap is particularly great for homicide and suicide. Other external causes of death that are very much more common in the East than in the West are drowning and deaths in fires. Alcohol plays a key role in all these causes. A study comparing homicides in the early and late 1990s, which collected information on both the victims and their killers, found that it was very common for both to be intoxicated [31]. Other research has shown a close correlation in time and place between deaths from alcohol poisoning and both homicide and suicide [32].

In addition to alcohol, death rates from unintentional injuries reflect many factors related to risk and its perception, and to the environment. Particularly in the CIS, there are few of the design features that enhance safety in the West. In many cases effective health care could save some of these lives, but it is either unavailable or of poor quality, especially in rural areas suffering from poor communications and transport infrastructure. A further problem is widespread corruption involving the police and agencies that should be enforcing safety standards.

Cardiovascular disease

Deaths from cardiovascular disease are also much more common in Eastern Europe than in the West. In Central and Eastern Europe this clearly reflects high levels of many traditional risk factors, such as a diet rich in saturated fats and high rates of smoking. Several of the countries which joined the European Union in 2004 experienced a marked decline in deaths from cardiovascular disease, beginning almost immediately after the transition in 1989. This is believed to reflect a change in the composition of fat in the diet following removal of subsidies and the opening of the retail sector to international trade [5].

The situation in the CIS is rather different. Deaths from ischaemic heart disease are much more likely to be sudden than in other parts of the world [33], and death rates remain extremely high. It is now apparent, from the research described above, that alcohol plays a major role in this situation, although almost certainly its effects are superimposed upon an underlying high level of risk due to smoking and poor diet.

While the conventional view is that alcohol, at least at 'moderate' consumption levels, exerts a protective effect on cardiovascular disease, there are specific dangers from episodic heavy drinking. Research has defined this in various ways, including frequent hangovers, getting into trouble with the police because of drinking, or frequent absence from work for alcohol related disorders; all these indicators of heavy drinking are consistently associated with a substantially increased risk of, especially, sudden cardiac death [34]. This is due to the different responses of lipids (Box 5.3), blood clotting, and myocardial function to binge drinking compared with regular moderate consumption.

An emphasis on the role of lipids has distracted attention from the other elements of thrombosis, first described by Virchow over a century ago [39]. These include changes in vascular endothelium, permitting lipid to accumulate, and changes in platelet and fibrinolytic activity, influencing the propensity of blood to clot [40]. Eastern European diets are characterized by large quantities of fat and very low levels of fruit and vegetables [41]. Correspondingly, antioxidant

Box 5.3 Differing lipid responses

Lipid levels, which are a major focus of attention in Western countries, seem to have less predictive value in this region. Thus, in a comparison of Russian and American populations, the protective effect of a given level of high-density lipoprotein (HDL) was much less in the former and it took much longer follow-up to become apparent [35]. *In vitro* studies of HDL from the same study found that samples from Russian blood had less effect on cholesterol metabolism in cultured fibroblasts than did HDL from the American samples [36]. While conventional risk factors explained all the variation in incidence of myocardial infarction in the INTERHEART study, they explained only 71 per cent in this region, and that research was limited to those surviving to hospital [37]. There is also evidence of differences in activity of lipids, perhaps because of the effects of cofactors [36]. Many victims of sudden cardiac death in this region display little evidence of atheroma at autopsy [38].

activity in blood, which is determined primarily by intake of micronutrients, is extremely low [42]. While changes in lipids are important, these other mechanisms may provide an explanation for the rapid reduction in cardiovascular deaths seen in some countries such as Poland [5] and the Czech Republic [4].

Finally, on the basis of what is known about the aetiology of cardiovascular disease in the West, it is unlikely that these explanations will be able to account for all the changes that have been observed, and further research is required to explore, in particular, the role of psychosocial factors.

Cancer

Cancer covers a multitude of diseases, each with their own risk factors. Here, we consider two examples, lung and cervical cancer. Death rates from lung cancer among men are extremely high, in some cases reaching levels never previously observed anywhere in the world. This reflects the very high prevalence of smoking in men throughout Eastern Europe [43], possibly encouraged by a shared experience of military service as teenagers. Death rates from lung cancer fell briefly during the 1990s, reflecting transiently lower levels of commencing smoking in the austere period of the late 1940s and early 1950s [44].

In contrast, smoking has always been relatively uncommon among women. This is now changing rapidly, and female smoking rates, especially among young women in major cities, are increasing rapidly [45]. A major factor is aggressive advertising by Western tobacco companies [46]. It is anticipated that lung cancer rates among women will soon start rising [47].

The policy response to tobacco has been, in general, very weak. The tobacco industry, which has aggressively targeted this region [46], has been able to ignore many health ministries that have extremely limited capacity, stretched further by a focus on health-care reform [48]. In some countries, the industry has effectively written laws on tobacco control for governments that lack any meaningful capacity [49], or has blocked the introduction of policies that would have been effective even though surveys indicate considerable public support for stronger measures against smoking [50]. Even where advertising is illegal, fines are often derisory. There are some exceptions. Poland has been able to implement a wide-ranging policy on tobacco [51], including a ban on advertising, that has led to a reduction in tobacco use.

Cervical cancer is also rather more common than in the West, a finding that is unsurprising given the high rates of sexually transmitted diseases and, until recently, the difficulty in obtaining barrier contraceptives [52]. Unfortunately, the few effective cervical screening programmes are rare exceptions, and screening is often opportunistic, with little quality control, and generally ineffective.

In brief, the pattern of cancer mortality in Eastern Europe is complex and changing. In the future, it is likely that deaths from some types, such as stomach cancer, will continue to decline, while others, such as breast and prostate, will come closer to those in the West.

Infectious diseases

As in the West, acute infectious diseases are no longer major causes of death. This reflected the high-level political commitment to disease control during the twentieth century, following Lenin's famous statement in response to outbreaks of typhus that 'If communism does not destroy the louse, the louse will destroy communism'. The Soviet system was particularly successful in reducing vaccine-preventable diseases, in part because of its pervasive system of monitoring and use of compulsion, although a breakdown of control systems in some countries following independence has allowed them to re-emerge [53]. In contrast, the lack of investment in infrastructure, with many rural hospitals lacking hot water even in the early 1990s, meant that other aspects of infection control were poor. This was exacerbated by adherence to outdated concepts of disease transmission and surveillance.

Infectious diseases causing concern are sexually transmitted diseases (STDs), HIV, and tuberculosis. STD rates rose rapidly in many countries in the 1990s. They have since fallen, although there are concerns as to whether this reflects a true reduction in incidence or a decline in notification, as treatment is increasingly provided privately. Rates of HIV infection are still low, in global terms, but are rising rapidly in many parts of the former Soviet Union [54]. At present, spread is primarily due to needle-sharing among addicts, but the epidemic is beginning to move into the wider population via sexual spread.

Rates of tuberculosis have also increased markedly in recent decades, especially among the large prison population where conditions are highly conducive to rapid spread and where treatment is often inadequate [55]. Research at an individual level in Russia demonstrates how imprisonment increases the risk of contracting tuberculosis 12-fold [56], and other research demonstrates a strong association between incarceration levels and tuberculosis incidence in former communist countries [57]. A matter of particular concern is the high rate of drug-resistant disease, reflecting poor prescribing practices [58]. The coexistence of HIV and resistant tuberculosis poses enormous challenges for the future, which have yet to elicit an effective response [59].

Finally, changes in land use related to the adoption of new agricultural practices, coupled with changes in human activity with greater recreational use of the countryside, are contributing to a shift in patterns of zoonotic infections,

such as an increase in leptospirosis in Bulgaria [60] and in tick-borr
litis in the Baltic States [61].

The underlying factors

One of the most striking features of mortality in Eastern Europe is the way that
death rates have been much higher in men than in women. Much of this can
be explained by differences in lifestyle, in particular use of alcohol and tobacco.
However, although they live longer, it is also clear that surviving women bear
a heavy burden of ill health, so that the gap in healthy life expectancy is actually
much smaller [62].

Lifestyle choices are heavily influenced by social circumstances, and they
can only be understood fully by considering the context in which they are
made. The social forces driving trends in mortality in this region are still
inadequately understood, although some parts of the picture are clear. Those
groups that have been worst affected have been so as a result of increasing
deaths from external causes and cardiovascular diseases. Consistent with
the findings discussed earlier, while deaths from causes linked directly with
alcohol have been numerically less important, they have shown the steepest
social gradients [63].

In Russia, at least, the rise in mortality in the early 1990s was greatest in
regions experiencing the most rapid pace of transition, as measured by employment turnover (the sum of hirings and firings) [64], and where measures of social
cohesion were weakest [65]. Subsequent research has shown how differences in
the scale of transition-related mortality can be explained by the extent to which
countries adopted mass privatization strategies, selling off large enterprises
rapidly, but also that the impact on mortality was, to some extent, mitigated by
social support structures, measured as membership of organizations such as
churches and trade unions [66]. This is consistent with other research showing
that members of such organizations enjoy better health, after adjusting for
other factors [67], and with the observation that the individuals most affected
by transition have been men with low levels of education [19], low levels of
social support, such as the unmarried [17,18], and low levels of control over
their lives [68]. Women may have had some degree of protection as they could
find fulfilling roles within the home [18], while men with low skills levels were
confronted with a feeling of impotence in a hostile and unresponsive world [69].

These findings paint a picture of societies in which young and middle-aged
men, in particular, face a world of social and economic disruption for which
they are poorly prepared [70]. For many, the opportunities are constrained by
low levels of education and a lack of social support. Poor nutrition and high

rates of smoking have already reduced their chances of a long life, but the easy availability of cheap alcohol provides a pathway to oblivion and then to premature death. The hazards of drunkenness are exacerbated in a society in which there are few on whom one can depend and where one is surrounded by a poorly maintained hazard-ridden environment.

The contribution of health care

There is now considerable evidence that timely and effective health-care interventions have played an important role in reductions in mortality in Western countries [71]. Research using the concept of avoidable mortality suggested that in 1988 about 25 per cent of the mortality gap between Eastern and Western Europe between birth and age 75 could be attributed to inadequacies in medical care [72], and a comparison of deaths from causes amenable to health care found that, while in the mid-1960s they were similar in Russia and the UK, they then fell markedly in the latter while remaining stubbornly high in the former [73]. This period was marked by impressive developments in drug discovery, technological advances, and the application of evidence-based practice, all impacting on Western countries but largely absent in the USSR.

While evidence of the contribution of health care to population health remains fragmentary, three broad patterns can be discerned within this region. Some countries, most often those that have been most successful in achieving economic growth, have been able to reform their health care systems relatively successfully. In others, mostly in the less developed parts of the CIS, while the basic infrastructure remains in place, some elements have effectively collapsed. In particular, there have been major problems with pharmaceutical supply. The third pattern is seen in those regions that have suffered from war and other conflict, where there has been widespread destruction of facilities.

While the specific impact of health care on measures of population health is often difficult to detect, there are several well-documented examples of where it has been identified [74,75]. Research on neonatal mortality has sought to separate the impact of health care from broader social determinants, with the former assessed by birthweight-specific survival and the latter by the overall birthweight distribution. Closing the remaining gap with the best-performing Western countries will require policies that address the social determinants of low birthweight. In the CIS, while there is also a need to address the high levels of low birthweight [76], there is also a need to tackle a combination of inadequate care [77] and, in some countries, fatalism leading to premature infants being left untreated.

Problems with drug supply affect all chronic diseases. The high levels of mortality among the elderly in some CIS countries may be a consequence of inadequate care and inadequate treatment of high blood pressure. As patients must pay for their own drugs, which can be very expensive, many patients with hypertension take treatment only when they are feeling unwell, a practice that is often endorsed by physicians. The converse problem also exists, with widespread use of inappropriate treatments, in many cases due to fee-splitting between physicians and pharmacists [78].

Shortage of drugs is also a factor explaining the increase in deaths from diabetes observed in many CIS countries. However, other factors are also important. There have been widespread shortages of equipment for monitoring blood glucose, few primary care physicians are trained to manage diabetes (so that care is provided by specialists in national or regional centres, often involving inpatient care), and there is inappropriate treatment of complications, such as the widespread use of amputation for leg ulcers [79,80].

Although the collapse in vital registration systems that has accompanied the breakdown of health-care delivery in areas beset by conflict means that very little information is available, it is almost certain that, apart from the more obvious direct effects of war, there will have been a substantial increase in mortality among those with chronic diseases requiring long-term treatment, including not only diabetes and hypertension but also conditions such as asthma and epilepsy.

The weak public health response

The public health challenges facing policy-makers in this region are enormous. Yet the public health response has been very weak. Why is this? An earlier analysis of the policy inaction on childhood injuries provides some clues [81]. One problem was that worsening health was invisible. Data on health trends presented to politicians is often limited to easily understood aggregate measures, such as life expectancy at birth. While this has the benefit of simplicity, it obscures the complex nature of mortality. For example, in the CCEE in the 1980s it was recognized that life expectancy was stagnating, but this concealed a substantial increase in mortality among young and middle-aged men which was counteracted by a steady fall in infant mortality [1]. This was only belatedly recognized in the early 1990s.

A second problem was a lack of public health capacity. Organizations responsible for public health were typically weak. The Soviet model sanitary–epidemiological system had been relatively effective in tackling communicable disease in the post-war period, but was unable to adapt to the challenge of non-communicable diseases. As in many countries, a career in public health was less enticing than many of the alternatives, thus attracting many of the weakest graduates, a situation exacerbated by undergraduate specialization in the USSR. An additional problem in some countries is corruption, with public health officials ideally placed to extract contributions from those whom they are regulating, such as food outlets.

Public health functions can, of course, reside in many other settings—within government, academia, and non-governmental organizations. In many countries these functions were also weak or, in the case of non-governmental bodies, virtually non-existent. With a few exceptions, such as Hungary, Czechoslovakia, Poland, and the Baltic States, statistical offices confined their activities to the minimum necessary to satisfy the reporting requirements of the WHO. In some places the academic public health community was somewhat stronger, but these were isolated examples.

The legacy of the past

There were specific problems in the Soviet Union, where access to ideas developed elsewhere was extremely limited [82] (the Baltic States were an exception as they were able to maintain contacts with the West, in the case of Estonia because of a close linguistic affinity with nearby Finland), and where the legacy of the past continued to exert an influence (Box 5.4). Marxist–Leninist teaching suggested that many of the emerging threats to health were transient, attributable to the transition to communism, and thus were expected to resolve spontaneously over time [83]. A rejection of experimental methods, linked with an absence of effective peer review and an extremely hierarchical academic structure, in which knowledge accumulated only with age, led to many

---

Box 5.4 A legacy from the past

In the Soviet Union access to ideas developed elsewhere was limited. Much of this was the legacy of a Ukrainian agriculturalist, Trofim Lysenko. He rejected Mendelian ideas, arguing that change in plants arose from adaptation to changing circumstances within a few generations. Although Lysenko was eventually discredited in the 1960s, his views remained widely held for several decades. The academic culture that allowed him to thrive was the same in which many senior Soviet public health scientists were trained, and where voicing a contrary view could easily lead to the Gulag, and thus to premature death [85]. While many of the particular beliefs that emerged from this system are now of historical interest, their true legacy is of a culture in which dissent and open debate, especially with those in senior positions, are often strongly discouraged.

ideas that had no scientific basis and which were often harmful [84]. The use of transfusions to treat undernourished Romanian children is an extreme example, but there are many more. Thus, expectant mothers in Russia can expect, routinely, to spend several weeks in hospital before giving birth, while they are administered numerous totally ineffective preparations, many by infusion [78].

A third issue was a lack of clear ownership. No-one was responsible for broadly defined population health. Finally, effective public health interventions often require working across sectors. However, the widespread use of highly centralized vertical programmes conspired against collaboration at local level, and central government ministries guarded their responsibilities jealously [86].

Recent progress

The situation has changed substantially since 1990, especially in the CCEE, where the process of European Union accession has required revision of many laws in areas that impact on public health, in particular in relation to health and safety and to food safety. Participation in European Union programmes has contributed to a valuable process of shared learning with colleagues in Western Europe. However, there are still problems in many parts of the CIS. A review of the Russian language literature on the determinants of trends in health in Russia found little evidence of awareness of relevant research published in Western journals or of modern epidemiological methods [87]. Analytical capacity remains weak. Many ministries of health have become even weaker than in the communist period. The sanitary–epidemiological system has remained relatively untouched by the process of reform, partly reflecting the low priority given to it by governments but also a reluctance to adopt new ideas, in some countries due to widespread corruption among a group that is invested with much discretionary power but with low wages and little accountability.

However, there are some encouraging signs even in the CIS. During the past few years some new streams of research have emerged in this region that is, at last, capturing the attention of policy-makers. One relates to the demographic crisis and its impact on recruitment to the armed forces. It is now apparent that the rapidly falling birth rate, coupled with the poor health of many recruits, is a serious threat to Russia's military strength [88]. The other is an exploration of the economic impact of the high toll of disability and premature death [89]. This research has shown how the poor health in this region impacts adversely on productivity and labour force participation. Projections indicate that, unless addressed, poor health will act as a serious drag on future economic growth [90].

Public health training initiatives

Expansion of public health training in this region has been a great success although, given the time lag between establishing a training programme and producing skilled specialists, the effects are only now being seen [91]. Much of the credit must go to the Open Society Institute, which provided funding to support schools of public health and public health associations, and to the Association of Schools of Public Health in the European Region, which led a programme of pairing schools in East and West, linked to a process of peer review. Additional support has been provided by the European Commission and the World Bank.

Several thriving schools of public health now exist with staff who have received training abroad teaching modern public health concepts. Some, such as the Hungarian School of Public Health in Debrecen, Hungary, the Andrija Stampar School of Public Health, in Zagreb, Croatia, and the Kaunas Medical Academy, in Lithuania, are now well established and use innovative learning methods, combining masters and doctoral level training with short courses. Increasingly, they are developing research infrastructures, such as the network of sentinel health-monitoring stations established by the Hungarian School of Public Health, that provide data for research and teaching, as well as facilitating close links with public health practitioners. Unfortunately, the situation is less encouraging in some other countries, in particular in the former Soviet Union outside Russia, where there are only a few isolated developments in countries such as Armenia, Georgia, and Kazakhstan, and generally very little capacity.

The new institutions that are emerging will only become effective if they can draw on appropriate locally relevant evidence on the causes of disease and the appropriate responses. As the preceding sections have shown, the many natural experiments that have taken place in Eastern Europe have provided important new insights on the determinants of health and disease. However, they have also illustrated some of the challenges facing public health researchers in this region.

Conclusion

The challenges to public health in Eastern Europe are considerable. Overall levels of health continue to lag well behind those in the West and are continuing to deteriorate in some places. Old threats, such as tuberculosis, are re-appearing and new ones, such as smoking among women and HIV, have emerged. But there are also many examples of success. Death rates from cardiovascular disease are falling rapidly in some countries. Transition-related increases in injury deaths have been brought under control. However, many of these successes owe more to wider societal changes, such as growing prosperity and opening of markets, than to specific public health policies. Unfortunately, the public health infrastructure remains weak in many countries.

Several needs are apparent. One is a larger number of people from a wide range of disciplines trained in modern public health. In some countries newly established schools of public health are already making a substantial contribution to this goal. These individuals need a secure career structure that rewards them sufficiently to ensure their retention and gives them the opportunity to use their newly developed skills to develop and implement the healthy public policies that are noticeable by their absence. These changes will only come about if politicians recognize the need to improve the health of their population, recognizing that progress is possible and necessary. The international community has a role to play in supporting these efforts and the research on which effective policies can be based.

References

[1] Chenet L, McKee M, Fulop N, *et al*. Changing life expectancy in Central Europe. Is there a single reason? *J Public Health Med* 1996; **18**: 329–36.

[2] Leon DA, Chenet L, Shkolnikov VM, *et al*. Huge variation in Russian mortality rates 1984–94: artefact, alcohol, or what? *Lancet* 1997; **350**: 383–8.

[3] Nolte E, Shkolnikov V, McKee M. Changing mortality patterns in East and West Germany and Poland. I: Long term trends (1960–1997). *J Epidemiol Community Health* 2000; **54**: 890–8.

[4] Bobak M, Skodova Z, Pisa Z, Poledne R, Marmot M. Political changes and trends in cardiovascular risk factors in the Czech Republic, 1985–92. *J Epidemiol Community Health* 1997; **51**: 272–7.

[5] Zatonski WA, McMichael AJ, Powles JW. Ecological study of reasons for sharp decline in mortality from ischaemic heart disease in Poland since 1991. *BMJ* 1998; **316**: 1047–51.

[6] Dolea C, Nolte E, McKee M. Changing life expectancy in Romania after the transition. *J Epidemiol Community Health* 2002; **56**: 444–9.

[7] Shkolnikov V, McKee M, Leon DA. Changes in life expectancy in Russia in the mid-1990s. *Lancet* 2001; **357**: 917–21.

[8] Rechel B, Schwalbe N, McKee M. Health in south-eastern Europe: a troubled past, an uncertain future. *Bull WHO* 2004; **82**: 539–46.

[9] Anderson B, Silver B. Issues of data quality in assessing mortality trends and levels in the New Independent States. In: Bobadilla J, Costello C, Mitchell F (eds). *Premature Death in the New Independent States*. Washington, DC: National Academies Press, 1997; pp. 120–55.

[10] Shkolnikov V, Mesle F, Vallin J. Health crisis in Russia. I: Recent trends in life expectancy and causes of death from 1970 to 1993. *Popul* 1996; **8**:123–54.

[11] Timaeus I, Chackiel J, Ruzicka L. *Adult Mortality in Latin America*. Oxford: Oxford University Press, 1996.

[12] Badurashvili I, McKee M, Tsuladze G, Mesle F, Vallin J, Shkolnikov V. Where there are no data: what has happened to life expectancy in Georgia since 1990? *Public Health* 2001; **115**: 394–400.

[13] Rechel B, Shapo L, McKee M. *Millennium Development Goals for Health in Europe and Central Asia*. Washington, DC: World Bank, 2004.

[14] Kuh D, Ben-Shlomo Y. *A Life Course Approach to Chronic Disease Epidemiology* (2nd edn). Oxford: Oxford University Press, 2004.

[15] Hirte L, Nolte E, Bain C, McKee M. Breast cancer mortality in Russia and Ukraine 1963–2002: an age–period–cohort analysis. *Int J Epidemiol* 2007; **36**: 900–6.

[16] McKee M, Shkolnikov V. Understanding the toll of premature death among men in Eastern Europe. *BMJ* 2001; 323: 1051–5.

[17] Hajdu P, McKee M, Bojan F. Changes in premature mortality differentials by marital status in Hungary and in England and Wales. *Eur J Public Health* 1995; **5**: 259–64.

[18] Watson P. Marriage and mortality in Eastern Europe. In: Hertzman CE, Kelly SE, Bobak ME (eds). *East–West Life Expectancy Gap in Europe: Environmental and Non-environmental Determinants*. Dordrecht: Kluwer Academic, 1996.

[19] Shkolnikov VM, Leon DA, Adamets S, Andreev E, Deev A. Educational level and adult mortality in Russia: an analysis of routine data 1979 to 1994. *Soc Sci Med* 1998; **47**: 357–69.

[20] White S. *Russia Goes Dry: Alcohol, State and Society*. Cambridge: Cambridge University Press, 1996.

[21] Szucs S, Sarvary A, McKee M, Adany R. Could the high level of cirrhosis in Central and Eastern Europe be due partly to the quality of alcohol consumed? An exploratory investigation. *Addiction* 2005; **100**: 536–42.

[22] Varvasovsky Z, Bain C, McKee M. Deaths from cirrhosis in Poland and Hungary: the impact of different alcohol policies during the 1980s. *J Epidemiol Community Health* 1997; **51**: 167–71.

[23] McKee M, Pomerleau J, Robertson A, *et al*. Alcohol consumption in the Baltic Republics. *J Epidemiol Community Health* 2000; **54**: 361–6.

[24] Pomerleau J, McKee M, Rose R, Haerpfer CW, Rotman D, Tumanov S. Drinking in the Commonwealth of Independent States: evidence from eight countries. *Addiction* 2005; **100**: 1647–68.

[25] McKee M. Alcohol in Russia. *Alcohol Alcoholism* 1999; **34**: 824–9.

[26] Lang K, Vali M, Szucs S, Adany R, McKee M. The composition of surrogate and illegal alcohol products in Estonia. *Alcohol Alcoholism* 2006; **41**: 446–50.

[27] McKee M, Suzcs S, Sarvary A, *et al*. The composition of surrogate alcohols consumed in Russia. *Alcohol Clin Exp Res* 2005; **29**: 1884–8.

[28] Gil A, Polikina O, Koroleva N, McKee M, Tomkins S, Leon DA. Availability and characteristics of nonbeverage alcohols sold in 17 Russian cities in 2007. *Alcohol Clin Exp Res* 2009; **33**: 79–85.

[29] Tomkins S, Saburova L, Kiryanov N, *et al*. Prevalence and socio-economic distribution of hazardous patterns of alcohol drinking: study of alcohol consumption in men aged 25–54 years in Izhevsk, Russia. *Addiction* 2007; **102**: 544–53.

[30] Leon DA, Saburova L, Tomkins S, *et al*. Hazardous alcohol drinking and premature mortality in Russia: a population based case-control study. *Lancet* 2007; **369**: 2001–9.

[31] Chervyakov VV, Shkolnikov VM, Pridemore WA, McKee M. The changing nature of murder in Russia. *Soc Sci Med* 2002; **55**: 1713–24.

[32] Pridemore WA, Chamlin MB. A time-series analysis of the impact of heavy drinking on homicide and suicide mortality in Russia, 1956–2002. *Addiction* 2006; **101**: 1719–29.

[33] Laks T, Tuomilehto J, Joeste E, *et al.* Alarmingly high occurrence and case fatality of acute coronary heart disease events in Estonia: results from the Tallinn AMI register 1991–94. *J Intern Med* 1999; **246**: 53–60.

[34] Britton A, McKee M. The relation between alcohol and cardiovascular disease in Eastern Europe: explaining the paradox. *J Epidemiol Community Health* 2000; **54**: 328–32.

[35] Perova NV, Oganov RG, Williams DH, *et al.* Association of high-density-lipoprotein cholesterol with mortality and other risk factors for major chronic noncommunicable diseases in samples of US and Russian men. *Ann Epidemiol* 1995; **5**: 179–85.

[36] Shakhov YA, Oram JF, Perova NV, *et al.* Comparative study of the activity and composition of HDL3 in Russian and American men. *Arterioscler Thromb* 1993; **13**: 1770–8.

[37] Yusuf S, Hawken S, Ounpuu S, *et al.* Effect of potentially modifiable risk factors associated with myocardial infarction in 52 countries (the INTERHEART study): case–control study. *Lancet* 2004; **364**: 937–52.

[38] Vikhert AM, Tsiplenkova VG, Cherpachenko NM. Alcoholic cardiomyopathy and sudden cardiac death. *J Am Coll Cardiol* 1986; **8** (1 Suppl A): 3A–11A.

[39] Virchow R. *Phlogose und Thrombose im Gefäßsystem: Gesammelte Abhandlungen zur Wissenschaftlichen Medizin.* Frankfurt: Staatsdruckerei, 1865.

[40] West SG. Effect of diet on vascular reactivity: an emerging marker for vascular risk. *Curr Atheroscler Rep* 2001; **3**: 446–55.

[41] Pomerleau J, McKee M, Robertson A, *et al.* Macronutrient and food intake in the Baltic Republics. *Eur J C lin Nutr* 2001; **55**: 200–7.

[42] Bobak M, Brunner E, Miller NJ, Skodova Z, Marmot M. Could antioxidants play a role in high rates of coronary heart disease in the Czech Republic? *Eur J Clin Nutr* 1998; **52**: 632–6.

[43] Gilmore A, Pomerleau J, McKee M, *et al.* Prevalence of smoking in 8 countries of the former Soviet Union: results from the living conditions, lifestyles and health study. *Am J Public Health* 2004; **94**: 2177–87.

[44] Shkolnikov V, McKee M, Leon D, Chenet L. Why is the death rate from lung cancer falling in the Russian Federation? *Eur J Epidemiol* 1999; **15**: 203–6.

[45] Perlman F, Bobak M, Gilmore A, McKee M. Trends in the prevalence of smoking in Russia during the transition to a market economy. *Tob Control* 2007; **16**: 299–305.

[46] Gilmore AB, McKee M. Moving East: how the transnational tobacco industry gained entry to the emerging markets of the former Soviet Union. I: Establishing cigarette imports. *Tob Control* 2004; **13**: 143–50.

[47] Bray I, Brennan P, Boffetta P. Projections of alcohol- and tobacco-related cancer mortality in Central Europe. *Int J Cancer* 2000; **87**: 122–8.

[48] Gilmore AB, Radu-Loghin C, Zatushevski I, McKee M. Pushing up smoking incidence: plans for a privatised tobacco industry in Moldova. *Lancet* 2005; **365**: 1354–9.

[49] Gilmore AB, McKee M, Collin J. The invisible hand: how British American Tobacco precluded competition in Uzbekistan. *Tob Control* 2007; **16**: 239–47.

[50] Danishevski K, Gilmore A, McKee M. Public attitudes towards smoking and tobacco control policy in Russia. *Tob Control* 2008; **17**: 276–83.

[51] Fagerstrom K, Boyle P, Kunze M, Zatonski W. The anti-smoking climate in EU countries and Poland. *Lung Cancer* 2001; **32**: 1–5.

[52] Levi F, Lucchini F, Negri E, Franceschi S, la Vecchia C. Cervical cancer mortality in young women in Europe: patterns and trends. *Eur J Cancer* 2000; **36**: 2266–71.

[53] Markina SS, Maksimova NM, Vitek CR, Bogatyreva EY, Monisov AA. Diphtheria in the Russian Federation in the 1990s. *J Infect Dis* 2000; **181** (Suppl 1): S27–34.

[54] Coker RJ, Atun RA, McKee M. Health-care system frailties and public health control of communicable disease on the European Union's new Eastern border. *Lancet* 2004; **363**: 1389–92.

[55] Stern V. *Sentenced to Die?: The Problem of TB in Prisons in Eastern Europe and Central Asia*. London: International Centre for Prison Studies, 1999.

[56] Coker R, McKee M, Atun R, *et al*. Risk factors for pulmonary tuberculosis in Russia: case–control study. *BMJ* 2006; **332**: 85–7.

[57] Stuckler D, Basu S, McKee M, King L. Mass incarceration can explain population increases in TB and multidrug-resistant TB in European and central Asian countries. *Proc Natl Acad Sci USA* 2008; **105**: 13280–5.

[58] Ruddy M, Balabanova Y, Graham C, *et al*. Rates of drug resistance and risk factor analysis in civilian and prison patients with tuberculosis in Samara Region, Russia. *Thorax* 2005; **60**: 130–5.

[59] Atun RA, Lebcir RM, Drobniewski F, McKee M, Coker RJ. High coverage with HAART is required to substantially reduce the number of deaths from tuberculosis: system dynamics simulation. *Int J STD AIDS* 2007; **18**: 267–73.

[60] Stoilova Y, Popivanova N. Epidemiologic studies of leptospiroses in the Plovdiv region of Bulgaria. *Folia Med (Plovdiv)* 1999; **41**: 73–9.

[61] Sumilo D, Bormane A, Asokliene L, Lucenko I, Vasilenko V, Randolph S. Tick-borne encephalitis in the Baltic States: identifying risk factors in space and time. *Int J Med Microbiol* 2006; **296** (Suppl 40): 76–9.

[62] Andreev EM, McKee M, Shkolnikov VM. Health expectancy in the Russian Federation: a new perspective on the health divide in Europe. *Bull WHO* 2003; **81**: 778–87.

[63] Chenet L, Leon D, McKee M, Vassin S. Deaths from alcohol and violence in Moscow: socio-economic determinants. *Eur J Popul* 1998; **14**: 19–37.

[64] Walberg P, McKee M, Shkolnikov V, Chenet L, Leon DA. Economic change, crime, and mortality crisis in Russia: regional analysis. *BMJ* 1998; **317**: 312–18.

[65] Kennedy B, Kawachi I, Brained E. The role of social capital in the Russian mortality crisis. *World Dev* 1998; **26**: 2029–43.

[66] Stuckler D, King L, McKee M. Mass privatisation and the post-communist mortality crisis: a cross-national analysis. *Lancet* 2009; **373**: 399–40.

[67] d'Hombres B, McKee M, Rocco L, Suhrcke M. Does social capital determine health? Evidence from eight transition countries. *Health Econ* 2009; in press.

[68] Bobak M, Pikhart H, Hertzman C, Rose R, Marmot M. Socioeconomic factors, perceived control and self-reported health in Russia. A cross-sectional survey. *Soc Sci Med* 1998; **47**: 269–79.

[69] Rose R. Russia as an hour-glass society: a constitution without citizens. *East Eur Constitut Rev* 1995; **4**: 34–42.

[70] Cockerham WC. Health lifestyles in Russia. *Soc Sci Med* 2000; **51**: 1313–24.

[71] Nolte E, McKee M. *Does Health Care Save Lives? Avoidable Mortality Revisited*. London: Nuffield Trust, 2004.

[72] Velkova A, Wolleswinkel-van den Bosch JH, Mackenbach JP. The East–West life expectancy gap: differences in mortality from conditions amenable to medical intervention. *Int J Epidemiol* 1997; **26**: 75–84.

[73] Andreev EM, Nolte E, Shkolnikov VM, Varavikova E, McKee M. The evolving pattern of avoidable mortality in Russia. *Int J Epidemiol* 2003; **32**: 437–46.

[74] Nolte E, Scholz R, Shkolnikov V, McKee M. The contribution of medical care to changing life expectancy in Germany and Poland. *Soc Sci Med* 2002; **55**: 1905–21.

[75] Becker N, Boyle P. Decline in mortality from testicular cancer in West Germany after reunification. *Lancet* 1997; **350**: 744.

[76] Danishevski K, Balabanova D, McKee M, Nolte E, Schwalbe N, Vasilieva N. Inequalities in birth outcomes in Russia: evidence from Tula oblast. *Paediatr Perinat Epidemiol* 2005; **19**: 352–9.

[77] Duke T, Keshishiyan E, Kuttumuratova A, *et al.* Quality of hospital care for children in Kazakhstan, Republic of Moldova, and Russia: systematic observational assessment. *Lancet* 2006; **367**: 919–25.

[78] Danishevski K, McKee M, Balabanova D. Prescribing in maternity care in Russia: the legacy of Soviet medicine. *Health Policy* 2008; **85**: 242–51.

[79] Hopkinson B, Balabanova D, McKee M, Kutzin J. The human perspective on health care reform: coping with diabetes in Kyrgyzstan. *Int J Health Plann Manage* 2004; **19**: 43–61.

[80] Balabanova D, McKee M, Koroleva N, *et al.* Navigating the health system: diabetes care in Georgia. *Health Policy Plan* 2009; **24**: 46–54.

[81] McKee M, Zwi A, Koupilova I, Sethi D, Leon D. Health policy-making in Central and Eastern Europe: lessons from the inaction on injuries? *Health Policy Plan* 2000; **15**: 263–9.

[82] McKee M. Cochrane on communism: the influence of ideology on the search for evidence. *Int J Epidemiol* 2007; **36**: 269–73.

[83] Deacon B. Medical care and health under state socialism. *Int J Health Serv* 1984; **14**: 453–80.

[84] Krementsov NL. *Stalinist Science.* Princeton, NJ: Chichester: Princeton University Press, 1997.

[85] Soyfer VN. The consequences of political dictatorship for Russian science. *Nat Rev Genet* 2001; **2**: 723–9.

[86] Varvasovszky Z, McKee M. An analysis of alcohol policy in Hungary. Who is in charge? *Addiction* 1998; **93**: 1815–27.

[87] Tkatchenko E, McKee M, Tsouros AD. Public health in Russia: the view from the inside. *Health Policy Plan* 2000; **15**: 164–9.

[88] Giles K. *Where Have All the Soldiers Gone? Russia's Military Plans versus Demographic Reality.* Swindon: Defence Academy of the UK, 2006.

[89] Marquez P, Suhrcke M, McKee M, Rocco L. Adult health in the Russian Federation: more than just a health problem. *Health Aff (Millwood)* 2007; **26**: 1040–51.

[90] Suhrcke M, Rocco L, McKee M. *Health: A Vital Investment for Economic Development in Eastern Europe and Central Asia.* Brussels: European Observatory on Health Care Systems, 2007.

[91] McKee M. A decade of experience in Eastern Europe. In: Foege W, Black R, Daulaire N (eds) *Leadership and Management for Improving Global Health.* New York: Jossey Bass/John Wiley, 2005; pp. 167–86.

Chapter 6

Improving Canada's response to public health challenges: the creation of a new public health agency

Sylvie Stachenko, Barbara Legowski, and Robert Geneau

Canada's experience with severe acute respiratory syndrome (SARS) in 2003 propelled federal public health authorities to scale up and coordinate appropriate policies and actions with respect not only to infectious agents, but also to chronic diseases and injuries, and their risk factors and determinants. While the federal government has made progress in this regard, sustaining a renewal process within Canada's decentralized public health configuration requires continued partnership building among numerous public health players.

This chapter highlights the historical context and current challenges of public health in Canada. It describes recent key institutional developments involving the new Public Health Agency of Canada and its contributions to leadership and to new investments that address domestic and global public health challenges.

The context for renewal

During the 1980s and 1990s, various reports repeatedly highlighted weaknesses in public health across Canada [1]. These reports warned that, as a system intended to serve the whole of the country, public health required increased investments in capacity at all levels of jurisdiction that share public health responsibility and better coordination among them. However, these recommendations received limited attention until the SARS outbreak in 2003.

The challenge of coordination: public health in a decentralized health system

Well before the SARS outbreak, evidence suggested that the challenges associated with intergovernmental cooperation for purposes of public health were not being met effectively. The lack of clear inter-jurisdictional interfaces was evident, particularly with infectious disease surveillance. The most dramatic and tragic manifestation of this was the compromised safety of blood supplies during the late 1970s and throughout the 1980s. Canada's public health system failed when 30,000 cases of hepatitis C and approximately 1000 cases of HIV were transmitted through the public blood supply [2,3].

In 1999, and again in 2002, the Auditor General of Canada raised critical questions about the federal/provincial/territorial (F/P/T) collaborative framework for infectious disease surveillance and outbreak management. A major concern was the lack of pan-Canadian legislation defining the roles and responsibilities of the F/P/T governments as well as the terms of inter-jurisdictional cooperation. Provinces and territories were under no obligation to report most communicable diseases to either the federal government or to other provinces/territories [4,5].

Historical context

The multi-jurisdictional nature of the public health system originates from Canada's founding constitutional framework of 1867, the British North America Act (now the Constitution Act). Overall, the Act assigns relatively narrow responsibilities for health to the federal government relative to those given to provinces and territories. The provinces are understood to have general jurisdiction over health care, with the exception of services to specific populations for which the federal government has responsibility. Jurisdiction over public health is less clear, apart from explicit federal authority over the control of infectious agents at the borders, assistance with public emergencies, and in international relations.

Over time, federal responsibilities have evolved to include a greater scope of action to address health threats at a national level. For example, in the 1919 post-war period, concern about the spread of influenza led the Government of Canada to create a national department of health through the Department of Health Act. This act centralized authority over several pieces of legislation on food and drug standards, and the control of infectious diseases [6]. The federal legal regime now includes modern quarantine legislation and a variety of acts related to public health protection that cover the import of human pathogens, food and drugs, medical devices, biologics, some environmental health matters, and consumer products. Since the Lalonde Report of 1974 and the

Ottawa Charter of 1986, the federal government has engaged in the overall promotion of population health and has regulated against threats to the general population (e.g. cigarette package warning labels).

Provincial and territorial involvement

Provincial involvement in public health has been explicit since the 1800s, when provincial legislation provided for the establishment of local boards of health, which were to be the first responders to local epidemics, quarantine, and immunization. As the science of public health evolved, the local boards gained infrastructure and addressed increasing numbers of infectious agents as well as maternal and child health. Today, provincial and territorial public health legislation covers several issues, ranging from safety of drinking water to road traffic safety, while municipal by-laws control local issues such as smoke-free space, insecticide and pesticide use, and land use for physical activity [8].

Since the constitutional framework around public health requires that all 14 jurisdictions (one federal, ten provincial, and three territorial governments), and often municipal governments or regional health authorities, be involved in decision-making on public health matters of a national concern, complexity is inherent in any consensus-seeking mechanism. The complexity is increased further by the diversity of provincial and territorial public health systems and capacities. In this context, federal efforts in public health are distinct from, and complementary to, activities of other jurisdictions. In some cases the federal role is explicit, while in others it is negotiated with provinces, territories, regional authorities and municipalities, requiring agreements to take collaborative action.

Erosion of public health capacity

Since the mid-1990s, public health experts had warned that the resiliency of Canada's public health system to respond to the emergence of new infectious agents was becoming increasingly compromised. In 1995, the federal government cut transfer payments to the provinces to reduce the federal deficit, and provinces in turn cut transfers to local governments, affecting services like public health [9]. While public health was losing resources across all the jurisdictions involved (municipal, F/P/T), concerns were rising about mad cow disease and West Nile virus [4]. In fact, governments were steadily committing virtually all new health expenditure to areas other than public health [4], and even the systems to protect the public from conventional threats were being eroded (Box 6.1).

From the broad population health perspective, a National Forum on Health in the mid-1990s tried to balance the national preoccupation with health care with the need to deal with population health determinants. Its recommendations

Box 6.1 Erosion of public health capacity

In 2000 seven people died from an *Escherichia coli* outbreak in Walkerton, Ontario, and in 2001 an outbreak of *Cryptosporidium parvum* occurred in the water supply for the community of North Battleford, Saskatchewan. Both incidents were attributed to several factors that compromised water safety supervision, among them provincial budget cutbacks and a lack of training and failsafe systems for reporting [10]. In the case of Walkerton, an additional contributing factor was the Ontario government's privatization of water testing in 1996, which failed to make reporting of positive tests for contamination mandatory [11].

Experts across the country had also expressed concerns about the lack of effective public health infrastructure in the provinces and territories with regard to vaccine-preventable diseases. Since the 1990s, several studies and reports have concluded that Canada's immunization coverage rates are still too low, in part because of geographical and socio-organizational factors which prevent access to immunization services [12,13].

led to significant institutional responses with regard to population health research and information, including the creation of the Canadian Institute for Health Information and the Canadian Population Health Initiative, and funding for health-promotion related research through several Canadian Institutes for Health Research [14]. Despite this response, in 2001 an F/P/T Advisory Committee on Population Health examined the health protection and promotion infrastructure in Canada and reported that, although regional variations in public health capacity existed, overall capacity to respond effectively to public health issues was lacking across the country [15].

The final catalyst for change: the SARS outbreak

In 2003, the outbreak of SARS in Toronto, Ontario, provided the necessary wake-up call to improve public health in Canada. The outbreak lasted approximately six months, until July 2003, by which time there had been 438 probable and suspected cases including 44 deaths, three of which involved health-care workers. More than 25,000 residents of the Greater Toronto Area had been placed in quarantine. SARS cost the province of Ontario an estimated $945 million in health care [16]. Even before the outbreak was contained, the Conference Board of Canada estimated a loss in national economic activity for 2003 of roughly $1.5 billion by the end of May, representing 0.15 per cent of Canada's actual GDP. Toronto was to feel two-thirds of the impact [17].

The alarming emergence of SARS in Toronto and the international attention it drew were the final catalyst for a thorough and critical examination of Canada's public health system. In October 2003, a National Advisory Committee on SARS and Public Health produced the Naylor Report, considered to be the most contemoporary impetus for the comprehensive renewal of Canada's public health system [4].

Pathways to improving Canada's response to public health challenges

Many of the Naylor Report recommendations addressed infectious agents and reiterated what experts had been saying over years of examination of Canada's public health system. In particular, the report identified the following priorities: developing a national strategy for surveillance and control of emerging and resurgent infections together with support for improved infrastructure, developing a national research agenda addressing infectious agents, strengthening capacity and flexibility to investigate outbreaks, and increasing federal leadership, coupled with additional resources [4].

Also in 2003, the Canadian Institutes for Health Research identified the following elements which needed to be achieved in order to improve Canada's public health system and have a strong coordinated response to public health challenges in the twenty-first century [15]:

- reaching a consensus on essential functions and corresponding infrastructure for the public health system;
- strengthening collaboration and partnership across jurisdictions and among players within the decentralized system;
- strengthening support for service delivery, including workforce development and public health research;
- establishing an exclusive national public health leadership position and enacting comprehensive pan-Canadian public health legislation detailing inter-jurisdictional cooperation;
- developing critical partnerships across sectors and jurisdictions.

Public Health Agency of Canada: providing a national focus

The creation of the new Public Health Agency of Canada (PHAC) in September 2004 was one step along the pathway to realizing the new vision for public health in Canada. The government of Canada created PHAC out of the Health Promotion and Protection Branch of the federal department of health (Health Canada). In December 2006, the Public Health Agency of Canada

Act (Bill C-5) came into force, providing a statutory basis for PHAC [8]. Under Bill C-5, PHAC administers the Quarantine Act and regulations on import of human pathogens [7]. Health Canada retains regulatory authority over various other public health matters including drug and alcohol abuse, pollution prevention for the protection of human health, food and drug safety, sales, and advertisement, pest control products, pesticide residues; and tobacco [18].

The Public Health Agency of Canada Act also created the position of Chief Public Health Officer (CPHO) with a unique dual role. First, as Deputy Head of the Agency, the CPHO is accountable to the Minister of Health regarding the daily operations of the Agency, advises the minister on public health matters, submits to the minister an annual report on the state of public health in Canada to be tabled in parliament, and engages other federal departments to manage threats to the health of Canadians. Secondly, as Canada's lead public health professional, the CPHO also has the legislated authority to communicate directly with Canadians and to prepare and publish reports on any public health issue. Dr David Butler-Jones was appointed as the first CPHO in 2004.

Sharing public health functions

In collaboration with its partners, the Agency leads federal efforts to mobilize pan-Canadian action to prevent disease and injury, and to promote and protect national and international public health [19]. To this end, PHAC shares the following six public health functions with other federal institutions, with provincial and territorial governments, and sometimes with regional, municipal, and county authorities.

+ Population health assessment
+ Health surveillance
+ Health promotion
+ Disease and injury prevention
+ Health protection
+ Public health emergency preparedness and response

Development of a strategic plan

One of PHAC's undertakings as a new entity was the development of a Strategic Plan for 2007–2012. The Plan confirms key federal leadership in quarantine, control of pathogens, and emergency and pandemic preparedness. For issues of a national concern that fall short of an emergency, the federal level adds value that is distinct from and complementary to activities of other jurisdictions. In particular, PHAC is positioned as a key player in knowledge translation by linking information, knowledge, and action in the field of public health. The Plan also places PHAC in a stewardship role to lead action on the social determinants of health to reduce health inequalities, particularly among aboriginal peoples and other vulnerable groups in Canada.

New mechanisms to support Canada's renewal of public health

Federal/provincial/territorial public health network

F/P/T mechanisms are the cornerstone of interjurisdictional collaboration in Canada. Post-SARS, another F/P/T mechanism was recommended specifically for public health. To this end, PHAC now coordinates the Pan-Canadian Public Health Network (Box 6.2), a new collaborative mechanism designed to enable the different levels of government and public health experts to respond in a coordinated manner to national concerns while respecting jurisdictional responsibilities for public health.

National collaborating centres

In keeping with its commitment to an improved knowledge-to-action approach, PHAC has also facilitated the establishment of a new mechanism for

Box 6.2 The Public Health Network Council

The Public Health Network is led by a council which includes senior public health representatives from each province and territory and from the federal government. It is co-chaired by the CPHO and a senior public health official from a province. Its mandate is to develop and implement collaborative pan-Canadian approaches to public health matters and to advise the Conference of F/P/T Deputy Ministers of Health. A Council of Chief Medical Officers of Health (CCMOHs) from the provinces and territories is also linked to the Network's structure. The CCMOH performs a scientific advisory role, reporting through the Public Health Network Council to the F/P/T Deputy Ministers of Health. Expert Groups report to the Public Health Network Council. They form the basis for F/P/T collaboration and are currently working on the following public health matters:

- communicable disease control;
- emergency preparedness and response;
- public health laboratories;
- public health surveillance and information;
- prevention and control of chronic disease and injury;
- population health promotion.

knowledge translation in public health through national collaborating centres. These arms-length centres are distributed across Canada, each intended as a national focal point and knowledge network hub for a different priority area of public health including environmental health, infectious disease, public health methodologies and tools, public policy, health determinants, and aboriginal health [20]. The centres were created to integrate information from various sources and, in this way, to strengthen knowledge translation and exchange between the research community, whether government funded or private, and the public health community, specifically public health policy-makers and practitioners.

Strengthening public health capacities

Towards integrated public health surveillance

As a core public health function, surveillance provides the building blocks to support the other major functions of public health. At the federal level in Canada, the mandate for routine collection of health statistics is shared principally between four organizations: Statistics Canada and the Canadian Institute for Health Information perform key roles, while PHAC and Health Canada also collect health status data. In addition, each province and territory collects its own population and public health data.

Post-SARS, PHAC compiled what were the major gaps and recommendations from past reviews of Canada's traditional health surveillance infrastructure, examining documents released between 1994 and 2007 and looking for direction as to where and how PHAC could best influence and lead a renewal and revitalization in surveillance. Several issues stem from the fact that current cross-jurisdictional cooperation associated with sharing surveillance information is largely based on voluntary agreements [9], highlighting the complexities inherent in a decentralized surveillance system.

Other notable issues are related to data standards and quality management, principles and priorities for surveillance, knowledge management capacity, knowledge translation, governance and accountability, funding, and system responsiveness with the overarching matter of change management [21].

The general recommendation from the reviews was for a geographically distributed, linked, and collaborative pan-Canadian surveillance system. Working towards this goal, PHAC has developed a new Surveillance Strategic Plan with the current priority being to strengthen the internal governance of surveillance efforts within PHAC to better support and coordinate inter-jurisdictional surveillance systems [22].

New core competencies for public health

Because public health practice in Canada is inherently diversified by virtue of the decentralized responsibilities for public health practice and training, an F/P/T Task Group on Public Health Human Resources recommended in 2005 that PHAC undertake a national process to review and validate core competencies for public health. This led to the release in 2007 of the Core Competencies for Public Health in Canada. These 36 core competencies reflect traditional requirements of public health professionals as well as new skills such as policy assessment and analysis, policy and programme planning, policy and programme implementation and evaluation, partnerships, collaboration and advocacy, diversity and inclusiveness, communications, and leadership. The recognition that these new skills are necessary reflects the expectation that future public health practitioners will become science integrators, using improved communication and negotiation skills to influence the institutions and interests that have the potential to push public policies that promote health onto political agendas.

These core competencies are intended for practitioners in a variety of settings, such as front-line providers, consultants, managers, and policy-makers. They also provide a tool to assess and create the best mix of competencies for a public health team or interdisciplinary organization. Work is currently under way to expand into discipline-specific competencies for seven professions related to public health: epidemiologists, health promotion practitioners, environmental public health professionals, nurses, physicians, dieticians, and public health dental practitioners [23]. In addition, the public health schools that are emerging in many universities across Canada are critical to advancing public health competencies in the country.

New investments

Infectious disease and emergency preparedness

PHAC is taking an all-hazards approach to emergency preparedness, covering emergency public health response to infectious disease outbreaks, natural disasters, explosions, and chemical, biological, or radiological/nuclear incidents. Preparedness planning involves provincial and territorial governments, other federal departments and agencies, and non-governmental organizations.

Preparedness for avian and pandemic influenza is being managed as a horizontal government initiative. In this regard, PHAC has established a Pandemic Preparedness Secretariat, acting as the focal point for the Government of Canada on human health aspects of avian and pandemic influenza, both domestically and internationally. At F/P/T levels, public health officials have collaborated to develop a Canadian Pandemic Influenza Plan for the Health Sector in consultation with non-governmental organizations, external technical experts, local governments, emergency planners, and bioethicists. The Plan maps out how the health sector is preparing for, and will respond to, pandemic influenza in Canada. It outlines the actions that should be taken during the different phases of a pandemic and clarifies the roles and responsibilities of the health sector at all levels of government [24].

In addition, a number of complementary initiatives have been designed to better prepare front-line physicians and public health professionals to rapidly detect and respond to suspected cases of influenza, and also to expand an influenza surveillance network that includes First Nations and Inuit communities.

At the international level, Canada is a signatory and a strong supporter of the revised WHO International Health Regulations (IHR). If Canada is to meet its IHR obligations, it needs effective intergovernmental collaboration [25]. To this end, PHAC is investing in the development of a new F/P/T information-sharing agreement and a plan of action to ensure rapid and effective responses to public health threats at both the national and international level. As a member of the Global Health Security Initiative, PHAC is also collaborating in a round-the-clock global emergency management system. Together with other federal agencies (Public Safety Canada, the Department of Foreign Affairs and International Trade, and the Canadian Food Inspection Agency), PHAC has contributed to the development of the North American Avian and Pandemic Influenza Plan [26].

In 2008, the Auditor General re-examined the state of infectious disease surveillance in Canada and concluded that progress has been made, with surveillance systems in place to detect and monitor existing and emerging infectious diseases in Canada. However, a clear emphasis was placed on the need to establish formal data-sharing agreements between the federal government and all provinces, and to develop corresponding protocols regarding the disclosure of personal information [27].

Mainstreaming health promotion

Since the 1980s, health promotion at the federal level in Canada has focused on community-based interventions outside the formal health system. These health promotion programmes targeted families and children who live in high-risk conditions, with federal funding directed to three key programmes that for the most part engage the social services sector: Community Action Programme for Children, the Canada Prenatal Nutrition Programme, and Aboriginal Head Start [28].

In contrast, the Canadian Heart Health Initiative (CHHI) was cross jurisdictional, engaging key F/P/T stakeholders in the formal public health system to build health promotion capacity at local and provincial/territorial levels. This resulted in partnerships and coalitions at local, provincial, and national levels, many of which became precursors to chronic disease and healthy living alliances. A case in point is the Chronic Disease Prevention Alliance of Canada, a network of national, provincial, and territorial organizations and alliances representing hundreds of groups across Canada [29].

These health promotion initiatives reflect several of the principles contained in the Ottawa Charter for Health Promotion [30] and the Bangkok Charter for Health Promotion in a Globalized World [31]: intersectoral approaches, strengthening community actions, building supportive environments, and developing personal skills. However, despite their successes, they were not sufficient by themselves to strengthen the position and status of health promotion within the traditional public health constituency, or to fundamentally reorient health services towards integrating health promotion, particularly at the primary health care level. This has led some experts to conclude that a discrepancy existed between Canada's international image as a leader in the field of health promotion and the Canadian experience within our own borders [32].

Health promotion: a core function

Since the enactment of Bill C-5, PHAC has been enabled with a stewardship role to strengthen public health, including health promotion as a core function. With this legitimization of health promotion in the PHAC mandate, the potential now exists for a more collaborative culture among public health and health promotion professionals, and, more importantly, for health promotion to become an integrating and unifying concept in public health policies and programmes [8,14].

Increasingly, new efforts to bring health promotion into the mainstream of public health practice and health care are emerging. At the federal level, the Integrated Strategy on Healthy Living and Chronic Disease, initiated by PHAC in 2005, provides a broad framework for linking action on the underlying determinants of health while at the same time ensuring a health-system response to address common risk factors for chronic disease [33]. The strategy has three interlinked pillars that uphold a continuum of actions involving health and other sectors. The first pillar calls for promotion of health by addressing the underlying conditions that lead to unhealthy eating, physical inactivity, and excessive weight. The second pillar aims at preventing major chronic diseases (e.g. cardiovascular disease, cancer, and diabetes) through focused and integrated action on their common risk factors. The third pillar focuses on supporting the early detection of chronic diseases and the prevention of the major disabilities related to them.

With regard to the major chronic diseases, the federal emphasis is on the development of a new national Heart Health Strategy [34], implementation of the Canadian Strategy for Cancer Control [35] and the National Diabetes Strategy [36], launch of the Lung Health Framework and scaling up chronic disease and risk factor surveillance systems.

Acting on the social determinants of health

To enable better informed actions on the broad determinants of health, PHAC has established a new focal point, effectively increasing the internal capacity to address complex public health issues, such as obesity, that require societal and intersectoral responses. In addition, through an Innovations and Learning Strategy, PHAC emphasizes that lessons learned should be captured and knowledge transfer products prepared for audiences within and outside the health sector.

A key vehicle for the dissemination of new knowledge is the Canadian Best Practices Portal for Health Promotion and Chronic Disease Prevention. This is an example of a readily available web-based resource which provides evidence-based information to public health practitioners and experts [37].

PHAC also supports the work of the F/P/T Advisory Committee on Population Health. The role of the Advisory Committee is to advise the Conference of Deputy Ministers of Health on national and inter-provincial strategies which should be pursued to improve the health status of the Canadian population and to provide a more integrated approach to health [38].

At the international level, PHAC contributed to the work of the WHO Commission on Social Determinants, assisted in the preparation of several case studies on intersectoral initiatives that address determinants of health in Canada and abroad, and is preparing a synthesis of the cases. Furthermore, PHAC established the Canadian Reference Group (CRG) to inform Canada's contributions to the WHO Commission. The CRG is composed of experts with knowledge and policy development expertise in the area of social determinants of health [39].

The CRG will also look for opportunities to provide information to a Canadian Senate Committee that is reviewing how the federal government could advance population health policy. The Committee is examining the impact of multiple factors and conditions on the health of Canada's population and is reporting on the major challenges to the development of population health policy that requires intersectoral action. Policy options will be prepared relevant to the federal government for improvement of overall health status and to reduce health disparities in Canada [40].

Conclusion

Public health in Canada is in the midst of renewal. While it is too soon to assess the contribution of PHAC towards improving the health of Canadians, some early lessons from its implementation can be drawn. First, the creation of a distinct Agency as a focal point dedicated to promoting a sound evidence-based approach to public health policy has attracted new investments from the federal government directed at both infectious and chronic disease issues. Second, in a highly decentralized health system as exists in Canada, a mechanism like the Public Health Network is proving to be essential to rally the efforts of F/P/T and local authorities towards common goals.

Building on the strengths of existing and new strategic partnerships, PHAC is moving towards a stronger stewardship role in the field of public health. In an era where multi-level and multi-sector initiatives are critical to the success of public health, the Agency is using its position as a focal point to play a brokering role. Ultimately, as the federal role in public health solidifies Canada is expected to have a stronger capacity to address domestic and global public health challenges.

Acknowledgements

The authors would like to thank Mr Brian Ward for his insightful comments and suggestions for improving this chapter, and Ms Gayle Fraser for the technical support provided.

References

[1] Mowat DL, Butler-Jones D. Public health in Canada: a difficult history. *Healthc Pap* 2007; **7**: 31–6.

[2] Wilson K. The Krever Commission—10 years later. *Can Med Assoc J* 2007; **117**: 1387–9.

[3] Health Canada. *Commission of Inquiry on the Blood System in Canada (Krever Commission)*. Ottawa: Health Canada, 1997.

[4] National Advisory Committee on SARS and Public Health. *Learning from SARS—Renewal of Public Health in Canada A Report of the National Advisory Committee on SARS and Public Health: The Naylor Report*. Ottawa: Health Canada & Public Health Agency of Canada, 2003.

[5] The Standing Senate Committee on Social Affairs Science and Technology. *Reforming Health Protection and Promotion in Canada: Time to Act*. Available online at: http://www.parl.gc.ca/37/2/parlbus/commbus/senate/com-e/SOCI-E/rep-e/repfinnov03-e.htm (accessed 14 December 2007).

[6] Department of Justice Canada. *Department of Health Act*. Available online at: http://laws.justice.gc.ca/en/ShowFullDoc/cs/H-3.2///en (accessed 14 December 2007).

[7] Public Health Agency of Canada. *The Quarantine Act: Questions and Answers*. Available online at: www.phac-aspc.gc.ca/media/nr-rp/2006/2006_10bk1_e.html (accessed 13 December 2007).

[8] Library of Parliament—Parliamentary Information and Research Service. *Bill C-5: Public Health Agency of Canada Act. Legislative Summaries.* Available online at: www.parl.gc.ca/common/bills_ls.asp?lang=E&ls=c5&source=library_prb&Parl=39&Ses=1.

[9] Deber R, McDougall C, Wilson K. Public health through a different lens. *HealthcPap* 2007; **7**: 66–71.

[10] Woo D, Vicente K. Sociotechnical systems, risk management, and public health: comparing the North Battleford and Walkerton outbreaks. *Reliab Eng Syst Safe* 2002; **80**: 253–69.

[11] O'Connor D. *Report of the Walkerton Inquiry. Part One: A Summary.* Toronto: Ontario Ministry of the Attorney General; 2002.

[12] Public Health Agency of Canada. *Final Report of Outcomes from the National Consensus Conference for Vaccine-Preventable Diseases in Canada.* Report No. CCDR 33S3. Ottawa: Public Health Agency of Canada, 2007.

[13] Guttmann A, Manuel D, Stukel TA, Desmeules M, Cernat G, Glazier RH. Immunization coverage among young children of urban immigrant mothers: findings from a universal health care system. *Ambul Pediatr* 2008; **8**: 205–9.

[14] Pinder L. *The federal role in health promotion: art of the possible. Health promotion in Canada: provincial, national and international perspectives.* In: Pederson A, O'Neil M, Rootman I (eds). Toronto: W.B. Saunders Canada, 2007; pp. 98–9.

[15] Frank J, Di Ruggiero E, Moloughney B. *The Future of Public Health in Canada: Developing a Public Health System for the 21st Century.* Ottawa: CIHR–Institute of Population and Public Health, 2003.

[16] CBC News. *The Economic Impact of SARS.* Available online at: www.cbc.ca/news/background/sars/economicimpact.html (accessed 20 November 2007).

[17] Conference Board of Canada. *Economic Impact of SARS.* Available online at: www.dfait-maeci.gc.ca/mexico-city/economic/may/sarsbriefMay03.pdf (accessed 20 November 2007).

[18] Health Canada. *About Health Canada—Acts.* Available online at: www.hc-sc.gc.ca/ahc-asc/legislation/acts-lois/index_e.html (accessed 14 February 2008).

[19] Public Health Agency of Canada. *Strategic Plan: 2007–2012, Information, Knowledge, Action.* Available online at: http//www.phac-aspc.gc.ca.

[20] Public Health Agency of Canada. *National Collaborating Centres.* Available online at: www.phac-aspc.gc.ca/php-psp/ncc_e.html (accessed 27 November 2007).

[21] Public Health Agency of Canada, Surveillance Strategy Working Group. *Surveillance Strategic Plan, Version 5.1 Appendix B Assessment of Past Reviews of Canada's Health Surveillance Infrastructure.* Ottawa: Public Health Agency of Canada; 2007.

[22] Public Health Agency of Canada, Surveillance Strategy Working Group, *Surveillance Strategic Plan, Version 5.1.* Ottawa: Public Health Agency of Canada; 2007.

[23] Public Health Agency of Canada. *Core Competencies for Public Health in Canada.* Available online at: www.phac-aspc.gc.ca/ccph-cesp/pdfs/cc-manual-eng090407.pdf (accessed 28 December 2007).

[24] Health Canada. *Pandemic Influenza.* Available online at: www.influenza.gc.ca/index_e.html (accessed 14 December 2007).

[25] McDougall C, Wilson K. Canada's obligations to global public health security under the revised International Health Regulations. *Health Law Rev* 2007; **16**: 25–32.

[26] Treasury Board of Canada Secretariat. *Public Health Agency of Canada: Section I—Overview.* Available online at: www.tbs-sct.gc.ca/dpr-rmr/2006–2007/inst/ahs/ahs01-eng.asp (accessed 28 November 2007).

[27] Office of the Auditor General of Canada. *Report of the Auditor General of Canada to the House of Commons*. Ottawa: Public Health Agency of Canada, May 2008; Chapter 5.

[28] Standing Senate Committee on Social Affairs, Science and Technology. *The Standing Senate Committee on Social Affairs, Science and Technology Continues its Study on Child Care in View of the OECD Report 'Starting Strong II'*. Available online at; www. parl.gc.ca/39/1/parlbus/commbus/senate/com-e/SOCI-E/press-e/05jun07-e.htm (accessed 20 November 2007).

[29] Chronic Disease Prevention Alliance of Canada (CDPAC). *Confronting the Epidemic of Chronic Disease*. Available online at: www.cdpac.ca/content.php?sec=0

[30] World Health Organization, Health and Welfare Canada, Canadian Public Health Association. *Ottawa Charter for Health Promotion: An International Conference on Health Promotion*. Available online at: www.phac-aspc.gc.ca/ph-sp/docs/charter-chartre/index-eng.php (accessed 28 December 2007).

[31] World Health Organization. *The Bangkok Charter for Health Promotion in a Globalized World*. Available online at: www.who.int/healthpromotion/conferences/6gchp/bangkok_charter/en/

[32] O'Neil M, Pederson A, Rootman I. Health Promotion in Canada: Declining or trans-forming? *Health Promot Int* 2000; **15**: 135–41.

[33] Public Health Agency of Canada. *Integrated Strategy on Healthy Living and Chronic Disease: Overview*. Available online at: www.phac-aspc.gc.ca/media/nr-rp/2005/2005_37bk1_e.html (accessed 14 December 2007).

[34] Public Health Agency of Canada. *Canada's New Government to Develop a New Heart Health Strategy*. Available online at: www.phac-aspc.gc.ca/media/nr-rp/2006/2006_09-eng.php (accessed 13 December 2007).

[35] Public Health Agency of Canada. *Centre for Chronic Disease Prevention and Control: Cancer*. Available online at: www.phac-aspc.gc.ca/ccdpc-cpcmc/cancer/cpac-accc_e. html (accessed 28 November 2007).

[36] Public Health Agency of Canada. National Diabetes Surveillance Association. Available online at: www.phac-aspc.gc.ca/ccdpc-cpcmc/ndss-snsd/english/index_e. html (accessed 27 November 2007).

[37] Public Health Agency of Canada. *The Canadian Best Practices Portal for Health Promotion and Chronic Disease Prevention*. Available online at: http://cbpp-pcpe. phac-aspc.gc.ca/(accessed 27 November 2007).

[38] Federal Provincial Territorial Advisory Committee on Population Health. *Intersectoral Action … Towards Population Health*. Ottawa: Health Canada, 1999.

[39] Public Health Agency of Canada. *Canada's Response to WHO Commission on Social Determinants of Health*. Available online at: www.phac-aspc.gc.ca/sdh-dss/crg-grc-eng.php

[40] Subcommittee on Population Health of the Standing Senate Committee on Social Affairs, Science and Technology. *Population Health Policy: Issues and Options* Available online at: http://www.parl.gc.ca/39/2/parlbus/commbus/senate/Com-e/SOCI-E/rep-e/rep10apr08-e.htm (accessed 27 May 2008).

Chapter 7

Public health in Latin America and the Caribbean

Cristiani Vieira Machado, Henri Jouval Jr, José Carvalho de Noronha, and Mario Roberto Dal Poz

Introduction

In the last decade of the twentieth century, Latin American countries faced significant economic, social and political changes. The countries were strongly influenced by both economic globalization and their marginal role in the new global economic and power arrangements. There were many positive changes in the political sphere, especially with the consolidation and expansion of democracy. However, the expectations of accelerated economic growth, improvements in social conditions, and reduction of inequalities after the intense slowdown of the 1980s (the 'lost decade') were not met. The enforcement of economic liberalization throughout the world led to many adverse changes in the region. Indeed, economic growth in most Latin American countries in the 1990s was lower than in the previous decades. External dependence deepened and productivity remained low. External and internal indebtedness increased in the region [1].

In the last five years (2003–2007), Latin America has registered the greatest increase in GNP per capita since the 1970s, although there is variation among countries [2,3]. In general, social data indicate a significant reduction in poverty in the region (Fig. 7.1), particularly because of the effect of demographic changes in employment rates and the implementation of government cash transfer programmes [2,4]. Nevertheless, unemployment rates are still high and poverty in the region is widespread. As shown in Fig. 7.1, in 2006 almost 200 million Latin Americans (36.5 per cent of the population of the region) lived in poor conditions and more than 70 million (13.4 per cent) could be considered indigent or destitute.

Moreover, inequalities between rich and poor countries not only globally but also within and between regions and countries are either increasing or

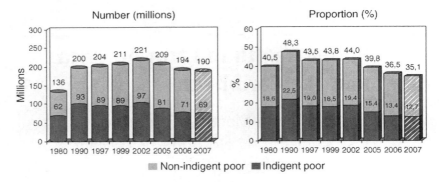

Fig. 7.1 Evolution of poverty and indigence in Latin America 1980–2007 (Note: Data for 2007 are estimates).
Source: Comisión Económica para América Latina y el Caribe (CEPAL), Panorama social de América Latina, 2007 (LC/G.2351-P/E), Santiago de Chile, November 2007, Cap. I, gráfico I.1. UN Publication S.07.II.G.124.

persisting at high levels [5]. Latin America and the Caribbean are no exceptions, and large inequalities are the trademark of the subcontinent. Some countries in the region are among those with the most unequal wealth distribution in the world. Although some Latin American countries have shown improvements in economic and social conditions since 2003, inequalities persist or have even become greater in others [2]. These inequalities have strong implications for social and health conditions.

Demographic changes

The Pan American Health Organization (PAHO) divies the Region of the Americas into the following sub-regions to allow comparisons of country groups:

- North America
- Latin America, comprising: the Andean Area, Brazil, Central American Isthmus, Latin Caribbean, Mexico, and the Southern Cone
- Non-Latin Caribbean.

A summary of population indicators by sub-regions is presented in Table 7.1. The overall population in the Region of the Americas was estimated at 910 million in 2007, nearly 14 per cent of the world's population. About 37 per cent reside in North America, and another third can be found in Brazil and Mexico. The remaining third is scattered among the other 43 countries and territories

Table 7.1 America's basic population and health indicators, 2007—selected indicators by PAHO sub-region

	Total population (million)	Annual population growth rate (%)	Urban population (%)	Total fertility rate (children/woman)	Life expectancy at birth (years)	Infant mortality 1997–2006 (per 1000 live births)	Estimated under five mortality in 2006 (per 1000 live births)
The Americas	910.9	1.1	79.3	2.2	75.3	17.7	22.4
North America	338.8	1.0	81.3	2.0	78.5	6.7	7.8
Latin America & The Caribbean	572.2	1.2	77.9	2.4	73.1	22.2	28.5
Latin America	565.2	1.2	78.5	2.4	73.5	22.2	28.5
Mexico	106.5	1.1	76.5	2.2	76.2	18.1	21.1
Central American Isthmus	41.0	1.9	55.2	3.2	72.3	29.6	35.9
Latin Caribbean	35.7	0.9	67.0	2.5	72.0	34.5	45.4
Brazil	191.8	1.3	85.2	2.2	72.4	22.6	30.0
Andean Area	124.6	1.3	76.2	2.5	72.4	23.2	30.3
Southern Cone	65.6	1.0	87.1	2.2	75.9	12.1	17.5
Non-Latin Caribbean	6.9	0.5	46.6	2.2	71.8	19.9	–

Source: Data from PAHO (2007) *Health Situation in the Americas. Basic Indicators 2007*. Available online at: http://www.paho.org/english/dd/ais/BI_2007_ENG.pdf (accessed March 2008).
Reproduced with permission from the Pan American Health Organization (PAHO). This table is based on data originally published on PAHO's website *Regional Core Health Data Initiative*. To obtain information about PAHO publications visit their website (http://publications.paho.org).

in the region. In the last few decades, the region has been marked by important demographic changes with regard to population growth, urbanization, and population ageing.

Population growth

The annual population growth in the Americas decreased from an estimated average of 1.6 per cent in 1980–1985 to around 1.2 per cent in 2006. The sub-regions with the slowest population increase were North America and the Non-Latin Caribbean. Brazil, Mexico, and the Andean Area showed large decreases in their population growth. One of the main causes for this phenomenon is the accentuated decrease in total fertility, which has diminished from 5.1 to 2.6 in Latin America and the Caribbean over a 30-year period, approaching 2.4 children per woman in 2007 [6].

Population distribution

Geographical trends in population distribution show higher growth in urban areas and lower growth in rural areas. In Latin America and the Caribbean, the urban population has grown from 58 per cent in 1950 to 78 per cent in 2007. However, there are large differences between the sub-regions, ranging from 47 per cent in the non-Latin Caribbean to 87 per cent in the Southern Cone [7]. Almost 20 per cent of the population is concentrated in the 20 largest cities of the region. However, there has been an important change in the concentration of people in metropolitan areas, where population growth has slowed. This phenomenon implies that medium-sized cities which can still respond to new demands will grow more rapidly, and the excessive growth pressure on the region's major cities will abate.

Life expectancy

Over the last two decades life expectancy at birth in the Americas has increased on average by 6.1 years, from an estimated 69.2 years in 1980–1985 to 75.3 in 2007 (78 years for women and 72 years for men). North America reached the highest levels of life expectancy at birth (78.5 years) in 2007. However, Brazil, the Caribbean, Central America, and the Andean Area still lag behind North America by more than 6 years [7].

Ageing

In 2006, more than 50 million people living in Latin America and the Caribbean were aged 60 years or older, representing 9 per cent of the region's population. The United Nations estimates that, by 2050, this percentage will reach 24 per cent [6], with important implications for health conditions and health system responses.

Health status in the region

Mortality

Apart from rare exceptions, mortality indicators have improved over the past seven five-year periods for all age groups in every country in the Americas. However, there are large variations between and within countries. These variations become obvious when differential mortality rates by age group and cause of death are compared among those countries presenting a similar economic development level, as determined by per capita income adjusted by their currency's purchasing power. For example, infant mortality in the Americas has decreased from an estimated 36.9 deaths per 1000 live births in 1980–1985 to 17.7 deaths per 1000 live births in 1997–2006. [7,8]. When countries are grouped in five levels of economic development, infant mortality shows a sustained downward trend in all the countries and territories of the Americas. However, the presence of inequalities in infant mortality among the groups of countries persists over time. The most recent data available for each sub-region showed an infant mortality of 6.7 deaths per 1000 live births in North America and of around 34.5 in Latin Caribbean (Table 7.1) [7].

Great progress has been made in the struggle against childhood diseases in the countries of the region. Poliomyelitis was eradicated in 1991, advances have been made in the eradication of measles and neonatal tetanus, the number of episodes of acute diarrhoeal disease has decreased, and there have been significant reductions in mortality from intestinal infectious diseases and acute respiratory infections. However, despite this progress, diarrhoeal diseases, acute respiratory infections, and malnutrition remain the leading causes of death in the population under 5 years of age in most of the middle- and lower-income countries of the region.

In some sub-regions of central America and the Latin Caribbean, mortality due to communicable diseases is still very high. In others, such as the Andean Area and Brazil, mortality due to external causes is of greater concern [8].

Communicable diseases

Despite substantial progress in reducing the importance of infectious diseases as mortality causes, there are still major challenges regarding the control of HIV/AIDS, tuberculosis, hanseniasis, malaria, dengue fever, and other conditions.

The number of people living with AIDS continues to increase in the Americas, but at a slower rate than in Africa, Asia, and Eastern Europe. The Caribbean has the highest rates and is second only to sub-Saharan Africa in the number of people by HIV/AIDS. The percentage of females with AIDS reported in the Americas increased from 6 per cent of all prevalent AIDS cases in 1994 to approximately 31 per cent in 2005, with this general trend repeated in all sub-regions [8]. All countries now have national programmes and surveillance systems. Massive research efforts have resulted in promising, but expensive and complex, treatment regimes. The relevance, magnitude, and positive results of the national policy for AIDS control in Brazil has motivated the country's efforts to reduce drug prices internationally.

Chronic non-communicable diseases

There has been a marked change in lifestyle in most of the countries as a result of urbanization, sedentary lifestyle, and stress, with an associated rise in the burden of non-communicable diseases. Population ageing also accounts for the importance of cardiovascular disease as a cause of morbidity and mortality in the majority of the countries.

Injury, an important cause of death in the region, is a growing problem, and has reached epidemic proportions in some countries. With almost 400,000 deaths due to road traffic injuries and a similar number due to homicides; these conditions were the two leading causes of death for the 15–44 age group, especially in men [8]. A high prevalence of mental disorders has been observed in all the countries, but only a small proportion of affected people receive appropriate treatment.

The environmental situation

Housing and basic domestic sanitation services are of paramount importance for health. In the Region of the Americas, marked inequalities are seen in exposure to environmental risks in all countries and territories, and between different population groups. Some of these inequalities are seen in rural areas and among specific groups which can be identified as more vulnerable (e.g. indigenous groups, African descendants, gold diggers, and fisherman). Other inequalities exist in urban areas populated by the poorest and most marginalized groups.

Water and sanitation

It is estimated that one out of every four people lacks access to safe water and basic sanitation services, and this need affects one out of every two people in the communities and areas in which socio-economic inequalities are most acute [8]. In 2004, there were about 54 million people without access to drinking water and 130 million people without access to improved sanitation facilities in Latin America and the Caribbean. The distribution of the population with poor access to drinking water and sanitation facilities by sub-region or country is presented in Table 7.2. Although the worst situation is observed in the Latin Caribbean, Brazil and the Andean Area countries account for a large

Table 7.2 Population without access to improved drinking water sources or to improved sanitation facilities by sub-region or country, Latin America and the Caribbean, 2004

	Population without access to improved drinking water sources			Population without access to improved sanitation facilities		
	Number (million)	Percentage of sub-region or country total population	Percentage of Latin America and Caribbean population	Number (million)	Percentage of sub-region or country total population	Percentage of Latin America and Caribbean population
Latin America & The Caribbean	54.0	9.8	100.0	130.1	23.5	100.0
Mexico	3.2	3.0	5.9	22.2	21.0	17.1
Central American Isthmus	4.2	10.7	7.8	10.7	27.2	8.2
Latin Caribbean	9.2	28.6	17.1	12.0	37.0	9.2
Brazil	18.4	10.0	34.0	46.0	25.0	35.3
Andean Area	14.4	11.9	27.7	31.2	25.8	24.0
Southern Cone	3.2	5.0	5.9	6.1	9.6	4.7
Non-Latin Caribbean	1.4	17.7	2.6	2.0	25.2	1.5

Source: Data from WHO/UNICEF Joint Monitoring Program for Water Supply and Sanitation Database, 2006. Available online at: http://www.wssinfo. org (accessed March 2008). Consolidation by sub-regions by the authors.

proportion of the region's population living without appropriate drinking water sources and sanitation facilities.

There are some signs of improvement. Eighty per cent of the region's population have an improved domestic drinking water supply. However, in rural areas only 45 per cent have domestic drinking water, compared with 90 per cent in urban areas [8]. Roughly 77 per cent of the total population have access to improved sanitation facilities (86 per cent of the urban population and 49 per cent or the rural population) [8]. This represents a modest growth of this service since 1980 when the total coverage was 59 per cent (78 per cent in urban areas and 28 per cent in rural areas) [9].

Even so, the situation is serious, because access to water and sanitation services is a prerequisite for improving public health. Diarrhoeal and parasitic diseases are among the leading causes of morbidity in children under five in the Americas. During the period 2000–2005, mortality attributable to acute diarrhoeal diseases among children under five was 3.7 per cent, and in the Andean Area this figure reached 7.8 per cent of total mortality in this age group. This proportion was also high (above 5.0 per cent) in Central America, Mexico, and Brazil. Approximately 70 per cent of all the waste produced daily in the region is collected, but only about half is disposed in sanitary landfills and controlled landfills; the rest ends up in open-air dumps or watercourses [8].

Pollution

Pollution, especially from industrial activities, burning of fuel, and transportation, is a growing problem which affects the entire population, although with varying degrees of exposure and risk. Poor areas are the most vulnerable because of their greater exposure to industrial and domestic waste. In urban areas, burning of fossil fuels to generate energy for home heating, motor vehicles, and industrial processes constitutes the main source of air pollution.

In summary, Latin American countries are facing significant changes in their demographic, social, and epidemiological profiles. The epidemiological transition is well advanced and new problems such as injuries and AIDS are important causes of death and morbidity. These changes do not reach all social groups uniformly, and inequalities persist among and within countries. Decreases in the proportion of many problems have not been sufficient to produce a drop in the absolute numbers of people affected by them.

Public policies and health systems

In Latin America and the Caribbean, public health policies and health systems vary enormously among countries, making comparative or integrated analyses a challenge.

Discussions on what should be understood by social welfare and in what institutional framework health policies should be formulated and implemented have grown in importance in Latin America and the Caribbean in a regional scenario dominated by the following [8]:

- questioning of the sector reforms carried out in the 1980s and 1990s;
- the absence of a social safety net capable of acting as the foundation for social development in a new context;
- commitment to the Millennium Development Goals (MDGs) by 2015;
- a growing concern over the problems of inequity, exclusion, and poverty that prevail in the countries of the region.

Segmentation, fragmentation, and exclusion are very common features of health systems in the region, although systems funding and organization vary among countries. Recently, the PAHO has been emphasizing a new approach to making changes in health systems, centred on the concept of social protection of health as a universal human right that is no longer contingent on employment or other individual or group characteristics.

Health policies and health systems can be analysed from many different perspectives. A possible approach to public health is discussion of the main functions of health systems, which can be summarized in four areas: financing, stewardship, regulation, and the delivery of health services. Analysing strategic areas of public intervention, such as health promotion, health status monitoring/epidemiological surveillance, health care, health professionals, and health products and technologies, offers another approach. These two broad approaches are described below.

Functions of the health systems

Financing

Public health expenditure is essential to improve health status and to reduce inequalities in access to health services. Health spending expressed as a percentage of GDP in Latin America and the Caribbean increased from 2.6 per cent in the 1980s to 3.6 per cent in 2005–2006, figures lower than those of Organization for Economic Cooperation and Development (OECD) countries (7.3 per cent and 8.6 per cent, respectively). In 2005–2006, health expenditure was between 1.3–4.5 per cent of GDP in Latin America and Caribbean countries. In the OECD countries with universal health coverage the same indicator varied between 7.5 and 10 per cent. The fact that countries spend relatively more or less of their GDP on health appears to be influenced more by national policy decisions regarding universal access and coverage and, to a lesser extent, by the way in which national health systems are organized and financed [8].

On average, private spending on health (the purchase of health goods and services) accounts for 52 per cent of national expenditure on health in the countries of the region, which is very high compared with OECD countries (Table 7.3). However, there are wide variations in the public–private composition of health financing. The countries with the highest public health expenditure as a percentage of GDP, such as Costa Rica and Cuba, generally have national health systems with universal or near universal coverage. High levels of private expenditure on health in some countries reflect an increase in direct household spending and growth in private insurers and prepaid medical plans. This trend poses a large challenge for health policies.

Some key measures to improve health status and reduce inequalities in access to health services are:

- increasing public spending on health, both in collective actions and health care;
- making improvements in the distributional effects of such spending;
- extending coverage of public health systems.

Table 7.3 National expenditure on health care in the Americas and other regions, 2004

	Per capita GDP (US$ PPP 2000)	National expenditure on health as percentage of GDP	Per capita national expenditure on health (US$ PPP 2000)	Public/private ratio
All regions and countries	8284	8.7	588	58/42
European Union	25,953	9.6	2552	74/26
America	18,149	12.7	2166	47/43
Canada	28,732	10.3	2669	71/29
United States	36,465	13.1	5711	45/55
Latin America & The Caribbean	7419	6.8	222	48/52
Argentina	12,222	8.6	1045	55/45
Brazil	7531	7.0	530	49/51
Costa Rica	8714	8.5	738	60/40
Cuba	3483	6.3	220	—[1]
Mexico	9010	5.5	497	44/56
Uruguay	8658	9.0	781	71/29

PPP, purchasing power parity

[1] Only public expenditure is considered.

Source: Data from PAHO (2007), *Health in the Americas*, pp. 314–16. Reproduced with permission from the Pan American Health Organization (PAHO). This table is based on data originally published *Health in the Americas* (PAHO 2007). Also see (http://publications.paho.org).

Stewardship

Many efforts have been made to achieve an operational concept of stewardship in health. The stewardship function in health policy is considered to be the exercise of substantive responsibilities and competencies that are incumbent on the state and that cannot be delegated. According to the WHO, a government has the capacity and obligation to take responsibility for the health and well-being of its citizens and to direct the health system as a whole. This responsibility should involve three fundamental aspects:

- ♦ providing vision and direction for the health system;
- ♦ collecting and using intelligence;
- ♦ exerting influence through regulation and other means.

The stewardship function is usually exercised by the national health authority, the Ministry of Health. However, in federal countries (e.g. Argentina, Brazil, and Mexico) and in those characterized by segmented health systems (e.g. Chile, Colombia), definitions of state institutions responsibilities and attributions are often complex and controversial.

In order to achieve the goal of improving the health of the people, health authorities must formulate appropriate policies and develop adequate planning, regulatory, and evaluative actions. In most Latin American and Caribbean countries, a critical problem is institutional weakness, a factor which influences the possibilities for economic and social development. The effective practice of public health requires many civil servants, but appropriately trained public health personnel are lacking in many levels of the administration. Specific governmental health careers have not been established, and because of current structural adjustment policies there is instability and high turnover among public health administrators. Unfortunately, the region faces a decrease in the incentives for working in governmental institutions and the labour conditions in the field are deteriorating.

In many countries, state reforms in the 1990s weakened the long-term planning capacities of national governments. Health sector reforms included health systems segmentation or fragmentation, privatization and decentralization [10]. In this context, the role of the national health authority has to be reformulated [11], and local health authorities and managers have to be trained to respond to the new functions. A larger number of trained public health staff are needed in newly established health administrative structures.

In recent years, redefinition of institutional roles and strengthening of the functions of the state have become priorities in the economic and the social spheres, including the health sector. Health legislation and other institutional rules which establish the legal framework for government action in health have been revised or developed in many countries. Some countries, such as Brazil, Chile, and Costa Rica, implemented concrete actions to strengthen the stewardship functions of the health authorities. However, the challenge of directing institution-building efforts towards enhancing the functions of planning, financing, and development of resources, public management, and knowledge persists.

Regulation

Some authors and agencies include regulation in the function of stewardship. In this chapter, it is considered separately because it involves a wide range of state actions that can be directed towards the following groups:

+ health authorities at different government levels;
+ health care providers;
+ health-related products;
+ specific health markets, such as prepaid private health plans.

In this sense, regulation includes normalization, coordination, supervision, control, and evaluation strategies which must be coherent with the general direction and public purpose of the health system. Regulation directed towards different government levels can be pertinent in decentralized health systems, particularly in unequal countries in which the national authority role must involve investments to reduce inequalities, redistribute resources, and efforts to achieve national health standards. In federal countries such as Brazil, these efforts comprise intergovernmental negotiation and definition of common priorities and goals.

Health care providers

Regulation of health care providers involves actions to ensure that the population can have appropriate and timely access to the necessary health services, standards are of high quality, and proper public payment mechanisms are defined. Increased participation of the private sector in the delivery of health services requires the strengthening of the regulatory capabilities of public health administrators, since inappropriate action can lead to an increase in health inequalities. Whereas most industrialized countries exercise strict control over private practice in the health sector, these regulations are underdeveloped in Latin American and Caribbean countries.

Health products

Regulation of health-related products comprises different actions directed towards preventing and reducing health risks in consequence of the utilization of a wide range of products, including food, drugs, cosmetics, etc. This very traditional public health function is structured in different ways in Latin American and Caribbean countries. Regional integration processes have brought new pressures to achieve transnational agreements and patterns of quality concerning health-related products.

Health markets

State regulation of health markets is essential, considering the intensity of economic interest in the health sector that can be exemplified by the expansion of private health insurance companies in the region. New roles for the private sector in health care delivery led to the production of a new set of laws and norms related to their functioning, mainly devoted to the protection of consumers' rights. A few countries, such as Brazil, have made some efforts to improve state regulation of these markets and instituted regulatory agencies to coordinate this new governmental role. However, as well as organizing private markets and protecting consumers' rights in the health sector, Latin American countries face important challenges in directing state regulatory action to reduce inequalities and promote citizenship in health.

Health care services

Health care services include those that respond to individual and collective needs covering the whole spectrum of care, ranging from health promotion and disease prevention to curative and palliative treatment, rehabilitation, and long-term care. The health care services delivery function is probably the most visible to the population because it embodies the purpose of the health care systems. According to PAHO [8], in Latin America the trend towards decentralization and a reduction in government intervention in the direct provision of health services has turned the ministries of health into coordinators of the management and delivery of services by public institutions rather than direct administrators of services. Therefore the function of harmonizing the provision of health services is particularly important in systems in which there are many public and private players whose activities must be channelled for the purpose of achieving common goals. Thus, the health authority must have the capacity to promote complementarities among different providers and to extend-health care coverage in an equitable manner.

Some critical aspects of this function are:

- coordination of different levels of health service (with respect to their character and complexity);
- improving accessibility for different population groups;
- quality assurance.

Social inequalities, the trademark of the region, have a strong influence in all these dimensions, and therefore planned governmental action must take this into consideration.

Strategic areas of public intervention in health

Health promotion

Improvements in health care technology and health service delivery are not sufficient to meet the challenges presented by the current health situation in the region. Recognition of the need to address the social determinants of health have revolutionized the debate on the effects of social processes on health and facilitated the emergence of an approach that promotes health through public policy formulation. A broader range of activities across many sectors is required to promote individual and collective health, involving environmental protection, investments in water supply and sanitation services, housing conditions, waste collection and disposal, and food protection. Health promotion policies also include health communication efforts and intersectoral strategies, such as the 'healthy municipalities' and the 'health promoting schools' initiatives that have been adopted in some countries. Although many countries have made efforts to propose new strategies in this field, fragmentation of social policies is still prominent, making it difficult to implement a comprehensive approach to health promotion at national level.

There are examples of specific policies that are very relevant. Norms and regulations for protection against toxic agents such as oil and asbestos have been presented in some countries. Since tobacco exposure is high in the majority of the countries, many governments have launched anti-tobacco initiatives including advertising restrictions. The Framework Convention on Tobacco Control was signed by 60 per cent of the nation states in the region. In recent years, some countries, such as Brazil and Uruguay, have made considerable advances in this area [8].

Health situation monitoring and epidemiological surveillance

Monitoring health status activities has been developed to some extent by most countries in the region, although not necessarily routinely or adequately. There is wide disparity among countries in national politics regarding health information and informatics, as well as in technological infrastructure, investment, and deployment of health information systems.

A survey of 24 Latin American and Caribbean countries by PAHO showed that nearly all of them conduct systematic health data collections, making use of standards defined at the national level, and that most of these data are related to epidemiological surveillance and the services provided [12]. However, many problems were identified in the utilization of information systems, such as duplication and gaps in the information, dubious quality, and little use of information by health policy-makers and managers.

Epidemiological surveillance relates to the capacity to conduct research and surveillance on epidemic outbreaks and patterns of communicable and non-communicable diseases, accidents, and exposure to toxic substances or environmental agents harmful to health. Since the 1990s, efforts have been made to restructure national epidemiological surveillance systems in the region; even so many of these systems are still inadequate. PAHO evaluates these surveillance systems regularly [13].

In June 2007, the International Health Regulations (2005) [14] entered in force. This agreement provides a new framework for coordination of the management of events which could constitute a public health emergency of international concern, and aims to improve the capacity of all countries to detect, assess, notify, and respond to public health threats.

Health care

Inequities in access to health services are a common feature in Latin American and Caribbean countries. Although health systems in many countries represent a major commitment of financial, organizational, physical, and human resources, they are still insufficient for the vast and diverse needs of the region's population. Scarcity of resources related to economic adjustment processes and recent reforms, such as the increasing participation of the private sector in the area, pose new equity challenges to health authorities.

Access to health care

In addition to the financial constraints and broader economic and social inequalities that affect health conditions and policies, accurate information on access to health services is rare. Thus it is difficult for health authorities to implement adequate strategies to increase health services delivery and reduce the inequalities in access. Existing data suggest that there are significant inequalities in access between regions in the same country, between urban and rural populations, and between different social classes. These inequalities can be observed at every level of service complexity. In many countries the coverage and quality of prenatal care varies greatly depending on the woman's social and educational status, despite efforts by health authorities to improve access to primary health care. Proper diagnostic facilities, such as imaging services, are scarce or inadequately distributed in most countries of the region, so that the opportunity for effective early intervention is sometimes reduced. The situation is even worse regarding more complex services which tend to be concentrated in the largest cities.

Improvements in access to health care in the region depend on many factors. Recently, WHO and PAHO have proposed a strategy of 'renewing' primary health care (PHC) in the Americas by adopting a comprehensive concept and framework. The position of these agencies is that that PHC renewal must be an integral part of health systems development and that basing health systems on PHC is the best approach for producing sustained and equitable improvement in the health of the peoples of the Americas [15].

Innovative health-care models

Some countries have made efforts to adopt innovative health care models, such as family doctors (i.e. Cuba) or family health programmes based on interdisciplinary teams (i.e. Brazil). Others have adopted policies which aim at augmenting coverage in specific population groups or diseases. However, considering that the majority of the region's population is poor, targeting alone will not improve equity in access to health services because of the overlap of many health interventions. Implementation of health policies that guarantee universal access to all system levels and specific strategies directed to the more vulnerable groups is required.

Population-based health services

With regard to the quality of population-based health services, most countries have licensing norms and regulations for health professionals, facilities, drugs, equipments, and devices. However, almost none have regular evaluation or quality improvement initiatives in place. Argentina, Colombia, Brazil, and Mexico are implementing systems of health care evaluation for accreditation purposes, but these are mostly directed towards hospitals. Some countries are adopting technical protocols or clinical guidelines to reduce the variation in practice among care providers and assist in ameliorating the quality and safety of the care delivered.

Human resources

Human resources development is one of the central elements in national health policies and health sector reforms. Since the 1990s, this area has experienced many changes, most of which derive from broad economic and political determinants, such as globalization and state reform processes. The most salient effect of sector reforms has not been a reduction in health personnel, but changes in the health sector's labour market and an increase in the flexibility of labour relations.

The availability of health professionals varies between and within countries. The concentration of health professionals in large cities and in some specialties is a problem in most of the countries. Unresolved issues in human resources development in the region include the limited capacity of authorities to plan and act upon human resources needs and to improve health personnel distribution, reduced budgets in public institutions resulting in a decrease in the numbers of public positions for health workers and a drop in their remuneration, and a scarcity of professionals with credentials required by public health systems and new health-care management models.

A survey conducted by PAHO in 28 countries in 2005 [16] showed that three-quarters did not have sufficient information about healthworkers, their occupations, and their skills. A few countries (e.g. Brazil, Chile, Guatemala, and Peru) had institutionalized national bodies or departments responsible for developing human resources policies in health care. In the last decade, many countries began to decentralize health services management, which led to radical changes in personnel administration in the public sector [8].

Public–private practitioners

Although public institutions remain the major health personnel employers in the region, an increasing number of health personnel are combining their public functions with private practice. Many countries have promoted reforms that deregulate or increase flexibility in labour relations, including the health sector. Changes observed in the sector include a reduced number of permanent positions in public health institutions, changes in remuneration, such as public wages contracts and introduction of productivity incentives, an increase in temporary contracts and third-party hiring, and creation of new types of private associations, such as professional cooperatives and other professional groups.

Health workforce: education and training

Other relevant issues in health personnel development are education and training of the health workforce. Educational institutions, particularly universities, do not usually cater for the needs of public health systems. For example, although in many countries there is an increasing demand for personnel capable of performing functions at the primary care level, universities tend to encourage specialization. Continuing education of health personnel is either insufficient or inappropriate in most countries. Recently, in many countries interactions between the institutions that train health professionals, the health services, and the ministries or departments of health have increased and have continued to develop. There are some examples of comprehensive strategies in

Chile and Brazil. Good progress has also been made in Bolivia, Costa Rica, Ecuador, Guatemala, Mexico, and Paraguay. In Cuba, health personnel are trained within health services, which function as professional training centres. Health professions and occupations are mainly regulated by professional bodies, although formal laws and norms are increasingly being produced in the region.

Health products and technologies

The appropriate provision of health care services demands the utilization of a wide range of products and technologies, such as medicines, vaccines, and different types of equipments. The availability of these supplies in the public health system depends on the relationship between health, science and technology, and industrial policies [17]. Unfortunately, the level of research, innovation, and industrial capacity is low in the majority of Latin American countries, and most of them depend strongly on imported health technologies.

The pharmaceutical industry is extensively globalized today. International companies are rapidly increasing their share of the Latin American market. National producers have the highest market share in Argentina (50 per cent of laboratories), followed by Chile with 43 per cent, Uruguay with 26 per cent, Brazil with 25 per cent, and Mexico with 12 per cent [8]. It is estimated that more than half of the region's inhabitants have difficulty in obtaining essential medicines; in 60 per cent of the countries of the region access to essential medicines in 2003 was less than 80 per cent [18]. Prices are the main barrier and access depends strongly on income. Two-thirds of financing for medicines in Latin America comes from household expenditures, and just one-third is paid by insurance plans or the government. This is strongly regressive, indicating the importance of improving public pharmaceutical financing and supply. Another barrier has been attributed to the fact that the fast pace of innovation in the industry is not responsive to the problems that prevail in less-developed countries and areas.

Almost all countries in the region have adopted new drug regulations, although the scope and strength of the regulatory capacities vary between them. Some countries, such as Argentina and Brazil, are putting forward policies to promote the use of pharmaceutical generics. Brazil has also advanced in the revision of intellectual property agreements for essential drugs, and in 2007 adopted for the first time the compulsory licensing of a patented drug for AIDS treatment. Many legislative initiatives are now in place to protect special population groups, such as children, adolescents, HIV-positive people, handicapped people, and the elderly.

In many countries, the list of essential medicines serves as a guide to the public sector in providing medicines. In the larger countries, such as Brazil and

Colombia, the responsibility for procuring most medicines has been transferred to the local level. The decentralization process creates certain problems
and in some cases leads to significant increases in the cost of medicines because
the economies of scale are lost, particularly for more expensive drugs.

In the last 10 years, the Latin American and Caribbean countries have
increased their dependence on imported vaccines produced outside the region,
as a consequence of the development of new products by transnational companies. Today, few countries in the region have the capacity to modernize their
technical infrastructure and installations to produce the combined vaccines
that are necessary to meet the demands of their immunization programmes.
Promising efforts have been made by Brazil, Colombia, Cuba, and Venezuela
concerning specific vaccines.

Conclusion: public health challenges

Market forces alone will not drive the appropriate response to cover either the
old or the emerging agenda of health problems in Latin America and Caribbean.
Governments will have to play a central role in articulating economic and
social policies oriented to re-engage a new era of development and to reduce
social and regional inequalities. Multilateral agencies have a role to play in
stimulating cooperation among countries and in finding ways to deal with the
debt burden, without imposing an extra burden upon socially and economically disadvantaged populations.

Comprehensive health policies and systems will be a crucial component of a
new development model for Latin American and Caribbean countries, since
the health sector generates many specialized jobs and utilizes many different
products and technologies relevant to regional and national economies. The
recognition of three different dimensions of health policy—social, economic,
and political [19]—indicate that efforts should be directed to: strengthening
national social protection systems, based on universal principles and more
integrated social policies, and investing in science, technology, and industrial
production of strategic health technologies. The overall goals are to reduce
external dependence and health system vulnerability, and to reduce health
inequalities among regions and social groups.

National social and health goals must underpin all economic policies and
adjustment policies should not compromise progress in social security and
welfare. Sound national social policies for the protection of the disadvantaged
should be developed and implemented in an integrated way, related to comprehensive universal policies. Health sector planning should be based on a
sound epidemiological basis and priorities set according to the needs of the
population. The effectiveness of proposed actions should always be taken into

account when designing strategies for coping with the complexities of current health problems.

Decentralization of activities continues to be a major administrative goal in the region. However, adequate coordination and regional and national objectives must guide the process. Increased accountability to the public, associated with community participation and social control, is crucial to the achievement of the best results of public health initiatives. Information systems which continuously feed policy makers and health professionals must be developed and improved. Development and engagement of health personnel are crucial in order to promote the required changes.

These objectives will necessitate a new wave of health reform initiatives that will require the leadership of health authorities at all political levels as well as mobilization of the public health community, health professionals, and the public at large. Recognition of health as a human social right should guide the process. The success or failure of health policies must, as always, be measurable in terms of the reduction of inequalities in health determinants, improved access to health services, and a sustained reduction of the burden of disease and suffering.

References

[1] Ocampo JM. The pending agenda. *ECLAC Notes* 2001;**15**: 2.

[2] Economic Commission for Latin America and the Caribbean. *Panorama Social de América Latina. Documento Informativo.* Santiago: ECLAC, 2007.

[3] Economic Commission for Latin America and the Caribbean. *Balance Preliminar de las Economías de América Latina y el Caribe 2007.* Santiago: ECLAC, 2007.

[4] Economic Commission for Latin America and the Caribbean. *La Protección Social de Cara al Futuro: Acceso, Financiamiento y Solidaridad.* Santiago: ECLAC, 2006.

[5] United Nations. *The Inequality Predicament. Report on the World Social Situation.* New York: United Nations, 2005.

[6] United Nations. *World Population Prospects: 2004 Revision. Highlights.* New York: United Nations, 2005.

[7] Pan American Health Organization. *Health Situation in the Americas. Basic Indicators 2007.* Available online at: http://www.paho.org/english/dd/ais/BI_2007_ENG.pdf (accessed 20 December 2007).

[8] Pan American Health Organization (2007). *Health in the Americas: 2007 Edition.* Washington, DC: PAHO, 2007.

[9] Pan American Health Organization (1997). *Mid-Decade Evaluation of Water Supply and Sanitation in Latin America and the Caribbean.* Washington, DC: PAHO, 1997.

[10] Almeida C (2000). Reforma de sistemas de servicios de salud y equidad en América Latina y el Caribe: algunas lecciones de los años 80 y 90. *Cad Saúde Públ* 2000; **18**: 905–25.

[11] Machado CV. *Direito Universal, Política Nacional: O Papel do Ministério da Saúde na Política se Saúde Brasileira de 1990 a 2002.* Rio de Janeiro: Editora do Museu da República, 2007.

[12] Pan American Health Organization. *Health in the Americas: 1998 Edition.* Washington, DC: PAHO, 1998.

[13] Pan American Health Organization. *Public Health Surveillance in the Americas: National Epidemiological Surveillance and Statistical Information Systems.* Available online at: www.paho.org/English/DD/AIS/vigilancia-en.htm (accessed 22 December 2007).

[14] World Health Organization. *International Health Regulations 2005.* Available online at: www.who.int/gb/ebwha/pdf_files/WHA58/WHA58_3-en.pdf (accessed 10 January 2008).

[15] World Health Organization. *Renewing Primary Health Care in the Americas. A Position Paper of the PAHO/WHO.* Washington, DC: PAHO, 2007.

[16] Pan American Health Organization. Regional consultation on the critical challenges for human resources in health in the Americas. Regional Meeting of the Observatory of Human Resources in Health. Critical Challenges for Human Resources in Health: A Regional View. Toronto, 2005.

[17] Gadelha CAG. Desenvolvimento, complexo industrial da saúde e política industrial. *Rev Saúde Públ* 2006; **40**: 11–23.

[18] Pan American Health Organization, Center for Pharmaceutical Policies, National School of Public Health. *Pharmaceutical Situation in Latin America and the Caribbean. Structure and Processes.* Rio de Janeiro: NAF/ENSP, 2006.

[19] Moran M. Three faces of the health care state. *J Health Politics Policy Law* 1995; **3**: 767–81.

Chapter 8

Public health in Africa

David Sanders, Ehi Igumbor, Uta Lehmann,
Wilma Meeus, and Delanyo Dovlo

Introduction

This chapter addresses public health issues relevant to sub-Saharan Africa
(SSA). SSA comprises 48 countries, 42 located in the mainland sub-regions of
Central, Eastern, Southern and Western Africa and six island nations. It
excludes the northern African countries of Egypt, Libya, Tunisia, Algeria,
Morocco and Western Sahara.

The chapter outlines the current health status in SSA in relation to progress
towards achieving the Millennium Development Goals (MDGs); trends in the
development of public health services, including health sector reforms, and
prospects for the future following some major new public health initiatives. It
concludes with an overarching challenge—the need for human capacity to
meet the health needs of SSA.

Health status

While improvements in health status in SSA have occurred over the last few
decades, the current situation on the continent is of great concern. Despite the
paucity and unreliability of health data, as shown in Annex 1, reversal of health
gains is evident from several health indicators for a number of countries in the
region [1].

Life expectancy—and the impact of HIV

In 2005, 11 of the 48 SSA countries had a lower life expectancy (LE) than in
1970, and 12 countries had seen an increase in infant mortality rate (IMR)
between 1990 and 2005. Twelve countries had shown an increase in under-five
mortality rate, and in half of the countries LE decreased between 1999 and
2005, probably through a combination of extreme poverty, the impact of the
HIV epidemic, the decline in health service provision, and conflict [1].

The majority of countries where LE has decreased have a high prevalence of HIV, affecting in particular the 15–45 age range. At the end of 2007, the number of HIV-infected people in SSA was estimated at 22.5 million, 70 per cent of the global total of HIV-infected people [2]. Approximately 2.8 million additional people were infected with HIV in 2006, surpassing the combined number of new infections in all other regions of the world. A total of 2.1 million deaths in the region were attributed to HIV, accounting for 76 per cent of global AIDS deaths. The crosslinks between the HIV epidemic, tuberculosis, and malaria are significant and threaten a continuing impact of the AIDS epidemic over the next decade and beyond. Its social and economic consequences are already widely felt, not only in the health sector but also in sectors dependent on human resources such as education, industry, agriculture, transport, and the economy in general.

Increase in conflicts

Thirteen of the 48 SSA countries have recently been or are still involved in conflict, and neighbouring countries are affected because of population movements across international borders. There is some indication of relief in the numbers of refugees in Western and Southern Africa, with reductions of 31 per cent and 18 per cent, respectively, recorded for 2006 [3]. This is 'primarily due to the successful voluntary repatriations to Liberia and Angola respectively' but is offset by an increase of over 80,000 new refugees in the Eastern African region in 2006 [3]. The breakdown of the delivery of most social services, including health care, is a frequent accompaniment of conflict. In fact, the 2006 State of the World's Children report states that, globally, most of the countries where one in five children die before five years of age have experienced major armed conflict since 1999 [4].

The double burden of disease

The past two decades have witnessed a resurgence and spread of 'old' communicable diseases once thought to be well controlled, for example cholera, tuberculosis, malaria, yellow fever, and trypanosomiasis, while 'new' epidemics, notably HIV/AIDS, threaten last century's health gains in many developing countries, especially in SSA. At present, co-infection of mycobacterium tuberculosis and HIV together with the unprecedented emergence of multidrug-resistant (MDR) and extensively drug-resistant (XDR) tuberculosis present a major public health concern in the region. In addition, nutritional status is showing no improvement, as demonstrated by stunting rates of 30 per cent and above in 29 SSA countries, of which 11 have stunting rates of 40 per cent and above [4].

The rise of chronic non-communicable diseases

At the same time, many countries are experiencing an 'epidemiological transition', with cardiovascular diseases, cancers, diabetes, other chronic conditions, and trauma replacing communicable diseases as leading causes of death. Poorer sectors of the population may experience high child mortality and morbidity as well as a high burden of non-communicable disease [5]. In South Africa, for example, children from poor families still suffer mainly from infectious diseases, whereas increasing rates of hypertension, chronic lung diseases, and diabetes affect the urban, and especially poorer, adult population [6].

Health services and health systems

Access to health services in SSA improved considerably during the period 1980–1990, but worsened in the 1990s as shown by Expanded Programme on Immunization (EPI) coverage data (Table 8.1). Despite the intensive polio vaccination campaigns and regular measles vaccination campaigns in more recent times, the EPI coverage data for the period 1999–2005 showed only modest improvements following the dip in coverage of all routinely administered antigens in the 1990s.

In addition, many countries have been unable to significantly reallocate resources from tertiary and specialized services to basic health services or find increased resources to moderate the imbalance, despite warnings given as early as the mid-1960s [7]. In Ghana, for instance, only 42 per cent of the health

Table 8.1 EPI coverage (percentage of fully vaccinated 1-year-old children)

	1980	1990	1999	2005
BCG				
World	58	79	81	83
SSA	46	72	65	76
DPT 3				
World	44	74	75	78
SSA	30	55	50	66
Polio 3				
World	46	75	76	78
SSA	25	54	50	68
Measles				
World	39	75	72	77
SSA	37	58	51	65

Sources: UNICEF, *State of the World's Children*: 1984 [12], 1994 [13], 2001 [14], 2005 [4].

budget was allocated to district level health service delivery in 2001, while the central Ministry of Health's budget allocation amounts to 16 per cent, tertiary facilities use almost 20 per cent and regional level services use 23 per cent of the national health budget [8]. Most SSA countries still spend less than an average US$10 per person on health care, i.e. 20–40 per cent below the minimum amount recommended by the World Bank as necessary to provide the basic package of health services [9].

Millennium Development Goals (MDGs)

In its 2000 Millennium Declaration, the United Nations set eight ambitious goals for development, called the Millennium Development Goals (MDGs), which presented an agenda for improving human condition worldwide by 2015. Targets in the MDGs include commitment to reduce poverty and hunger, ill-health, gender inequality, and lack of education, to improve access to clean water supplies, and to reduce environmental degradation [9].

Growing poverty

In stark contrast with the rest of the developing world, progress in eradicating poverty and improving living standards remains 'stubbornly slow' in SSA with depressing indices [10]. For example, in 2006 the number of people living on less than US$1 a day had nearly doubled compared with 1981 [10].

Growing inequality in mortality experience

GDP data are aggregates that do not show the increasing gap between the rich and the poor within countries. Disaggregation of infant, under-five mortality, and life expectancy data reveals that the gap in mortality rates between rich and poor countries has widened significantly over the past decades: the relative probability of dying for children under five in developing countries compared with wealthy countries increased from a ratio of 5.7 in 1960 to 14.5 in 2003 [11]. Similarly, improvements in child health status have been slower in SSA as shown in Table 8.2 [12–14].

Education of girls and women

Education indicators show that a sizeable percentage of women in SSA are still functionally illiterate. Despite efforts to make primary education accessible to all children, it was estimated that 40 per cent of boys and 45 per cent of girls did not attend school in 2006. More than a third of those who enter primary school will not reach grade five, and about 80 per cent of all children of secondary school age will not attend secondary school [4].

Access to water and hygienic sanitation

Although there have been some improvements, access to a safe water supply is poor, with only 44 per cent of rural SSA (comprising 60 per cent of the SSA

Table 8.2 Decline in infant mortality rate and under-five mortality rate, 1960, 1981, 1999, and 2005

Indicator	Infant mortality rate				Under-5 mortality rate			
	1960	1981	1999	2005	1960	1981	1999	2005
World	127	78	57	52	198	91	82	76
SSA	156	126	107	101	258	203	173	169

Sources: UNICEF, *State of the World's Children* 1984 [12], 1994 [13], 2001 [14], 2005 [4].

population) having access to adequate water supplies in 2004 [4,12–14]. The same applies to access to good sanitation, particularly by rural populations. A review of global progress in meeting the MDG water and sanitation targets has highlighted a deteriorating trend, especially in SSA, and qualifies it as 'the urban and rural challenge of the decade' [15]. Over the period 1990–2004, the number of people without access to drinking water and sanitation increased by 23 per cent and over 30 per cent, respectively [15].

Summary

Gains in health status in SSA and access to health and related services have been slower than in other developing regions despite the efforts related to the Millennium Development Project. Africa is 'off-track' in meeting the health-related MDGs of reducing child mortality, improving maternal health, and combating infectious diseases [9], and at current rates of progress SSA will not achieve any of the MDGs. Given the much lower starting point of SSA countries, it is disturbingly apparent that some of the gains of the past 20 years are being reversed. These developments are partly explained by public health policy and governance trends in a context of economic globalization. In the following sections we briefly outline how public health policies and services have evolved in SSA since the end of the colonial period and how they have been influenced by globalization.

Trends in the development of public health services

Changes in health policies and their context in SSA

The economic and political history of SSA has been linked to the world economy for the past 500 years, starting with the slave trade in the sixteenth century. Colonization tightened and formalized these ties and European administrative systems dislodged, suppressed, and reinvented indigenous systems and traditions. Newly independent African states took over fragmented colonial state machinery, which had to be Africanized with an extremely weak human resource base. For instance, in Tanzania in 1962 only 16 of 184 physicians, one of 84 civil engineers, and two of 57 lawyers were Africans [16]. In a number of countries rebuilding and restructuring attempts ground to a halt during the 1970s oil crisis and the worldwide economic recession which followed. This recession was precipitated by the stringent financial policies adopted by the northern countries (particularly the USA and the United Kingdom) from the early 1980s, involving tight credit, high interest rates, and reductions in government spending. The resulting economic slowdown was passed on to low- and middle-income countries through reduced demand for exports and cuts in foreign aid. Together with deteriorating terms of trade, this led to a reversal in the flow of capital, with low- and middle-income countries becoming net exporters of capital and acquiring huge debts.

The current oil and food crisis may well hold the greatest threat yet for SSA. As the region experiences significant short- and long-term price increases in many staple foods, livelihoods and even survival for many in the population are threatened. Indeed, the MDG Africa Steering Group warn that the recent rise in food prices puts 'great pressure on African economies and is threatening to unravel hard-won progress in fighting hunger and malnutrition' [9]. Suffice it to state that the prices of healthy foods have increased at a much faster rate than those of non-healthy foods, and this is compounded by increases in prices of other basics such as household energy, rent, and transport.

Health sector policies in post-colonial SSA

As a rule, newly independent African states inherited patchy and highly uneven health care systems which they sought to restructure in different ways. While many tried to build health systems that would better serve disadvantaged areas, the majority of government and international funding continued to emphasize curative urban services [17]. There were exceptions, such as Tanzania, following the 1967 Arusha Declaration, and later Mozambique in the early years of the Frelimo government [18], both of which promoted a strategy emphasizing community-based health care. A significant post-colonial development was the expansion of rural health centres, staffed by auxiliaries such as medical and health assistants, which improved health service coverage. However, by the 1980s these early efforts to reshape health care delivery and governance were severely undermined by the economic recession which resulted in a dramatic shortage of resources to invest in health care, education, and social services.

The era of primary health care

These setbacks contributed to a growing realization internationally that the provision of health care for all would need a fundamental and systemic rethinking of strategies [19]. This culminated in the 1978 Alma Ata Declaration on Primary Health Care (PHC) which stressed the need for community-based affordable and accessible health care for all. The Declaration also placed health within its social, economic, and political context, calling for an equitable distribution of resources. However, the following years saw a move to 'selective primary health care' [20], with a continued focus on vertical programmes and selected technical interventions, eschewing comprehensive, multisectoral, and integrated health care provision. This trend was reinforced by the prevailing conservative political ideology of the 1980s which de-emphasized the broader determinants of health such as income inequalities, the environment, and community development, and emphasized health care technologies [21].

There were some significant successes in selective PHC, particularly in the 1980s. The most impressive achievements have been in child health care provision with the vigorous promotion of selected 'child survival' technologies such as growth monitoring, oral rehydration therapy (ORT), breastfeeding, and immunization. Of these, immunization improved most dramatically in the 1980s. More recently, there has been a revival of EPI as, evidenced by the substantial decline in the number of non-immunized children (defined as children who had not received the third dose of DTP-3 by their first birthday) from 1.4 million in 2002 to less than 900,000 in 2004 [22].

Selective PHC was reinforced by the World Bank's 1993 World Development Report *Investing in Health* [23] which emphasized the importance of health to development. Based on calculations of burden of disease, it specified the most cost-effective health interventions, and formulated a core package of health services to be provided at the different levels of care. The identification of core packages has become a rationing mechanism to control the cost of health services provided by the state. This reflected the World Bank's wider economic and fiscal policies, encouraging privatization of health-care delivery and cutting back state services. However, an assessment at the start of the twenty-first century is sobering (Box 8.1).For example, a systematic review has pointed out the lack of evidence for the effectiveness of DOTS (directly observed treatment, short course) for tuberculosis in the absence of well-functioning health services and community engagement [24]. Real and sustainable improvements in the health status of a population are only seen when core service activities such as DOTS are embedded in a more comprehensive approach (which includes paying attention to social equity, health systems, and human capacity development) [25,26].

Globalization, health, and health services in SSA

Increased mobility of capital and labour and cheaper costs of communication have accelerated the pre-existing economic, political, and social interdependence

Box 8.1 Vaccination campaigns: a problem of sustainability?

Apart from modest increases in vaccination coverage in countries in SSA, evaluations have raised questions about the sustainability of mass vaccination campaigns [27], the effectiveness of health-facility-based growth monitoring [28], and the appropriateness of ORT when promoted as sachets or packets without a corresponding emphasis on nutrition, water and sanitation [17]. For example, although Ethiopia had managed to increase polio vaccination coverage to approximately 80 per cent in 2001 from less than 10 per cent in 1992, largely as a result of vaccination campaigns, a total of 37 polio cases in four out of the 11 regions of the country have been reported since December 2004. Previously polio-free countries have reported reinfection in the last 2 years: Somalia reported a total of 215 confirmed cases in 14 out of the 19 regions in 2006 even though it was declared polio free in 2002; Kenya subsequently reported one case of polio in October 2006 which, through genetic sequencing, was noted to be imported from Somalia and originated in Northern Nigeria which is notoriously polio endemic. Namibia experienced a largely adult outbreak in 2006 with 34 suspect cases reported, and in 2007 the Democratic Republic of Congo and Chad also reported cases of polio [29].

which characterizes the modern phase of globalization. The most important early interventions which further integrated developing countries into the global economy, primarily through the imposition of stringent debt repayments and the liberalization of trade, have been Structural Adjustment Programmes (SAPs) promoted by the International Monetary Fund (IMF) and the World Bank. SAPs have also resulted in significant macro-economic policy changes, public sector restructuring, and reduced social provisioning, with mostly negative effects on education, health, and social services for the poor. A review of available studies on structural adjustment and health in Africa for a WHO commission states: 'The majority of studies in Africa, whether theoretical or empirical, are negative towards structural adjustment and its effect on health outcomes' [30].

More recently, other instruments of globalization have further undermined the ability of governments of developing countries to provide health care for their populations (Box 8.2).

Box 8.2 WTO and TRIPS

The development of agreements under the World Trade Organization (WTO), notably the Agreement on Trade-Related Intellectual Property Rights (TRIPS) and its interpretation by powerful corporate interests and governments, have threatened to circumscribe countries' health policy options. The best known case relates to the legal battle around the attempt by South Africa to secure pharmaceuticals, especially for HIV/AIDS, at a reduced cost. In 1997 Nelson Mandela signed into legislation a law aimed at lowering drug prices through 'parallel importing', i.e. importing drugs from countries where they were sold at lower prices, and 'compulsory licensing', which would allow local companies to manufacture certain drugs, in exchange for royalties. Both provisions are legal under the TRIPS agreement as all sides have agreed that HIV/AIDS is an emergency. This was confirmed during the WTO meeting in Doha in 2001. The US administration did not bring its case to the WTO but instead, acting in concert with the multinational pharmaceutical corporations, brought a number of pressures (e.g. threats of trade sanctions and legal action) to bear on the South African government to rescind the legislation. This followed similar successful threats against Thailand and Bangladesh [31]. However, an uncompromising South African government, together with a vigorous campaign mounted by local and international AIDS activists and progressive health Non Governmental Organizations (NGOs), forced a climbdown by both the US government and the multinational pharmaceutical companies [32], resulting in a rare, but important, victory.

The provisions of the WTO, particularly TRIPS and the General Agreement on Trade in Services (GATS), hold many threats for the health of developing countries' economies and their citizens [33,34]. This was succinctly noted in a speech by President Museveni of Uganda: 'It [globalization] is the same old order with new means of control, new means of oppression, new means of marginalization'[35].

Reforming health sector governance

The rapidly changing economic policy environment has been accompanied by an equally unstable organizational and governance environment. The development of district health systems was followed in the early 1990s by the concept of health sector reform (HSR) which introduced a comprehensive framework for government health sector policy development, strategies, structures, and systems under conditions of increasing fiscal austerity. In most cases, the HSR package includes the following components [19,36]:

+ measures aimed at improving performance of the civil service;
+ decentralization of management responsibility and/or provision of health care to local level;
+ measures aimed at improving functioning of national ministries of health and broadening health financing options (e.g. user fees, insurance schemes, introduction of managed competition between providers of clinical and support services);
+ working with the private sector through contracting, regulating, and franchising different service providers.

Whereas decentralization of the management of health services to districts began in the 1980s, other components of HSR have been introduced more recently. To date 46 countries in SSA have embarked on HSR. The contexts and contents of their health reform programmes have varied from one country to another [33,36]. In Ghana for example, the key principles enunciated in the Medium Term Health Strategy revolved around improving equity of access to health services, improving the efficiency with which resources for health are allocated and utilized, improving the effectiveness and quality of interventions, and incorporating and coordinating all stakeholders, consumers, and service providers in decisions for prioritizing services and utilizing resources [37]. These principles partly respond to significant pressure to shift aspects of service delivery to NGOs and other private sector providers. However, their implementation has been piecemeal and of limited success in promoting greater health equity [37]. Furthermore, health reforms in SSA have been influenced largely by the poor performance of health systems, particularly with regard to the quality of health services [33].

Human resources for health: a key challenge

The deteriorating economic environment and unstable organizational context have also impacted very negatively on the health workforce, leading to deterioration in the quality of health care. Key problems in SSA include the following.

+ Inherited professional cadres and health care structures fashioned for Western health systems, which were inappropriate for African health needs.
+ Inability to build adequate capacity within ministries of health and health services to manage new strategies and systems in a constantly changing policy environment.

◆ Increasing workloads of health workers caused by fiscal constraints, exacerbated by governments attempting to meet the Highly Indebted Poor Countries (HIPC) completion point for debt repayment. This resulted in ceilings for public sector wage bills which were often accompanied by recruitment bans, restructuring of services, and the impact of the HIV/AIDS epidemic;

◆ Low productivity and motivation of health workers due to the above factors, leading to poor service delivery and high rates of absenteeism and migration out of the system.

Inappropriate professional cadres and structures

Africa suffers from very low ratios of health workers to population [38]. Furthermore, the orientation of many health professionals remains more appropriate to the service needs of wealthy countries and better-off populations. As in wealthy countries, public health remains a marginal area of professional health activity; the number of health personnel with any significant public health training is miniscule [39].

In many SSA countries, tertiary health facilities (teaching and specialist hospitals) have continued to retain a high proportion of the health budget. These general trends in resource allocation have contributed to a maldistribution of staff, who prefer to work in well-resourced tertiary care facilities and in urban areas. Eventually, as these facilities have also deteriorated, they have joined the brain drain into the private sector or to other countries [40].

To achieve better coverage of essential services of their populations, 'task shifting' is increasingly considered as a promising intervention for strengthening health service coverage by improving the strategic skill mix in national health-care systems. This is mainly achieved by two processes: (1) shifting tasks from one cadre of health care worker to an existing, often lower-level, cadre; (2) shifting tasks to a new cadre developed to meet specific health-care goals [40]. For example, countries such as Tanzania, Malawi, and Mozambique introduced country-specific cadres such as medical assistants/assistant medical officers and clinical officers to whom were delegated some of the tasks carried out by doctors. These cadres were better retained in rural areas and in primary health care services. Other countries such as Ethiopia developed cadres such as field surgeons to deal with the consequences of war who have been integrated into the health system. Despite the impact these cadres have made in improving the coverage of services in underserved areas, their training and development have often not received adequate investment [40].

Inability to develop appropriate capacity

Capacity problems have been experienced at various levels. Few health workers have had training in areas of public health such as health systems management at the district level (e.g. planning, budgeting, financial and human resource management, monitoring, and evaluation). For example, capacity problems have been blamed for the slow implementation of reforms in Ethiopia [41], necessitating use of external technical assistance. The WHO-supported 'Strengthening District Health Systems' initiative in Ghana and Zambia is one recent effort to bridge the gap between planning and implementation in districts. However, such initiatives have often highlighted the lack of supervisory support needed to sustain implementation.

Attempts have also been made to restructure ministries of health in order to prepare them to give better support to the operational levels. Despite restructuring efforts, human resource development and retention have suffered in many countries, blunting the implementation or achievement of health goals. Retention and motivation have become major issues for service delivery in Africa, and it is recognized that most reform initiatives have tackled human resources issues mainly from the viewpoint of reducing costs by cutting staffing levels. An independent review of the Zambian health reforms [42] noted that human resource issues were not treated as a major priority. The resulting increase in workload and the perceived shift of resources and patients to the private sector have exacerbated staff frustration.

The brain drain of health professionals

The haemorrhage of health professionals from their home countries is the single most serious problem facing African health ministries today. A recent study noted that 'international medical graduates constitute between 23 and 28 per cent of physicians in the United States, the United Kingdom, Canada, and Australia, and lower-income countries supply between 40 and 75 per cent of these international medical graduates'[43]. Disturbingly, nine of the 20 countries with the highest emigration factors are in SSA.

'Brain drain' occurs from low income countries both to wealthy countries and to relatively better-off middle-income countries. For example, South Africa, despite its own emigration problems, is the recipient of large numbers of doctors from other African countries. In 1999 it was noted that 20 per cent of doctors (approximately 6000) on the South African Medical Register were expatriates [44], and in 2002 it was reported that 50 per cent of doctors in Namibia were expatriates [45]. The brain drain has affected some countries very severely [46–48]. A 2003 WHO survey on the migration of health workers in the Africa Region reported that more than 30 per cent of the stock of doctors in source countries had emigrated to more 'developed' countries: health workers from the Democratic Republic of Congo worked in Canada and France, and also in Senegal and Cote d'Ivoire; doctors from Tanzania worked in the UK and the USA, and also in Botswana, Kenya, and Namibia [45].

The recipient countries of the 'brain drain' are mostly (rich) OECD countries that make significant savings by attracting professionals from low-income countries where remuneration packages remain insufficient to retain skilled staff. The United Nations Conference on Trade and Development (UNCTAD) has estimated that developed countries save US$ 184,000 in training costs for each professional aged 25–35 years [48]. In fact, evidence further suggests that recipient countries produce fewer health professionals than required/planned since they are certain that they can recruit from countries where push factors, including the workloads and despair associated with the HIV/AIDS epidemic, are significant [48,49] (Box 8.3). The savings for the wealthy countries are significant and in effect amount to poorer countries donating to richer countries, contributing to widening the gap between rich and poor countries. Agreements to manage the process and the numbers, as well as the involvement of the 'exporting' countries in the recruitment and selection process, are necessary to ameliorate the situation and ensure some remittance of earnings. The UK and South African governments recently signed a memorandum of understanding with strategies aimed at reducing the seepage of doctors from South Africa to the UK. However, the effectiveness of this agreement in limiting migration is questionable.

Box 8.3 HIV/AIDS and human resources in Africa

The HIV/AIDS epidemic sweeping the continent is affecting the health workforce significantly. These effects include reduction in trained personnel through death, as indicated by the higher than usual death rates among some health personnel in Malawi [40] as well as a reduction in human resource production capacity. Other effects expressed anecdotally include 'burn-out' and high rates of early leavers from the services, absenteeism to attend funerals, and illness, all of which are aggravated by the existing service conditions in many countries. A national survey of health personnel, patients, and facilities in South Africa conducted in 2002 showed that 15 per cent of health workers were living with HIV, 16.2 per cent had been treated for stress-related illnesses with two-thirds taking sick leave, and a third reported low work morale due to stressful working conditions, heavy patient workload, staff shortages, and low salaries [49].

Summary

Economic decline, structural adjustment, and health sector reform, combined with the consequences of the HIV epidemic and continued conflict in a number of countries, have adversely affected the capacity of SSA health systems to provide comprehensive health services for their populations. Health human resource requirements are unmet in terms of both coverage and relevant skills. Moreover, many SSA countries continue to be embroiled in conflicts resulting in complex emergencies which affect livelihoods and increase demand for health care, while health service delivery is disrupted.

Prospects for the future

Global Health Initiatives: opportunity and threat for SSA

In recognition of the growing global health divide between North and South and the crisis imposed by HIV/AIDS and the resurgence of tuberculosis and malaria in the South, development assistance models collectively described as Global Health Initiatives (GHIs) have emerged [50–52]. These include such initiatives as the US President's Emergency Plan for AIDS Relief (PEPFAR), the World Bank's Multi-country AIDS Programme (MAP), the Global Alliance for Vaccines and Immunization (GAVI), and the Global Fund to Fight AIDS, Tuberculosis and Malaria (GFATM).

Whilst these initiatives are a welcome source of new and substantial funding to cash-strapped Southern governments, the rationale for and effects of such new resources provided through these funding platforms need to be understood in the light of the mixed experience of health policy implementation over the past 20 years (outlined above). For example, not long after the inception of the GFATM, concern had arisen '… that this new public–private partnership fund would (yet again) be donor-led. As a result undue emphasis would be put on supplying drugs rather than building up capacity to implement and sustain effective treatment and preventive programmes' [50].

This view is reinforced by reviews of health systems in Africa which indicate that 'Programmes to tackle important diseases will not be sustainable in the long-run unless effective health services are in place. International aid should therefore support system development and improve the delivery of health services' [9]. These concerns are reminiscent of the critical response from within the Health for All movement to selective PHC, and are supported by worrying evidence concerning the sustainability of the selected child survival interventions which received external resources and for which great progress was achieved in the 1980s. A sustainable response to the considerable health challenges of SSA must include a development strategy which addresses the strengthening of seriously weakened health systems. It is encouraging that following GAVI's lead, a number of GHIs, including the GFATM, have agreed to allocate a higher proportion of their funds to 'health system development' [52].

Sector Wide Approaches as a mechanism to reduce donor imposition

Sector Wide Approaches (SWAps) are a response to the limitations of development assistance and the practical expression of partnerships between governments and donors. Their aim is twofold: first, to facilitate the efficiency of resource generation, allocation, and utilization; secondly, to improve the effectiveness of service delivery by encouraging governmental leadership of policy formulation and priority setting for the sector, recognition and involvement of all stakeholders in the sector (especially development partners) in policy development, implementation, and monitoring, and better coordination of all resources of the sector. SWAps particularly aim to give governments a stronger role in coordinating external support and allowing a sustained partnership between government and all its partners [53].

A number of countries (Burkina Faso, Ethiopia, Ghana, Mali, and Mozambique) have made progress in the development of comprehensive health plans which include clear targets for the medium term [54]. The ability of SWAps to respond better to national priorities will probably depend on the capacity and ability of countries to retain control of the process and to implement plans adequately and manage the allocated funds competently. In March 2005, over 100 countries committed to the Paris Declaration of increasing efforts in 'harmonisation, alignment and managing aid for results with a set of monitorable actions and indicators'. Of the 12 indicators identified for measuring these objectives, 11 had targets for 2010; the impact of attaining these on the SSA region remains to be seen.

A strategy for health systems development

Countries which have achieved the greatest and most durable improvements in health tend to be those with a commitment to equitable and broad-based development, and to health systems that are comprehensive and engage related sectors. Good empirical evidence for this comes from a number of countries, including some poor developing countries, for example the 'Good Health at Low Cost' models of Sri Lanka, China, Costa Rica, and Kerala State in India. These countries have demonstrated that investment in the social sectors, and particularly in women's education, health, and welfare, can have a significant positive impact on the health and social indicators of the whole population [25].

The World Bank's Poverty Reduction Strategy Papers (PRSPs) were introduced as the basis for financing comprehensive poverty reduction strategies in
HIPCs. PRSPs are aimed at strengthening country ownership of poverty reduction strategies, broadening representation of civil society in the design of strategies, and improving coordination among development partners so as to focus
the resources of the international community on achieving results in reducing
poverty. However, as Verheul and Rowson [55] suggest:

> Systems to collect data to monitor poverty reduction are crude, government policies
> fragmented, and public servants demoralized. Countries such as Rwanda do not have
> their own technical capacity to collect and analyze data, while the scant national budg-
> ets of Benin or Mali offer little real prospect of reform.

These are some of the challenges that confront initiatives such as Ghana's
Poverty Reduction Strategy (GPRS), Ethiopia's Sustainable Development and
Poverty Reduction Programme (SDPRP), Kenya's Economic Recovery Strategy
for Wealth and Employment Creation (ERS), Senegal's Poverty Reduction
Strategy Paper (PRSP), and Uganda's Poverty Eradication Action Plan
(PEAP).

The need for integrated and sustainable comprehensive health systems providing comprehensive health care is of continuing and pressing relevance to the
challenge of health development in SSA [56]. Comprehensive health care comprises curative and rehabilitative components to address health problems and
their effects, a preventive component to address the immediate and underlying
causative factors which operate at the level of the individual, and a promotional
component which addresses the more basic social determinants that require
intersectoral actions and, increasingly, actions to address global factors that
impact negatively on health determinants [57].

Approaches to programme development

The principles of comprehensive programme development apply to all health
problems, whether HIV, tuberculosis, diabetes mellitus, or malaria. Much
experience has been gained internationally in the development of comprehensive and integrated programmes to combat under-nutrition; these experiences
can provide useful lessons for other programmes [58].

The specific combination of actions making up a comprehensive programme
will vary from situation to situation. The inclusion of a set of efficacious health
service activities should constitute the core of a comprehensive control strategy, for example DOTS for tuberculosis, early treatment of sexually transmitted
diseases, anti-retroviral drugs for AIDS, promotion of condom usage and prevention of mother to child transmission for HIV, and effective prophylaxis and
treatment and impregnated bed-nets for malaria. For these activities to be

sustained they need to be embedded within functioning health systems and complemented by relevant health promotion policies and activities in health-related sectors (e.g. improved housing and nutrition for tuberculosis, increased female economic independence for HIV prevention [59], and environmental improvements for malaria).

The development of comprehensive and integrated health systems requires transformation of both management and practice. A broadening and deepening of public health competencies is urgently required. A key first step is capacity development through training and guided health systems research which must be practice-based and problem-oriented, and must draw upon and simultaneously re-orientate educational institutions and professional bodies [60]. The successful development of decentralized health systems will require targeted investment in infrastructure, personnel, and management and in information systems. For instance, in South Africa the University of the Western Cape developed a model Health Information System Programme (HISP) which was adopted by the Department of Health for implementation throughout the country after it proved successful in the districts of one province. The Ministries of Health of Mozambique, Malawi, and Ghana have also adopted the HISP. Similarly, the innovations undertaken in Tanzania through the Tanzania Effective Health Interventions Project (TEHIP) demonstrate the importance of health systems research in improving district health development and management [61].

Development of human resources

The WHO Regional Office for Africa views the development of human resources (HR) as a priority and developed the Regional Strategy for Development of Human Resources for Health in 1998 [62]. Countries have been assisted to develop HR plans and policies, and a number of tools, advocacy packs, and guidelines have been developed. Prioritizing HR development has been identified as a global target, as is evident from the activities of the Joint Learning Initiative [63] on human resources for health and subsequently the Global Health Workforce Alliance [64]. It demands the 'cooperation and shared intent between the public and private sector parties which fund and direct educational establishments; between those who plan and influence health service staffing; and between those able to make financial commitments to sustain or support the conditions of service of health workers' [65].

Conclusions

The shift in focus from selective disease-specific interventions to a more comprehensive health systems approach implies a shift in policy emphasis, time horizons, and scale and duration of investment. To secure sustained investment in the health and social sectors and the equity essential for a healthy society, evidence suggests that a strong organized demand for government responsiveness and accountability to social needs is crucial [66]. Tacit recognition of this important dynamic informed the Alma Ata call for strong community participation. To achieve and sustain the political will to meet all people's basic needs and to regulate the activities of the private sector, a process of participatory democracy, or at least a well-informed movement of civil society, is essential. 'Strong' community participation is important not only in securing greater government responsiveness to social needs but also in providing the active, conscious, and organized population so critical to the design, implementation, and sustainability of comprehensive health systems.

The new and substantial funding that has recently become available through GHIs presents an opportunity to African countries to mount a large-scale response to their health crises. However, unless these resources contribute to the development of infrastructure, human capacity, and management processes and are increasingly replaced by countries' own financing, which ultimately will depend on their fiscal health, the response is likely to have only a short-term impact on Africa's pressing health problems.

References

[1] Sanders DM, Todd C, Chopra M. Confronting Africa's health crisis: more of the same will not be enough. *BMJ* 2005; **331**: 755–8.

[2] UNAIDS. *Report on the Global AIDS Epidemic 2008*. Available online at: http://www.unaids.org/en/KnowledgeCentre/HIVData/GlobalReport/2008/2008_Global_report.asp

[3] UNHCR. *2006 Global Trends: Refugees, Asylum-seekers, Returnees, Internally Displaced and Stateless Persons*. Available online at: http://www.unhcr.org/statistics.html

[4] UNICEF. *State of the World's Children 2006: Excluded and Invisible*. New York: UNICEF, 2006. Available online at: http://www.unicef.org/sowc06/

[5] Frenk J, Bobadilla JL, Sepulveda J, Lopez Cervantes M. Health transition in middle-income countries: new challenges for health care. *Health Policy Plan* 1989; **4**: 29–39.

[6] Department of Health Medical Research Council, OrcMacro. South Africa Demographic and Health Survey 2003. Pretoria: Department of Health, 2007.

[7] King M (ed). *Medical Care in Developing Countries. A Symposium from Makerere*. Oxford: Oxford University Press, 1966.

[8] Addai E, Gaere L. Capacity-building and systems development for Sector-Wide Approaches (SWAps): the experience of the Ghana health sector. Lagos, Ghana: MOH and DFID, 2001 (unpublished).

[9] MDG Africa Steering Group. *Achieving the Millennium Development Goals in Africa: Recommendations of the MDG Africa Steering Group*. United Nations: New York, 2008. Available online at: http://www.mdgafrica.org/

[10] World Bank. *World Development Indicators 2006*. Washington, DC: World Bank, 2006. Available online at: http://devdata.worldbank.org/wdi2006/contents

[11] Collins J, Rau B. *AIDS in the Context of Development*. Programme on Social Policy and Development, Paper No. 4. Geneva: UNRISD, 2000.

[12] UNICEF. *State of the World's Children 1984*. Oxford University Press, 1983.

[13] UNICEF. *State of the World's Children 1994*. Oxford University Press, 1993.

[14] UNICEF. *State of the World's Children 2001. Early Childhood*. Oxford University Press, 2001.

[15] WHO/UNICEF. *Meeting the MDG Drinking Water and Sanitation Target: The Urban and Rural Challenge of the Decade*. Available online at: http://who.int/water_sanitation_health/monitoring/jmpfinal.pdf

[16] Iliffe J. *A Modern History of Tanganyika*. Cambridge: Cambridge University Press, 1979.

[17] Werner D, Sanders D. *Questioning the Solution: The Politics of Primary Health Care and Child Survival*. Palo Alto, CA: Healthwrights, 1997.

[18] Zwi A, Mills A. Health policy in less developed countries. *J Int Dev* 1995; 7: 302–3.

[19] Sanders D. PHC 21—Everybody's business. Main background paper for PHC 21—Everybody's Business: An International Meeting to Celebrate 20 Years after Alma Ata. *WHO Report WHO/EIP/OSD/00.7*. Geneva: WHO, 1998.

[20] Rifkin SB, Walt G. Why health improves: defining the issues concerning 'comprehensive primary health care' and 'selective primary health care'. *Soc Sci Med* 1986; 23: 559–66.

[21] Chopra M, Sanders D, McCoy D, Cloete K. Implementation of primary health care: Package or process? *SAMJ* 1998; 88: 1563–5.

[22] Arevshatian L, Clements CJ, Lwanga SK, *et al*. An evaluation of infant immunisation in Africa. Is a transformation in progress? *Bull WHO* 2007; 85: 421–500.

[23] World Bank. *Investing in Health. World Development Report*. Washington, DC: World Bank, 1993.

[24] Volmink J, Garner P. Systematic review of randomised controlled trials of strategies to promote adherence to tuberculosis treatment. *BMJ* 1997; 315: 1403–6.

[25] Halstead SB, Walsh JA, Warren K (eds). *Good Health at Low Cost*. New York: Rockefeller Foundation, 1985.

[26] Fitzroy H, Briend A, Fauveau V. Child survival: should the strategy be redesigned? Experience from Bangladesh. *Health Policy Plan* 1990; 5: 226–34.

[27] Hall AJ, Cutts FT. Lessons from measles vaccination in developing countries. *BMJ* 1993; 307:1293–5.

[28] Chopra M, Sanders D. Is growth monitoring worthwhile in South Africa? *SAMJ* 1997; 87: 875–8.

[29] Global Polio Eradication Initiative. *Global Case Count*. Available online at: http://www.polioeradication.org/casecount.asp

[30] Breman A, Shelton C. Structural adjustment and health: a literature review of the debate, its role players and the presented empirical evidence. *WHO Commission on Macroeconomics and Health Working Paper WG 6:6*. Geneva: WHO, 2001.

[31] Bond P. Globalisation, pharmaceutical pricing, and South African health policy: managing confrontation with US firms and politicians. *Int J Health Serv* 1999; 29: 765–92.

[32] Sidley P. Drug companies sue South African government over generics. *BMJ* 2001; 322: 447.

[33] Lambo E, Sambo LG. Health sector reform in sub-Saharan Africa: a synthesis of country experiences. *East Afr Med J* 2003; **80** (6 Suppl): S1–20.

[34] See http://www.globalexchange.org/campaigns/wto/OpposeWTO.html

[35] *SA Business Day*, 23 August 2000.

[36] Cassels A. Health Sector Reform: key issues in less developed countries. *J Int Dev* 1995; **7**: 338.

[37] Ministry of Health, Ghana. *Medium Term Strategic Framework for Health Development in Ghana 1996–2000*. Lagos, Ghana: Ministry of Health, 1995.

[38] Crisis in Human Resources for Health in the African Region. African Health Monitor, January–June, 2007. WHO Regional Office for Africa. http://www.afro.who.int/press/periodicals/healthmonitor/jan-jun2007.pdf (accessed 15 February 2009).

[39] Ijsselmuiden CB, Nchinda TC, Duale S, Tumwesigye NM, Serwadda D. Mapping Africa's advanced public health education capacity- the AfriHealth project. *Bull WHO* 2007; **85**: 914–22.

[40] Dovlo D. Using mid-level cadres as substitutes for internationally mobile health professionals in Africa: a desk review. *Hum Resour Health* 2004; **2**: 7.

[41] Foster M, Brown A, Norton A, Naschold F. *The Status of Sector Wide Approaches: Centre for Aid and Public Expenditure (CAPE)*. London: ODI, 2000.

[42] WHO/UNICEF/World Bank. *Independent Review of the Zambian Health Reforms*. Vol. 1: Main Report. Geneva: WHO/UNICEF/World Bank, 1996.

[43] Mullan F. The metrics of physician brain drain. *N Engl J Med* 2005; **353**: 1810–18.

[44] Commonwealth Secretariat. *Migration of Health Workers from Commonwealth Countries. Experiences and Recommendations for Action*. London: Commonwealth Secretariat, 2001.

[45] WHO. *Survey on Migration of Health Workers in the African Region*. Brazzaville: WHO Regional Office for Africa, 2003.

[46] Dovlo D, Nyonator F. Migration of graduates of the Ghana Medical School: a preliminary rapid appraisal. *Hum Resour Health Dev J* 1999; **3**: 40–51

[47] Bach S. International mobility of health professionals: brain drain or brain exchange? *UNU-WIDER Research Paper No. 2006/82*. Available online at: http://www.wider.unu.edu/publications/rps/rps2006/rp2006-82.pdf

[48] Meeus W. 'Pull' factors in the international migration of health professionals, an analysis of developed countries' policies influencing migration of health professionals. Cited in: Sanders D, Lloyd B (2005) Human resources: international context. In: Ijumba P, Barron P, (eds). *South African Health Review 2005*. Durban: Health Systems Trust, 2005; pp 76–87. Available online at: www.hst.org.za/publications/682 (accessed 17 December 2007).

[49] Shisana O., Hall E., Maluleke KR., et al. The Impact of HIV/AIDS on the Health Sector. National Survey of Health Personnel, Ambulatory and Hospitalized Patients and Health Facilities, 2002. Cape Town: Human Sciences Research Council, 2003. Available online at: www.hsrcpublishers.co.za

[50] Richards T. The new global health fund (editorial). *BMJ* 2001; **322**: 1321–2.

[51] Hanefeld J, Spicer N, Brugha R, Walt G. *How Have Global Health Initiatives Impacted on Health Equity?* Health Systems Knowledge Network. Available online at: http://www.who.int/social_determinants/resources/csdh_media/global_health_initiatives_2007_en.pdf (accessed 17 December 2007).

[52] WHO. *Opportunity for Global Health Initiatives in The Health System Action Agenda*. Working Paper No. 4. Geneva: WHO/EIP/healthsystems/2006.1, 2006.

[53] Cassels A. *A Guide to Sector-Wide Approaches for Health Development. Concepts, Issues and Working Arrangements*. Geneva: WHO/ARA/97. 12, 1997.

[54] Dubbeldam R., Bijlmakers L. *Sector-Wide Approaches for Health Development. Dutch Experiences in International Co-Operation*. The Hague: Netherlands Ministry of Foreign Affairs, 1999.

[55] Verheul E, Rowson M. Poverty reduction strategy papers. It's too soon to say whether this new approach to aid will improve health. *BMJ* 2001; **323**: 120.

[56] WHO/UNICEF. *Report of the International Conference on Primary Health Care. Alma-Ata, USSR*, 6–12 September 1978. Geneva: WHO.

[57] Labonte R, Schrecker T. *Globalisation and Social Determinants of Health: Analytic and Strategic Review Paper 2006*. Available online at: http://www.who.int/social_determinants/resources/globalization.pdf

[58] Mason JB, Sanders D, Musgrove P, Soekirman, Galloway R. 2006 Community health and nutrition programs. In: Jamison DT, Breman JG, Measham AR, *et al.* (eds). *Disease Control Priorities in Developing Countries* (2nd edn). Oxford University Press/World Bank, 2006; pp. 1053–1074.

[59] Pronyk PM, Hargreaves JR, Kim JC, *et al.* Effect of a structural intervention for the prevention of intimate-partner violence and HIV in rural South Africa: a cluster randomised trial. *Lancet* 2006; **368**: 1973–83.

[60] Sanders D, Chopra M, Lehmann U, Heywood A. Meeting the challenge of Health for All through Public Health Education: a response from the University of the Western Cape. *SAMJ* 2001; **91**: 823–9.

[61] de Savigny D, Kasale H, Mbuya C, Reid G. *FixingHealth Systems*. Ottawa: International Development Research Centre, 2004.

[62] WHO. *Regional Strategy for the Development of Human Resources for Health. AFR/RC48/10*. Harare: WHO Regional Office for Africa, 1998.

[63] Joint Learning Initiative. *Human Resources for Health. Overcoming the Crisis*. Cambridge, MA: Global Health Initiative/Harvard University Press, 2004.

[64] Global Health Workforce Alliance. *Strategic Plan*. Geneva: WHO, 2006.

[65] WHO. *The World Health Report 2006: Working Together for Health*. Geneva: WHO, 2006.

[66] Mosley H. In: Halstead SB, Walsh JA, Warren K (eds). *Good Health at Low Cost*. New York: Rockefeller Foundation, 1985.

Annex 1

Changes in health indicators, Sub Saharan Africa:

	Under–5 mortality rate		Infant mortality rate		Life expectancy at birth (years)		
	1990	2005	1990	2005	1970	1999	2005
Angola	260	260	154	154	37	48	41
Benin	185	150	111	89	43	54	55
Botswana	58	120	45	87	52	45	34
Burkina Faso	210	191	113	96	39	45	48
Burundi	190	190	114	114	44	43	44
Cameroon	139	149	85	87	44	54	46
Cape Verde	60	35	45	26	57	70	71
Central African Republic	168	193	102	115	42	45	39
Chad	201	208	120	124	38	48	44
Comoros	120	71	88	53	48	60	64
Congo	110	108	83	81	46	49	53
Congo, Democratic Republic of the	205	205	129	129	45	52	44
Côte d'Ivoire	157	195	103	118	44	47	46
Djibouti	175	133	116	88	40	51	53
Equatorial Guinea	170	205	103	123	40	51	42
Eritrea	147	78	88	50	43	51	55
Ethiopia	204	164	131	109	40	44	48
Gabon	92	91	60	60	44	52	54
Gambia	151	137	103	97	36	48	57
Ghana	122	112	75	68	49	61	57
Guinea	240	150	145	98	37	47	54
Guinea-Bissau	253	200	153	124	36	45	45
Kenya	97	120	64	79	50	51	48
Lesotho	101	132	81	102	48	54	34
Liberia	235	235	157	157	46	50	42
Madagascar	168	119	103	74	45	58	56
Malawi	221	125	131	79	40	40	40

	Under–5 mortality rate		Infant mortality rate		Life expectancy at birth (years)		
	1990	2005	1990	2005	1970	1999	2005
Mali	250	218	140	120	42	54	48
Mauritania	133	125	85	78	43	54	53
Mauritius	23	15	21	13	62	72	73
Mozambique	235	145	158	100	42	42	42
Namibia	86	62	60	46	47	48	46
Niger	320	256	191	150	38	49	45
Nigeria	230	194	120	100	43	50	44
Rwanda	173	203	103	118	44	41	44
Sao Tome and Principe	118	118	75	75	–	–	63
Senegal	148	136	90	77	41	53	56
Seychelles	19	13	17	12	–	–	–
Sierra Leone	302	282	175	165	34	39	41
Somalia	225	225	133	133	40	48	47
South Africa	60	68	45	55	53	52	46
Sudan	120	90	74	62	43	56	57
Swaziland	110	160	78	110	46	61	30
Tanzania, United Republic of	161	122	102	76	45	48	46
Togo	152	139	88	78	44	49	55
Uganda	160	136	93	79	46	42	49
Zambia	180	182	101	102	46	41	38
Zimbabwe	80	132	53	81	50	43	37

Sources: UNICEF, *State of the World's Children* 1984 [12], 1994 [13], 2001 [14], 2005 [4].

Chapter 9

Public health in China: history and contemporary challenges

Liming Lee and Jun Lv

Introduction

Over the past 50 years China has made great progress in the prevention and control of communicable diseases, far in excess of what would have been expected at its stage of economic development. Demographic transitions have taken place in most of the cities and economically developed areas in China and the society has evolved from its historical norm in which young people made up the majority, to a society with a rapid increase in the middle-aged and elderly populations.

China now faces serious new public health challenges. While the 'older infectious diseases' are still prevalent in most parts of China, particularly in the economically underdeveloped areas, new infectious diseases, such as HIV/AIDS, severe acute respiratory syndrome (SARS), and human cases of avian influenza (H5N1), are threatening public health. As China develops into an ageing society, chronic non-communicable diseases (NCDs) now form the majority of the disease burden. Injuries and mental health issues also pose a tremendous economic and social burden for the Chinese people. Rapid development with industrialization and urbanization has resulted in inevitable negative effects on the health of the Chinese people. Health inequalities are widening. The maintenance of vaccination programmes and primary health care has become more difficult in poor and remote areas.

In this chapter, we briefly review the history of public health in China, discuss the emerging challenges, describe some of the responses to these public health challenges, and outline the prospects for public health in China.

History and development of public health in China

Prevention is an integral part of traditional Chinese medicine which considers two aspects of disease states: pathogenic factors and body resistance. In giving priority to strengthening body resistance, conventional wisdom encourages a regular life, a healthy diet, exercise, and harmony in mental and emotional activities. There is an ancient Chinese philosophy that encourages prevention: the best doctors care for people without sickness.

Western medicine was introduced into China by Christian missionaries in the 1830s. The establishment of the Peking Union Medical College (PUMC) in 1917 by the Rockefeller Foundation provided the base for educating the new elite in Western medicine. In 1921, a public health department was established within PUMC with the aim of providing epidemiological data and a focus for population-based health care [1]. Between 1932 and 1937 Professor Chen Zhi-qian (C.C. Chen), a medical graduate of PUMC working in Ding County, established an early example of public health activities integrated with the primary health-care system [2]. The public health practice in Ding County included health education, establishment of a health-care system, environmental health, immunization, maternal and child health, diet and nutrition, and family planning.

Health reforms after 1950

In 1949, China faced the daunting task of post-war infrastructure reconstruction, a severe shortage of resources, and the threat of bacteriological warfare. China formed a social movement called the Patriotic Health Campaign (PHC), which included elimination of rats, sanitary construction, clearing the environment, and sewage disposal. As a part of the early PHC, the government declared war on 'four pests': flies, mosquitoes, mice, and sparrows. People were instructed to clean their houses, schools, and workplaces, as well as to practise personal hygiene techniques every day. The PHC, together with the 'barefoot doctor' system described below, successfully controlled many serious epidemics of communicable diseases, such as cholera, plague, and malaria [3,4]. These campaigns continued throughout the 1960s and 1970s as the dominant form of public health intervention.

In the 1950s, China adopted the public health system of the former Soviet Union, setting up epidemic prevention stations (EPSs) all over the country and establishing public health schools separate from medical schools. Core public health activities included epidemic prevention and infectious disease control, occupational health and safety, environmental health, food hygiene, school health, radiation protection, health inspection, public health laboratory services, and health education. The responsibility for NCD prevention and control was added to the work of the EPSs in the mid-1990s.

The rural health service revolution

Chairman Mao Zedong, in his 'Directive on Public Health', on 26 June 1965, said that the title of the Ministry of Health should be changed to the 'Ministry of Urban Health', or 'Ministry of Health for Pampered Urbanites', as urban dwellers, constituting only 15 per cent of the population, had become the main beneficiaries of the existing system of health care. He stressed the importance of improving the state of health and hygiene in the countryside and decided that a third of the medical workers and administrators from the cities should start working in the rural areas to improve hygiene and reverse the situation where the large peasant population had no access to medical services or medicine. To implement Mao's 'June 26 directive' by training medical workers to serve the vast rural population, large numbers of substandard medical staff or health professionals with perceived political problems were dispatched to the countryside.

Before national economic reform started in 1978, the communes in rural China provided health care through a three-tier system that was managed and financed locally (Box 9.1). After economic reforms in the rural areas, this health-care system collapsed as the system of communes collapsed [5]. Starting in 1993, the Chinese government tried to partly re-establish the system. A rural

Box 9.1 Early organization of rural health

The part-time barefoot doctors in health clinics, as the first tier in the rural health system, provided preventive and primary care:

- administering the water and sewage systems;
- making improvements in wells, toilets, livestock areas, stoves and environment; giving vaccinations;
- controlling infectious diseases;
- collecting information on epidemics;
- providing simple medical treatment and temporary medical rescue.

For more serious illnesses, they referred patients to the second-tier commune health centres, which might have 10–30 beds and an out-patient clinic serving a population of 10,000–25,000 and which were staffed by junior doctors. The most seriously ill patients were referred by the commune health centres to the third-tier county hospitals staffed with senior doctors. The 'cooperative medical system' (CMS) that organized the barefoot doctors and provided other medical services to the rural population was part of the commune system and was financed by the communes' welfare funds. Thus the CMS served the dual role of a supplier and a collector of insurance funds for the farmers to pay for the services. This system ensured access to basic health care among the rural population.

health financing system, known as the New Cooperative Medical System (NCMS), was re-established in 2003.

Recent initiatives in public health

In January 2002, the Chinese Centre for Disease Control and Prevention (China CDC), based on the Chinese Academy of Preventive Medicine (CAPM), was officially established. It filled the vacancy of a national institute of disease control and prevention and was a key step in building a new type of national system for disease control and prevention. The task of the China CDC embodies the notion of comprehensive profiles of human health and is compatible with the international standard to prevent and control the following three groups of diseases identified by the WHO:

- communicable diseases, maternal and perinatal conditions, and nutritional deficiencies
- non-communicable conditions
- injuries.

From the viewpoint of population dynamics, preventing and controlling diseases must cover various groups in the population from birth to death, with emphasis on women and children, working-age population, ageing population, and the medically vulnerable (disabled and migrant) to ensure prevention and health-care services at all stages of life [6]. In addition, the new institution also inherited the traditional areas of health protection through the working of the five public health services which were copied from the former Soviet Union:

- occupational health
- environmental hygiene
- nutrition and food safety
- school health
- radiation health and safety.

A four-tier network of disease control services (national, province, city, and county) was also established and managed at different levels.

Challenges for public health in China

Ageing of the population

The doubling of life expectancy from 35.0 years before 1949 to 74.0 for women and 71.0 for men in 2005 [7] highlights health improvements in China. In the past 50 years, the Chinese population has rapidly expanded in size, increasing from 594 million in 1953 [8] to 1.323 billion in 2005 [7], despite the implementation

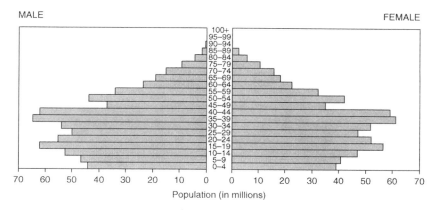

MALE

FEMALE

Population (in millions)

Fig. 9.1 China's population pyramid in 2007 (Source: U.S. Census Bureau, International Data Base.)

of the one-child policy since the 1970s. China's population pyramid in 2007 (Fig. 9.1) shows that the base is much smaller than the middle-aged group and reflects the very low fertility level reported in China today. In contrast, the upper end of China's age distribution has increased in both absolute number and in its relative proportion of the total population in the past 50 years, reflecting the combination of low fertility and improvements in longevity [9].

China has become an ageing society with 78.6 per cent of the population over the age of 15 years. By the end of 2004, there were 143 million people over 60 years old, accounting for 11 per cent of the total population [10]. Although the Chinese population is currently younger than those of many Western European countries and the USA, its aging process will accelerate and surpass their speed of ageing [9]. China is facing a much more compressed timetable in dealing with the ageing process and its associated challenges.

The issue of population ageing has been considered by the Chinese government. In October 1999, the China National Working Commission on Ageing (CNWCA) was established as an advisory and coordinating organization of the State Council. CNWCA consists of 26 members, including most of the government ministries [11]. The government focused on:

- developing and improving policies and legislative systems for elderly;
- establishing a social security system for elderly people, medical security, social relief, and social welfare;
- speeding up the construction of infrastructure that could benefit the lives of elderly people;
- developing a socialized service for the elderly.

Although the government has paid significant attention to the ageing problem, it will be a long road from government documents and pilot testing to daily practice.

Increasing burden of non-communicable diseases

Since 1949, the mortality rates from communicable diseases, maternal and perinatal conditions, and nutritional deficiencies have fallen dramatically. This achievement, together with the improvement in longevity, revealed the contribution of chronic NCDs to the overall disease burden. Table 9.1 shows the leading causes of death in China 2006 [12] based on the mortality surveillance system. Chronic NCDs accounted for an estimated 79 per cent of the estimated 10.3 million deaths in 2005, and 70 per cent of the total disability-adjusted life years (DALYs) lost [13]. The major causes of death in China are cardiovascular disease (32 per cent of deaths, 13 per cent of DALYs lost), cancer (20 per cent of deaths, 11 per cent of DALYs lost), and chronic respiratory disease (17 per cent of deaths, 7 per cent of DALYs lost) [13].

The economic consequences of NCDs for China are serious. In 2006, the estimated losses because of coronary heart disease, stroke, and diabetes (reported in 2005) was US$1 billion. If no preventive action is taken up to 2015, the accumulated losses in GDP between 2006 and 2015 may be as much as US$14 billion, representing a loss of around 0.1 per cent of the projected GDP for this period. This amount is substantial considering that it has not included all chronic diseases [14].

Table 9.1 Leading causes of death in China, 2006 (crude rates per 100,000 and percentage of all deaths)

	City			County	
Cause	Mortality (1/100,000)	Percentage	Cause	Mortality (1/100,000)	Percentage
1. Malignant neoplasm	144.6	27.3	1. Malignant neoplasm	130.2	25.1
2. Cerebrovascular disease	93.7	17.7	2. Cerebrovascular disease	105.5	20.4
3. Heart disease	90.7	17.1	3. Respiratory disease	84.9	16.4
4. Respiratory diseases	69.3	13.1	4. Heart disease	71.8	13.9
5. Injury & poisoning	32.4	6.1	5. Injury & poisoning	46.1	8.9

Source: Ministry of Health, PRC, 2007

The prevalence of common causes of non-communicable diseases

Tobacco use

China is the largest tobacco producer and consumer in the world, accounting for more than a third of the global total on both counts. The production and sale of tobacco in China increased significantly between 1949 and 2006 and the increase is continuing. The National Nutrition and Health Survey in 2002 showed that the smoking prevalence among Chinese adults aged 18 years and older was 25.8 per cent (men, 53.9 per cent; women, 3.1 per cent) [15]. There are more than 350 million smokers in China, and about 540 million Chinese, two-thirds of whom are children under 15 years, suffer the effects of passive smoking [16].

Tobacco use poses a significant economic burden in terms of both direct costs such as health care and indirect costs related to productivity losses resulting from disease, disability and premature death, passive smoking, fires, and environmental pollution. According to the China Centre for Economic Research [17], Chinese smokers cost the national economy at least RMB 250 billion (US$35 billion) in 2005. This is likely to be an underestimate because of the paucity of available data. The profit from the production and sale of tobacco in 2005 was RMB 240 billion, suggesting that the social costs of smoking are higher than the revenue obtained.

China signed the WHO Framework Convention on Tobacco Control (FCTC) in November 2003 and ratified the convention in October 2005. However, without strong government leadership to implement the FCTC provisions, it will be difficult to reduce tobacco use. In China, tobacco is perceived as an important source of income for the government, generating about RMB 388 billion (US$53.5 billion) from profits and taxes in 2007, and accounting for about 8 per cent of the country's fiscal revenues [18]. At the regional level, particularly in the tobacco-dependent provinces such as Yunnan and Guizhou, tobacco production has played a very important role in government finance and provincial development.

WHO has introduced the MPOWER package of six proven policies, including monitoring tobacco use and prevention policies, protecting people from tobacco smoke, offering help to smokers who want to quit tobacco use, warning about the dangers of tobacco, enforcing bans on tobacco advertising, promotion, and sponsorship, and raising taxes on tobacco [19]. China is falling behind expectations in most of these areas (Box 9.2).

Changes in dietary patterns and nutrition status

Rapid economic growth in China over the past 20 years has led to dramatic improvements in the nation's nutrition and health status. Parallel with rising

Box 9.2 Cost of cigarettes in China

There are about 224 different brands of cigarettes, with a retail cigarette pack price range for popular brands of RMB2–40. The large number of brands and the large price differences provide substantial scope for smokers to switch type of cigarettes rather than adjusting the quantity consumed in response to changes in price. For this reason it is possible that increasing cigarette prices may no longer be an effective policy tool [20]. Apart from failing to reduce consumption, such a measure might be counterproductive if, as seems likely, lower-quality cigarettes are more harmful to health. One solution would be progressive increases of the price of all cigarettes. The price of the most popular brand is 1.92 international dollars, and only 3 per cent of the annual per capita income is needed to buy 100 packs [19].

consumption of meat, poultry, eggs, and other animal products, China has achieved a sharp decline in all indicators of under-nutrition. Nevertheless, about 14.3 per cent of China's children under 5-years-old are stunted and 7.8 per cent are underweight [21].

However, China is also facing a major new public health problem of over-nutrition. There has been a marked transition from a predominantly cereal-based diet to a diet high in saturated fat, animal source foods, sugar, and refined foods (i.e. increased 'energy density' of diet) over the past 20 years. The changes in dietary patterns are not limited to urban areas, or to wealthier strata of the population. Research in China has found increasing intakes of animal foods and oils in large rural regions. Thus, China is one of a growing number of developing countries facing what has been dubbed 'the double burden of malnutrition', i.e. persistence of under-nutrition together with a rapid rise in over-nutrition.

Table 9.2 shows the major dietary sources of energy and proteins in the Chinese population in 2002 [21]. Grains accounted for almost half of all the sources of energy in the urban population and 61 per cent in the rural population. The daily mean percentage of calories from total fat is higher in urban areas than in rural areas [21]. Pork is still the major animal protein source among the Chinese. The consumption of other sources of protein (e.g. beef, lamb, poultry, fish, dairy products, and beans) remains low.

Physical inactivity

According to the National Nutrition and Health Survey in 2002, three different levels of occupational activity, i.e. light, moderate, and vigorous intensity, each

Table 9.2 Major dietary sources of energy in the Chinese population, 2002

	Total	Urban	Rural
Percentage of calories from foods (%)			
Grains	57.9	48.5	61.4
Potatoes	2.0	1.4	2.2
Beans	2.6	2.7	2.6
Animal food	12.7	17.6	10.8
Pure energy-rich foods (e.g., oils, sugar)	17.2	19.3	16.4
Percentage of calories from key nutrient (%)			
Total fat	29.6	35.0	27.5
Percentage of protein from foods (%)			
Animal food	25.3	35.8	21.3

accounted for about a third of energy expenditure among Chinese adults. More than half the workers sit or stand during most of their working time [22]. Women still do the majority of housework; Chinese women spend 2.5 hours and men 0.7 hours each day on domestic tasks [22]. The estimate for the prevalence of regular leisure-time physical activity among urban Chinese adults aged 18 years and over was 15.1 per cent [15]. Young adults are less physically active than the elderly.

The number of motor vehicles in China, especially privately owned vehicles, has increased rapidly. In March 2007, there were about 0.11 billion privately owned motor vehicles in China, accounting for 76 per cent of the total. There are about 0.15 billion motor vehicle drivers in China. As urbanization and technological expansion continue, the commuting patterns shift from active commuting on foot or bicycle to more passive forms of motorized transportation [22].

Some intermediate risk factors

Between 1992 and 2002, the prevalence of overweight and obesity increased in all gender and age groups and in all geographical areas of China. Based on the WHO body mass index (BMI) cut-off points (i.e. obesity defined as BMI ≥ 30 kg/m^2 and overweight as $25 \leq$ BMI < 30 kg/m^2), the combined prevalence of overweight and obesity increased from 15 to 22 per cent in adults aged ≥ 18 years. The Chinese obesity standard (i.e. obesity defined as BMI ≥ 28 kg/m^2 and overweight as $24 \leq$ BMI < 28 kg/m^2) shows an increase from 20 to 30 per cent. The annual rate of increase was highest in men aged 18–44 years and women aged 45–59 years [23]. In general, men, urban residents, and high-income groups showed the greatest increase.

The prevalence of hypertension (140/90 mmHg or above or on treatment) increased overall from 14.4 per cent in 1991 to 18.8 per cent in 2002 among adults aged ≥18 years; in adults aged 35–74 years, it increased from 19.7 to 28.6 per cent [23]. The prevalence of dyslipidemia (i.e. hypercholesteraemia, hypertriglyceridaemia, low HDLC, or mixed) was 18.6 per cent. The prevalence of impaired fasting glucose and diabetes mellitus among people aged ≥18 years was 1.9 per cent and 2.6 per cent, respectively [21].

Prevention of non-communicable diseases

The prevention of NCDs in China dates back to the end of the 1950s. The preventive practices at an early stage were mainly spontaneous developments by medical doctors and scientific researchers. These practices gradually developed from hospital-based secondary and tertiary measures (e.g. early diagnosis and treatment) to community-based primary measures (e.g. health education). Most of these activities were research oriented. Government did not play a role in NCDs prevention until the middle of 1990s. A specific Division of Non-communicable Disease Control and Management was established in the Ministry of Health in 1995, and the National Centre for Chronic and Noncommunicable Diseases Control and Prevention was established in China CDC in 2002. As one of most important aspects of government initiatives, the Division of NCDs organized a National NCDs Comprehensive Community-Based Intervention Demonstration Program (1997–2002) to search for suitable strategies, measures, and models to prevent NCDs in China. Up until 2002, 31 communities successively became demonstration sites, covering 27 provinces throughout China. Unfortunately, this programme became inactive after 2002 because of lack of funding. Currently, the Ministry of Health is promoting the National Healthy Lifestyle Initiative (2007–2015). In addition, some professional societies have recently published Chinese guidelines on the prevention and treatment of hypertension, dyslipidaemia, overweight and obesity, and Chinese dietary guidelines.

Efforts to control NCDs are still scattered and mainly operate on a piecemeal basis despite the huge potential for prevention (Box 9.3). Most of the local Centres for Disease Control and Prevention (CDCs) lack adequate sustained funding for routine NCDs prevention and control work. The focus of various measures has been on proximal determinants of health and what can be undertaken by the health sector, rather than on the more complex issues of the broader social forces that also affect health. Government underplays its key role of ensuring collaborative action in favour of individual-oriented effort, and the health sector continues to focus on immediate issues pertaining to health care. Lack of a coherent policy and a legal framework impedes the

Box 9.3 Preventing 9 million NCD deaths

The potential for prevention of chronic diseases in China is huge, and is a vital and highly cost-effective investment. Asaria *et al.* [24] selected two interventions: reduce the salt intake in the population by 15 per cent and implement four key elements of the WHO Framework Convention on Tobacco Control (FCTC). They showed that, over 10 years (2006–2015), 4.5 million deaths could be prevented by implementing these interventions, at a cost of less than $0.20 per person per year (as of 2005), equivalent to 0.9 per cent of government spending on health. Lim et al [25] showed that an opportunistic screening-based multidrug regimen for the prevention of cardiovascular disease in high-risk individuals could prevent almost 4.8 million deaths in China over the next 10 years. This intervention alone could prevent almost a fifth of deaths from cardiovascular disease. The 10-year financial resources needed to scale up this intervention would be equivalent to an annual cost of about $1 per head.

sustainable development of NCDs prevention efforts. In addition, one crisis after another (e.g. SARS, human *Streptococcus suis*, hand–foot–mouth disease, earthquakes) has gained attention at the expense of chronic disease prevention. A national policy and relevant legislation is urgently required in order to prevent and control chronic NCDs.

The persistence of communicable diseases

Despite achievements in the control of communicable diseases, China still faces challenges. In 2006, viral hepatitis and pulmonary tuberculosis ranked as the top two most commonly reported communicable diseases [12] in China.

Viral hepatitis

Viral hepatitis, especially hepatitis B, is one of most prevalent communicable diseases and causes huge economic and social burdens in China. The overall prevalence of HBsAg is 9.1 per cent [26], and 30 million people have chronic (lifelong) infections [27]. These chronically infected persons are at high risk of death from cirrhosis of the liver and liver cancer, which kill about 0.3 million people annually [27]. HBsAg is preventable with safe and effective vaccines. In 2002, China added hepatitis B as a routine childhood immunization. However, the disease burden in current adults will remain for a long time.

Tuberculosis

China is one of 22 countries with high rates of tuberculosis (TB), with the total number of cases ranking second in the world after India. In 2005, 1,319,328 people developed TB (100 per 100,000), of whom 593,311 were smear-positive (45 per 100,000). There were 2,736,852 (208 per 100,000) people living with TB in 2005 and the TB mortality rate was about 16 per 100,000 [28]. China reached the global TB targets of 70 per cent case detection and 85 per cent treatment success by the end of 2005, but must now determine how to sustain these achievements and ensure the quality of TB services throughout the country. In addition, there is an urgent need to scale up the management of multi-drug-resistant tuberculosis (MDR-TB). China must also confront the challenge of TB among internal migrants, ensuring that all patients are diagnosed, treated, and reported.

HIV/AIDS

In January 2006, the Chinese government, together with WHO and UNAIDS, jointly estimated that at the end of 2005 there were approximately 650,000 people living with HIV/AIDS in China (range, 540,000–760,000), and an estimated 75,000 of these were living with AIDS (range, 65,000–85,000). In 2005, there were an estimated 70,000 new HIV infections (range, 60,000–80,000) and an estimated 25,000 AIDS deaths (range, 20,000–30,000) [29]. The majority of people living with HIV still do not know their status [29]. New HIV cases are being transmitted primarily through intravenous drug use and sex. The HIV/AIDS epidemic continues to rise in China and is spreading from high-risk groups to the general population.

Emerging diseases

In 2003, the SARS epidemic showed that a new or unfamiliar pathogen would have profound national and international implications for public health and socio-economic security. China identified the first SARS case and reported about two-third of the global cases. While there is still much to learn about SARS, traditional public health interventions (e.g. surveillance, quarantine, and isolation, together with social mobilization techniques used during the Patriotic Health Campaign) played a significant role in containing its spread. SARS disappeared as quickly as it appeared—next came avian influenza. The possibility of avian influenza changing and infecting humans has given rise to the fear of a new human influenza pandemic. By the end of February 2008, China had confirmed 27 human cases of avian influenza, of whom 17 died [30]. Although this epidemic was less severe than that in some Southeast Asian countries, the most important question is whether China is sufficiently prepared to handle a potential epidemic in the future, even with traditional public health interventions.

Other diseases

The performance of the Expanded Programme on Immunization (EPI) for other routine vaccine preventable diseases is declining. Vaccination coverage no longer continues to increase as expected. Some regions are showing a decrease and no longer attain the goal of >85 per cent coverage. As with NCDs, one of the most important reasons is inadequate financial support from the government, in striking contrast with the attention paid to TB, HIV/AIDS, and some emerging diseases.

Mental health and injury issues

For a long time mental health and injury issues were at the periphery of and separate from public health practice. In 2002, 'Long-term (2002–2010) Planning for Mental Health Prevention and Control in China' was issued by the Ministry of Health, the Ministry of Civil Affairs, the Ministry of Public Security, and the China Disabled Persons' Federation. In 2004, a 'Directive Opinions on Strengthening Mental Health Prevention and Control' was issued by these four sectors and the Ministries of Education, Justice, and Finance. In 2007, the Ministry of Health released 'Report on Injury Prevention in China'. These reports indicate that these two issues have gradually been recognized by the Government. However, they still need more public health action and resource investment.

Mental health

Poor family environment and social ethos, inappropriate education style, unhealthy media function, and increasing pressures to study have encouraged the development of a 'psychologically fragile generation'. The main mental health problems are learning problems, emotional problems (such as unstable mood, depression), moral character problems (such as discipline-violating behaviour, crimes), smoking, heavy drinking, and drug abuse [31,32]. A survey of adolescent mental health in 22 provinces showed that approximately 13 per cent of Chinese adolescents had apparent mental and behavioural problems. The prevalence rate among students in elementary school and high school was 22–32 per cent. The prevalence rate among college students was 16–25 per cent. These rates have been increasing in recent years [33].

Pressure due to intense social competition and family responsibility are major challenges to psychological tolerance, especially for women. Suicide is a health problem among young adults in China. China is one of the few countries where suicide rates are higher among women than among men [34], particularly in rural areas. City women, in contrast with rural women, reported more negative moods and subjective discomfort which greatly affected their quality of life.

When reaching old age, more and more people live with chronic illness. Meanwhile, life events that influence mental health also occur more often. These events include severe disease and self-trauma, retirement, unemployment, economic difficulty, severe illness of family members, emigration of family members, loss of spouse, and family conflict. Women have a survival advantage but no health advantage over men. A survey on elderly support systems in rural areas of nine provinces in China showed that two-thirds of women had lost their spouse, compared with less than a quarter of men [35].

Injury

Injury is the fifth leading cause of death overall and the leading cause of death in the age group below 45 years [36]. With motor vehicle production tripling in the past decade, motor vehicle crashes have become the leading cause of deaths due to injury, followed by suicide, drowning, poisoning, and falls. These five causes account for 70 per cent of injury-related deaths. It is estimated that each year in China, injury claims about 0.70–0.75 million lives, 9 per cent of all deaths, and results in 62 million hospital admissions [37]. The annual productive years of life lost (PPYLL) because of injuries is 12.6 million, more than for any disease group; this is equivalent to the loss of 12.6 million labourers per year, which is more than the total number of new entrants to the labour force each year (9.7 million) [36]. The estimated annual economic cost of injury is about RMB 65 billion (US$9 billion) for direct costs such as health care and RMB 6 billion for indirect costs related to productivity losses. Despite the importance of injury as a public health problem in China, few resources have been deployed to support injury prevention and control programmes.

Impact of urbanization and industrialization

Environmental pollution

China is paying a heavy environmental price for its progress in industrialization. According to the Worldwatch Institute's *State of the World 2006* report, acidification now affects some 30 per cent of China's cropland, and the estimated damage to farms, forests, and human health is US$13 billion. China has just 8 per cent of the world's fresh water to meet the needs of 22 per cent of the planet's population. Of 412 sites on China's seven main rivers that were monitored for water quality in 2004, 58 per cent were found to be too polluted for human consumption. China's smog, caused mainly by emissions from power plants, vehicles, and other human activities, is seriously affecting urban air quality. In a 2003 World Bank survey of air pollution in 100 cities worldwide, more than 80 per cent of the Chinese cities listed had sulphur dioxide or nitrogen dioxide emissions above the WHO threshold, according to the Worldwatch Institute's *Vital Signs 2005* report. Globally, China is home to 16 of the 20 cities with the most polluted air. Environmental pollution accidents have occurred frequently in recent years. In 2004, the State Environmental Protection Administration of China received 67 reports of emergency environmental pollution accidents, which resulted in a direct economic loss of more than RMB 0.55 billion (US$76.5 million).

In recent years, pollution control has been high on the government agenda and investment in environmental protection increased significantly. However, the speed of treating pollution is far slower than the development of pollution. Trends in environmental pollution and devastation of natural ecosystems cannot easily be reversed. The government acknowledged in the 11th Five-Year Plan (2006–2010) Report that no breakthrough progress was made in some of the root environmental problems during the 10th Five-Year Plan (2001–2005) [38]. The economic losses as a result of environmental pollution (e.g. the impact of acid rain (droplets containing sulphur or nitrogen oxides) on crops, medical bills, lost work from illness, money spent on disaster relief following floods, and the implied costs of resource depletion) may account for as much as 10 per cent of China's GDP. The 2005 World Environmental Sustainability Index (ESI) ranked China 133rd out of 146 countries, indicating that China's environment has deteriorated to a dangerous degree. Environmental pollution and ecological destruction have inflicted colossal economic losses and put the public's health and social stability in jeopardy.

In 2007, 18 national ministries, committees, and other authorities jointly issued the China National Environment and Health Action Plan (2007–2015) to push forward efficient protection of environment and health, and to promote the sustainable development of economy and society [39].

Occupational health and injury

Occupational hazards are shifting from urban industrial areas to rural areas, from eastern China to central and western China, and from large and medium-sized industrial enterprises to medium- and small-sized industrial enterprises. There are about 0.7 billion people working in 16 million industries whose health is threatened by various occupational exposures in China. The incidence of occupational illnesses, especially among young adults, shows an increasing trend. Most of the patients have a low income and do not have medical insurance. Particularly serious and fatal accidents, especially accidents in mines, are out of control.

Increasing problems of food and drug safety

China has long suffered adverse publicity related to its lax enforcement of food and drug safety. China's chronic food safety problems are an international concern. Illegal use of farm chemicals, veterinary drugs, and food additives, and excessive pesticide residue content in food products have caused a rapid increase in related diseases. Recent drug-related incidents, such as the adverse reactions to antibiotic drug Xinfu manufactured in Anhui, have resulted in deaths and injuries blamed on shoddy or counterfeit drugs and food products. To address these problems, China will spend more than US$1 billion improving food and drug safety by 2010, and the regulator will be given stronger oversight powers.

Increasing health inequalities

Despite the great improvement in Chinese health, health inequalities undermine its development gains. China was ranked 188th out of 191 member states in terms of 'fairness of financial contribution' and was regarded as one of the most unfair countries on the 'financial burden' of health systems in the *World Health Report 2000* [40]. The health inequalities between urban and rural areas relate to uneven levels of economic development. The United Nations Development Programme's 2005 Human Development Report cited China as an example of a country where inequality is increasing. Because of the slow development of health care in rural areas, improvement in rural life expectancy lags far behind that of the cities. The difference in life expectancy between the urban and rural populations increased from 3.5 years in 1990 to 5.7 years in 2000 [41]. This type of inequality can be seen in many health indicators [42].

Financial difficulties, poor medical insurance coverage, and an unequal allocation of medical resources are the main reasons why the rural population, especially the poor, are unable to make use of medical services. There are large inequalities in the allocation of health resources between cities and rural areas in China. In the cities there are 5.2 medical personnel per 1000 residents, whereas in rural areas there are only 2.4 per 1000 residents. Even these figures understate the inequalities since they take no account of the quality of the personnel; 44.8 per cent of the urban population and 79.0 per cent of the rural population had to pay their medical expenses from their own pockets in 2003 [43]. Because of the income gap, the ratio of medical expenses to total income is far higher for farmers than for city dwellers. In addition, rural migrant workers are not covered by the medical insurance system in cities because they do not have permanent resident status. Many of the sick do not seek medical treatment because of the cost. This is a source of an emerging inequality among populations in urban areas [44].

The new pilot system, NCMS, is aimed at improving access to health-care services for the rural population and providing financial risk protection to patients with serious illnesses. This system is organized, guided, and supported by the government, but has voluntary rural resident involvement. It is financed by a combination of individual payments of fees, collective sponsorship, and government subsidies [45]. By the end of September 2007, NCMS had developed in 2448 counties of 31 provinces (roughly 85.5 per cent of all counties nationwide) and covered 726 million farmers with an 86 per cent enrolment rate [46]. The new system has shown some good results. More than half (58%) of rural families that had joined the system made claims by 2006 and were reimbursed a quarter of their total medical expenses (average of USD107). However, there are improvements that can be made to ensure that the system is sustainable. [47].

Fragile public health infrastructure

Over RMB 10.5 billion was invested in building disease prevention and control institutions by the Chinese government in the period from September 2002 to the end of 2005. Nevertheless, these efforts do not adequately address the deeper systemic problems which leave the population vulnerable. It is impossible for a chronically under-funded and neglected system to be repaired by increased funding on a crisis-by-crisis or programme-by-programme basis. As stated by the executive director of the American Public Health Association [48]:

> In the absence of a robust public health system with built-in surge capacity, every crisis also forces tradeoffs—attention to one infectious disease at the expense of another, infectious disease prevention at the expense of chronic disease prevention and other public health responsibilities.

This is what is now happening in China. It is important to repair and support the foundation of the public health system as a whole.

Fragmented public health information system

As early as 1950, China established the National Notifiable Infectious Diseases Reporting System. This system has played an important role in the control and prevention of infectious diseases in China. Since the 1980s, China has been establishing a National Disease Surveillance Points (DSP) System. This system includes 145 points, covering about 10 million people (around 1 per cent of the Chinese population). Information is collected on births, deaths, morbidity of notifiable diseases, and behavioural risk factors.

After the SARS crisis, the Internet-based (real-time dynamic) National Notifiable Infectious Diseases Reporting System began to function, covering 37 notifiable infectious diseases. The reporters, from hospitals, township health centres, local CDCs, medical institutes, or other units, can send the case report or the report of epidemic situation directly to this system via the Internet. This system greatly improves the timeliness, completeness, and accuracy of the reports, and the capacity for early detection, diagnosis, and response to outbreaks of communicable disease. Many other reporting or information systems (e.g. public health emergencies, 20 disease-specific enhanced surveillance activities, in-hospital mortality, health risk factors, vaccination, disasters) are also beginning to rely on Internet-based reporting platforms,.

Despite the rapid progress of these information systems, there are still many problems. Lack of coordination and integration among the dozens of surveillance systems result in the partial duplication of system constructions and reporting efforts. Under-reporting, inaccurate reporting, delayed reporting, and absence of reporting continue to be problematic. The small budgets, lack of equipment, and inadequate capacity, especially at the primary level, do not meet the needs of modern surveillance systems. Only a few people have permission to access the data, so that the use of surveillance data is at low level. Epidemiologists are unable to use the current information system to improve their research, and medical care workers are unable to use it to keep their services up to date. The system also fails to transform the data retrieved from these systems into information that can be used to develop public policy and inform decisions.

Public health workforce

The workforce, arguably the most important input to any health system, has a strong impact on overall health system performance. However, there are critical shortages of trained and skilled health workers in China. Paradoxically, these shortages often coexist with many unemployed new graduates from medical universities. In addition, China suffers from a maldistribution of the workforce characterized by urban concentration and rural deficit. Many health workers face daunting working environments—low wages, insufficient social recognition, and little attention to continuing professional development.

Meanwhile, public health education lags behind and plays an insufficient supportive role in the development of public health systems. Most of the public health schools have out-of-date curricular content and learning methods. The essential public health functions and the core competency requirements for public health professionals have not been clarified in China. In addition, the incentives for faculty and staff in the academic training institutions are often heavily weighted in favour of research and service delivery, to the detriment of teaching. There is little motivation for faculties to innovate.

Public health organization

The law is a traditional public health tool for disease prevention and health promotion. It has been crucial in addressing many public health problems, and many of the greatest public health successes have relied strongly on legal instruments. Ten laws and dozens of ordinances and codes on public health have been promulgated in China. These laws cover control of infectious diseases, food and health, family planning, drug management, blood donation, prevention and control of occupational diseases, maternal and child health care, national border health and quarantine, Red Cross Society, and practising physicians. Unfortunately, there is no unified and rigorous legal system which can support efficient operation of the public health system in China. A firm legal basis for the public health system is urgently required.

Measurement of performance is not new, nor is the concept foreign to most health departments. What is not being done is a comprehensive systematic performance evaluation. China does not have national performance standards. Outdated management practices mean that the public health system lacks direction.

Urgent need for evidence-based decision-making

It is commonly assumed that evidence-driven policy development and decision-making is superior to policy made 'on the run' or as a result of short-term political pressure, funding availability, the difficulties in making changes, and subjective preferences. Evidence-based public health is being promoted in China. However, it is still in the early stages. More and more people are using the term 'evidence-based' in speeches or articles. However, putting this idea into practice in China faces many obstacles. There is a lack of local evidence of sufficiently high quality to support evidence-based practice. Also, some people misunderstand the meaning of 'evidence-based' and are practising a false and dangerous decision-making process, i.e. adopting 'evidence' which supports the opinion of decision-makers. Too often, a desirable policy is determined by ideological or political considerations and then scientific justification is sought for it, often employing faulty science. The appropriate and effective approach is that science informs public health, which then leads to political change. As China has limited resources, it is particularly important to encourage evidence-based decision-making and to invest in effective public health and health promotion strategies.

Conclusion

China has achieved great success in public health in the past 50 years. However, there will be even more serious challenges in the future. The development of public health in China in the near future can be regarded with cautious optimism. China is actively drawing lessons from other countries in pursuit of a path that is suited to local conditions. One of the ways to address these major challenges will require the incorporation of the underlying social, cultural, and economic factors into public health interventions. Creation of an enabling environment, including the development of regulatory and legal systems, and complementary policies in sectors such as agriculture and education is necessary, and this requires strong government leadership. There is a central effort to improve the performance of health systems. Government has the responsibility for defining strategic directions, and legislative and regulatory frameworks for health systems. The government is key to ensuring collaborative actions in partnership with a wide range of groups from many sectors to promote population-wide health improvements.

References

[1] Brown E. *Rockefeller Medicine Men: Medicine and Capitalism in America*. Berkeley, CA: University of California Press, 1979.

[2] Chen ZQ. *Medicine in Rural China: A Personal Account*. Chengdu: Sichuan People's Press, 1997.

[3] Wang RT. Critical health literacy: a case study from China in schistosomiasis control. *Health Promot Int* 2000; **15**: 269–74.

[4] Horn J. *Away with All Pests*. New York: Monthly Review Press, 1969.

[5] Chow G. *An Economic Analysis of Health Care in China*. CEPS Working Paper 132. Available online at: www.princeton.edu/ ceps/workingpapers/132chow.pdf (accessed October 2007).

[6] Lee LM. The current state of public health in China. *Annu Rev Public Health* 2004; **25**, 327–39.

[7] WHO. *Core Health Indicators: China*. Available online at: www.who.int/whosis/database/core/core_select_process.cfm (accessed February 2008).

[8] National Bureau of Statistics of China. *1953 Chinese Population Census*. Available online at: www.stats.gov.cn/tjgb/rkpcgb/qgrkpcgb/t20020404_16767.htm (accessed October 2007).

[9] Kincannon CL, He W, West LA. Demography of aging in China and the United States and the economic well-being of their older populations. *J Cross Cult Gerontol* 2005; **20**: 243–55.

[10] China National Committee on Aging. *Research Report of Chinese Population Aging Trend*. Available online at: www.cnca.org.cn/default/iroot1000610000/4028e47d16ec2 fd901171963a2690382.html (accessed February 2008).

[11] China National Working Commission on Aging. Available online at: http://en.cnca.org. cn/en/iroot1007010000/4028e47d18a6b95c0118b05f581f0204.html (accessed May 2008).

[12] Ministry of Health PRC. *Chinese Health Statistical Digest 2007*. Available online at: www.moh.gov.cn/newshtml/19165.htm (accessed October 2007).

[13] Wang L, Kong L, Wu F, Bai Y, Burton R. Preventing chronic diseases in China. *Lancet* 2005; **366**: 1821–4.

[14] Abegunde DO, Mathers CD, Adam T, Ortegon M, Strong K. The burden and costs of chronic diseases in low-income and middle-income countries. *Lancet* 2007; **370**: 1929–38.

[15] Wang LD. *Report of National Nutrition and Health Survey in 2002*. Beijing: People's Medical Publishing House, 2005.

[16] Ministry of Health. *2007 Report on China's Smoking Control*. Available online at: www.moh.gov.cn/open/web_edit_file/20070529161216.pdf (accessed October 2007).

[17] China Centre for Economic Research. *Cost Estimation of Smoking in China*. http:// news.xinhuanet.com/fortune/2006–11/17/content_5341465.htm (accessed Feb 2008).

[18] State Tobacco Monopoly Administration. *Taxes, Profits Generated by China's Tobacco Industry up 25% in 2007*. Available online at: http://english.peopledaily.com. cn/90001/90776/90884/6338222.htm (accessed February 2008).

[19] WHO. *WHO Report on the Global Tobacco Epidemic 2008:The MPOWER Package*. Geneva: WHO, 2008.

[20] Franks P, Jerant AF, Leigh JP, *et al*. Cigarette prices, smoking, and the poor: implications of recent trends. *Am J Public Health* 2007; **97**: 1873–7.

[21] Li LM, Rao KQ, Kong LZ, *et al*. A description on the Chinese national nutrition and health survey in 2002. *Chin J Epidemiol* 2005; **26**: 478–84.

[22] Chinese Center for Disease Control and Prevention. *The Report of National Nutrition and Health Survey in 2002*. Available online at: www.chinacdc.net.cn/n272442/ n272530/n3246177/11031.html (accessed in October 2007).

[23] Wang Y, Mi J, Shan XY, Wang QJ, Ge KY. Is China facing an obesity epidemic and the consequences? The trends in obesity and chronic disease in China. *Int J Obes* 2006; **31**: 177–88.

[24] Asaria P, Chisholm D, Mathers C, Ezzati M, Beaglehole R. Chronic disease prevention: health effects and financial costs of strategies to reduce salt intake and control tobacco use. *Lancet* 2007; **370**: 2044–53.

[25] Lim SS, Gaziano TA, Gakidou E, *et al*. Prevention of cardiovascular disease in high-risk individual in low-income and middle-income countries: health effects and costs. *Lancet* 2007; **370**, 2054–62.

[26] Liang XF, Chen YS, Wang XJ, *et al*. A study on the sero-epidemiology of hepatitis B in Chinese population aged over 3 years old. *Chin J Epidemiol* 2005; **26**: 655–8.

[27] Zhuang H. National epidemic of hepatitis B and the challenge we are facing. *Chin J Infect Dis* 2005; **23**(Suppl), 2–6.

[28] WHO. *Global Tuberculosis Control: Surveillance, Planning, Financing*. Report WHO/HTM/TB/2007.376. Geneva: WHO, 2007.

[29] Ministry of Health PRC, Joint United Nations Program on HIV/AIDS, and World Health Organization. *2005 Update on the HIV/AIDS Epidemic and Response in China*. Available online at: www.casy.org/engdocs/2005-China%20HIV-AIDS%20Estimation-English.pdf (accessed October 2007).

[30] WHO (2008). *Cumulative Number of Confirmed Human Cases of Avian Influenza A/ (H5N1) Reported to WHO*. Available online at: www.who.int/csr/disease/avian_influenza/country/cases_table_2008_02_05/en/index.html (accessed February 2008).

[31] Ha S. Research progress on mental health problems in adolescent. *J Inner Mongolia Univ Nationalities* 2003; **17**: 250–4.

[32] Jing J. It is imperative to develop mental health related research of children and adolescents. South China. *J Prev Med* 2002; **28**: 7–9.

[33] China Internet Information Centre (2003). *30 Million Adolescents in China were in Mental Sub-Health*. Available online at: http://www.china.com.cn/chinese/kuaixun/261608.htm (accessed October 2007).

[34] Phillips MR, Li X, Zhang Y. Suicide rates in China, 1995–99. *Lancet* 2002; **359**: 835–40.

[35] Jiang JM. Analysis of disabled elderly in the rural areas of China. *Mod Prev Med* 2001; **28**: 119–20.

[36] Zhou Y, Baker TD, Rao K, Li G. Productivity losses from injury in China. *Inj Prev* 2003; **9**: 124–7.

[37] Ministry of Health PRC. *Ministry of Health Announce the Report of Injury prevention in China*. Available online at: www.moh.gov.cn/newshtml/19781.htm (accessed October 2007).

[38] Ministry of Environmental Protection of the People's Republic of China. *11th Five-Year Plan (2006–2010) Report*. Available online at: www.sepa.gov.cn/plan/hjgh/sywgh/gjsywgh/200801/t20080118_116458.htm (accessed May 2008).

[39] PR China. *China National Environment and Health Action Plan (2007–2015)*. Available online at: www.wpro.who.int/NR/rdonlyres/13A55C9E-9383–47E8–9F24-F23FDA48F066/0/NEHAPfinaledition.pdf (accessed May 2008).

[40] WHO. *World Health Report 2000*. Available online at: www.who.int/entity/whr/2000/en/whr00_en.pd (accessed Oct 2007).

[41] China Development Research Foundation (2005). *China Human Development Report 2005*. Available online at: www.undp.org.cn/downloads/nhdr2005/NHDR2005_complete.pdf (accessed October 2007).

[42] Ministry of Health PRC. *Chinese Health Statistical Digest 1996–2007*. Available online at: www.moh.gov.cn/menunews/C30302.htm (accessed October 2007).

[43] Centre for Health Statistics and Information MOH (2004). *An Analysis Report of National Health Services Survey in 2003*. Beijing: Peking Union Medical College Press.

[44] Li J, Zhang K, Tian L. Multiple Facets of China's Health Inequality. *Lancet* 2006; **36**: 1397.

[45] Wang Y. Development of the new rural cooperative medical system in China. *China World Econ* 2007; **15**: 77.

[46] Ministry of Health. Speech of the Head of the Ministry of Health at Annual National Health Conference, 7 January 2008. Available online at: www.ccms.org.cn/third-xwxx.asp?id=213 (accessed May 2008).

[47] Ministry of Health. Ministry of Health announced the situation on pilot operation of new cooperative medical system. Available online at: www.gov.cn/xwfb/2006–09/28/content_401003.htm (accessed May 2008).

[48] Benjamin G. Testimony of the Centers for Disease Control and Prevention (CDC) Coalition concerning the public health budget for fiscal year 2004. Available online at: www.apha.org/advocacy/priorities/comments/legislativetestbudget2004.htm (accessed October 2007).

Chapter 10

Public health in India

Puja Thakker and K. Srinath Reddy

Introduction

With a total population of 1.1 billon, India has almost one-sixth of the global population. Rapid economic growth in recent years places it alongside China (Chapter 9) as one of the emerging economic powers of the twenty-first century. However, the health of the Indian population lags behind the high profile that the country has achieved in other spheres. As the health transition transforms the determinants of health, altering the dynamics of development and modifying the patterns of diseases, India is experiencing the burden of infectious, nutritional, and chronic diseases coexisting with an unacceptably high death toll from endangered pregnancies and fatal injuries.

Major advances in global health will require progress of public health in India through appropriate and adequate investment of financial and human resources and strengthening of health systems. In this chapter we profile the health scenario of India, briefly describe the health system, and outline some of the major health programmes and new initiatives which are addressing the complex health challenges confronting the country.

Current health profile

India's population has experienced significant health gains in the six decades since Independence in 1947. The average life expectancy has risen from 37 years in 1951 to 63 years in 2004, and fertility rates have declined concurrently from 5.8 to 3.2 per 1000 women [1]. During this period, the infant mortality rate (IMR) has fallen from 140 to 58 deaths per 1000 live births [1], and the maternal mortality rate (MMR) has also declined from nearly 1300 to 301 per 100,000 live births [2]. Smallpox and guinea worm disease have been eradicated, and polio is soon to follow suit, currently endemic in only two of India's 35 states and Union Territories [3].

A closer look at regional data for India reveals wide differences in health status that are masked by national aggregates. Kerala (IMR, 14 per 1000; MMR,

Table 10.1 Progress towards the Millennium Development Goals in India

Indicator	Baseline 1990	Recent status (2005–2007)	MDG Target 2015
Prevalence of underweight children under 5 years of age (%)	53	43	27
Proportion of population undernourished (%)	62	35	31
Under-5 mortality per 1000 live births	123	74	41
Infant mortality per 1000 live births	84	56	28
Maternal mortality per 100,000 live births	570	301	142
Population with access to improved drinking water sources			
Urban (%)	89	95	95
Rural (%)	64	83	82
Population using improved sanitation facilities			
Urban (%)	45	59	72
Rural (%)	9	22	72

Data sources: UNSTATS [7]; National Health and Family Survey-III [5]; authors' calculations

110 per 100,000) and Tamil Nadu (IMR, 31 per 1000; MMR, 76 per 100,000) [4,5] compare favourably with several middle-income countries and already exceed the Millennium Development Goals which India aims to achieve by 2015 (Table 10.1). At the other end of the spectrum are Uttar Pradesh, Orissa, and Madhya Pradesh whose indicators are only marginally better than those of sub-Saharan Africa. The other states fall between these two extremes.

Large pockets of the population in rural and tribal areas are extremely poor, and have remained untouched by socio-economic advances. This population continues to suffer from a high burden of pre-transitional conditions, marked by high rates of maternal mortality, malnutrition, and infectious diseases. There are also segments of the population, such as urban slum dwellers and workers in the unorganized sector, who, moving between urban and rural India, suffer from several communicable diseases and are also exposed to newer risk factors such as cardiovascular and pulmonary diseases, accidents, addictions, mental disorders, and HIV [6]. Within individual states, the rural areas lag far behind their relatively more developed urban counterparts. India is at various stages of the health transition at the same time, exhibiting what can more aptly be described as an epidemiological polarization. The formidable challenge of the dual burden, and the deep inequities that exist, demand the full attention of public health practitioners, policy-makers and researchers if India is to meet its Millennium Development Goals by 2015 (Table 10.1).

Dual burden of disease

India accounts for 20 per cent of the global disease burden but only 16.5 per cent of the world's population [8]. Communicable diseases, nutritional deficiencies, and maternal and pregnancy-related health conditions still account for nearly 50 per cent of the disease burden and more than a third (37 per cent) of the estimated 10.3 million deaths that occurred in India in 2004 [9] (Fig. 10.1). Chronic non-communicable diseases, such as heart disease, stroke, cancer, diabetes, and chronic obstructive pulmonary disease (COPD), currently account for 53 per cent of the total deaths, and cardiovascular diseases alone will soon become the leading cause of death [8]. The remaining deaths are due to injuries, both intentional and unintentional.

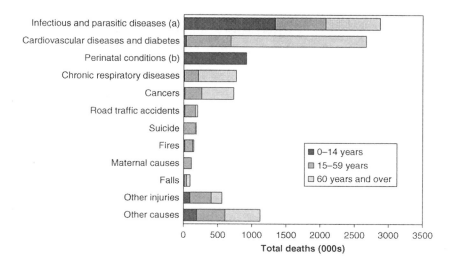

Fig. 10.1 Estimated deaths due to selected disease and injury causes, by broad age group, India, 2004.
(a) Includes acute respiratory infections. (b) Includes conditions arising in the perinatal period (such as prematurity, birth trauma, and neonatal infections) but not all deaths occurring in the neonatal period (first 28 days).
Source: Patel *et al.* [9].

Unfinished agenda of communicable diseases

Malaria remains a threat and has been a concern for policy makers since the 1950s. Initial attempts at malaria eradication were very successful, bringing the caseload down from an estimated 75 million to 100,000 by the 1960s [10]. However, malaria resurfaced as a result of technical, financial, and operational inadequacies of the implementing agencies, and there were 6.45 million cases in 1976 [11]. Although malaria accounts for only a few thousand deaths each year in India, according to the National Vector Borne Disease Control Programme (NVBDCP) estimates, there were at least 1.4 million cases in 2007, of which nearly half were the more virulent *Plasmodium falciparum* type [12].

Tuberculosis (TB) too has been a major public health challenge in India since the beginning of the twentieth century. The annual incidence of TB in India accounts for 1.9 million of the total 8.8 million cases worldwide, nearly one-fifth of the global burden [13]. According to WHO estimates, TB account-ed for approximately 309,000 deaths in 2004 [14]. Of growing concern is the increase in cases of multidrug-resistant TB (MDR-TB) and extensively drug resistant TB (XDR-TB). The spread of HIV and consequent opportunistic TB infections has further weakened efforts to control the disease.

Approximately 2.5 million people in India are living with HIV, accounting for a quarter of the estimated 10.7 million HIV cases outside sub-Saharan Africa [15]. According to WHO estimates, there were approximately 126,000 deaths from HIV in 2004 [14]. In addition, tropical diseases suchas kala azar, dengue, chikunguniya, lymphatic filariasis, and Japanese encephalitis continue to affect the population, especially the poor.

Maternal and child health

Despite significant gains in mother and child survival in recent years, morbid-ity and mortality are still greater than those attained by other countries with a similar economic profile. WHO estimates suggest that approximately 111,000 maternal deaths and 920,000 perinatal deaths occurred in 2004 [14]. According to the recent National Family Health Survey [5], only 15 per cent of Indian women received all recommended types of antenatal care, and 36 per cent of Indian mothers were found to be moderately anaemic. Almost four out of five children aged between 6 months and 3 years were reported as anaemic, 43 per cent of those under 5 years of age were found to be underweight, and only 44 per cent of children between 12 and 23 months had received full vaccination. Low immunization rates, in conjunction with weakened immu-nity from malnutrition, leave children even more vulnerable to the threat of infectious diseases.

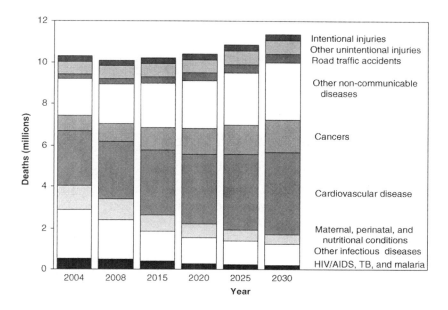

Fig. 10.2 Projected deaths by cause, India, 2004–2030.
Source: Patel *et al.* [9].

Rise of non-communicable diseases

Although deaths from communicable diseases are expected to decline, ageing of the population juxtaposed with an increasing exposure to risk factors such as tobacco use and diets high in salt, fat and sugar portend a rise in the burden of non-communicable disease in the future (Fig. 10.2).

Cardiovascular deaths are projected to rise from 2.7 million in 2004 to 4.0 million in 2030, and cancer deaths from 730,000 in 2004 to 1.5 million in 2030 [9]. Overall, chronic diseases are projected to account for just under three-quarters of all deaths in India in 2030. In addition, the estimated share of deaths due to injuries (10.7 per cent in 2004 according to WHO estimates) is estimated to rise to 30 per cent by 2030; most of this increase is attributable to road traffic injuries.

Estimates of age-specific chronic disease death rates are 60–100 per cent higher in India than in high-income countries. Two-thirds of the disease burden in India is concentrated in those aged 15 years and older; in this age group, chronic diseases were responsible for 62 per cent of the disease burden and injuries for 16 per cent (Fig. 10.1). The large number of people with diabetes (more than 40 million in 2007) makes India the largest diabetic population in the world; this number is expected to rise to 70 million by 2025 [16].

Mental health conditions are also increasing [8]. Unipolar depressive disorders and COPD were among the top 10 causes of disability. Officially reported suicides have quadrupled from 40,232 in 1981 to 118,112 in 2006, with an annual incidence rate of 108 per million [17].

An overview of India's health system

Delivery and financing of health services

The state-funded public health system is a three-tier network of health sub-centres at the village level, primary health centres (PHCs) at the block level, and community health centres (CHCs) or general hospitals at the district level. The CHCs and general hospitals are large in-patient facilities providing secondary and tertiary care, while the more widespread sub-centres and PHCs provide an array of primary preventive and curative services at the village level. In lieu of PHCs, urban areas have urban health centres (UHCs) and general hospitals, with a much wider coverage area. Together, these three tiers provide a complete range of health services to the population.

India currently spends 1.3 per cent of GDP on health [18]. Public health spending in India is one of the lowest in the world, comparing unfavourably even with other low- and middle-income countries. The level of out-of-pocket spending in India has remained virtually unchanged, at 77 per cent, since 1999 [19]. There is a gross mismatch between India's target of universal primary health care and the resources that are allocated for the attainment of this goal. With recent schemes such as the National Rural Health Mission, launched in 2005, and the National Urban Health Mission, launched in 2008–2009, the government aims to increase its current share of 17 per cent of total health spending [18] to 25 per cent by 2010 [20]. Social protection schemes, such as a health insurance scheme providing financial protection for nearly 35 million workers in the unorganized sector who are below the poverty line, are currently under development.

Human resources

India faces a severe shortfall in human resources for health. There are over 165 medical colleges in the allopathic system of medicine which produce close to 20,000 doctors each year, nearly 75 per cent of which are from government institutions. However, the public health system benefits little from them, as nearly 80 per cent of those graduating from government institutions join the private sector or migrate abroad [21]. There is an average of one physician per 1600 population [22]. This ratio is even lower for rural areas, the worst being West Bengal and Madhya Pradesh, which have an average of one physician per 40,000 rural population [23]. The nurse-to-population ratio is also unsatisfactory at one nurse per 750 population, compared with the international norm of one nurse per 150–200 population [22]. Auxiliary nurse midwives (ANMs), equivalent to the public health midwives who have been key to the reduction of maternal mortality in Sri Lanka, have thus far been the primary providers of maternal care at the village level. The introduction of a link worker, an accredited social health activist (ASHA) under the aegis of the NRHM, has substantially augmented the workforce at the primary care level. The ASHA (literally meaning 'hope') is now a crucial element of the rural public health system, contributing significantly to activities specifically aimed at improving maternal and child health indicators.

Public health policies and programmes: development and progress

When India gained independence in 1947, the majority of the population had little or no access to formal health services. The scant Western medicine facilities that existed had largely been put in place by the British and were reserved mainly for the ruling and elite classes during the colonial regime. As Western medicine became more popular among the affluent class, indigenous systems of medicine, which had historically thrived on their contributions, withered because of decreased demand and lack of state support, leaving the underprivileged masses with very poor access to care.

A Health Survey and Development Committee, widely known as the Bhore Committee, was set up in 1946 shortly before Independence, to evaluate the status of health conditions and health services in India. It found that mass access to health care was gravely inadequate, especially at a time when rates of malnutrition and under-nutrition were high, and communicable diseases were increasing. They urgently called for, *inter alia*, the establishment of a national health service that would ensure universal primary health care for all. The three-tier public health system as we know it today was the most direct outcome of this egalitarian recommendation. The report of the Bhore Committee is one of the founding doctrines of health policy in India even today.

Independent India's early commitment to a socialist state provided a vision for universal primary health care, but that was not translated into an operational reality. For several decades after Independence, the emphasis of national health policies was on the provision of essential clinical services, and public health services were not prioritized for resource allocation. As the economic policies veered towards the 'market' model, and the 'mixed economy' of the early years was influenced by neo-liberal recommendations for reform, the state became less committed to its role of a provider of health services. Technocentric approaches to family planning, disease control, and disease prevention, as well as progressive privatization of health care, prevented public health from adequately asserting its influence until recently.

However, the technocentric approach has had successes. The smallpox eradication mass campaign was instrumental in the eradication of the deadly disease, and an aggressive Pulse Polio vaccination campaign, which has dramatically reduced the incidence of acute flaccid paralysis cases in recent years, is in full swing. The population control programme that was started in 1956, now a family planning initiative, has been socially influential in reducing fertility, with 10 states already at or below the replacement level of 2.1 children per woman [5]. National level programmes targeting the control of specific communicable diseases for TB (Revised National Tuberculosis Control Programme), malaria (National Anti Malaria Programme), leprosy (National Leprosy Eradication Programme), and HIV/AIDS (National AIDS Control Programme), among several others, are actively combating the threat of infectious diseases. While concerted action within several of these vertically fragmented disease programmes has helped make much progress in the short term, the long-term sustainability of these achievements is questionable because of the lack of interdisciplinary understanding or a multisectoral approach to health policy and planning. Episodes of resurgence of infectious diseases—the plague epidemic of 1994, the upsurge of malaria in 1995, and the dengue fever outbreak in 1996—attest to this.

Despite some success, chronic disease programmes have also lacked an integrated and comprehensive approach to their implementation. Although far fewer in number compared with communicable disease initiatives, programmes such as the National Cancer Control Programme, the National Blindness Control Programme, the National Programme on Speech and Hearing, the National Iodine Deficiency Disorders Control Programme, and the National Mental Health Programme have been set up for the containment of chronic diseases. A pilot phase of the newly designed National Programme for the Prevention and Control of Diabetes, Cardiovascular Diseases, and Stroke was initiated in January 2008.

This narrow vision of health in the policy domain arose partly from the entrenched belief of economic planners that economic development was sufficient to improve health, as a passive consequence of improved living conditions. Through the Structural Adjustment Programmes propagated by the

World Bank in the 1990s, policy-makers consciously shifted their focus from comprehensive care to 'selective' primary care embodied by these vertical health programmes. Disease-specific programmes were also attractive to politicians because they not only provided political leverage for addressing popular concerns, but also appeared to demand fewer resources than the more costly alternative of investing in permanent comprehensive care facilities [24]. It is only recently that the bi-directionality of health and economic development has become widely accepted, and the importance of addressing the social determinants of health has been recognized.

A few initiatives, such as the Integrated Child Development Services (ICDS) and the National Rural Health Mission (NRHM), have broken through this apathy towards public health. The ICDS, launched in 1974, was the first scheme of its kind, addressing several upstream determinants affecting child development, ranging from nutrition and education to psychological well-being. It is the largest maternal and child development scheme in the world, costing nearly US$1 billion each year. The beneficiaries are primarily children under 6 years of age and pregnant and lactating mothers from underprivileged backgrounds. The services, rendered by an Anganwadi Worker (AWW) at a village centre known as an 'Anganwadi', include the provision of supplementary nutrition, preschool education, immunization, health check-ups for prenatal care, referral services, and nutrition and health education. The success of this scheme has been attributed to its holistic approach to child development through intersectoral collaboration across multiple government departments. The ICDS has resulted in a significant decline in the severe grades of malnutrition [25], and even improved performance in primary school [26].

The NRHM is one of the most celebrated initiatives in recent years to gain centre stage within the health sector. It was launched in April 2005 to address the largely unmet needs of the rural population, (who comprise 75 per cent of the total population), by scaling up all health service facilities. The NRHM was also an attempt by the state to increase public spending on health from the meagre 0.9 per cent of GDP to 2–3 per cent by 2012 [20]. The launch of the NRHM is a significant step towards an integrated response to India's public health challenges (Box 10.1).

A more integrated framework for disease surveillance systems has also been adopted. Surveillance has historically been instrumental in several of India's public health achievements. Sentinel surveillance was vital to the success of the smallpox eradication campaign. Surveillance was also a key element of the national programmes for malaria, tuberculosis, and HIV/AIDS, as well as in the early detection of acute flaccid paralysis for polio eradication. A formal surveillance system, the Integrated Disease Surveillance Programme (IDSP),

Box 10.1 The National Rural Health Mission (NHRM): a public health success story

Under the overarching framework of the NRHM, several existing vertical disease programmes converge, in terms of human resources and operations, for joint delivery through the rural public health system. Outside the health sector, the NRHM calls for convergent action across different departments, such as rural development, education, water and sanitation, and woman and child development, at every level of governance. A key feature of the framework provided by the NRHM is its emphasis on decentralization and community participation, through the transfer of decision-making authority and the devolution of funds to the local level (the merits of which were initially demonstrated by Kerala's decentralized planning exercise in 1996). Thus far, this approach has enabled local medical officers to respond more appropriately to the needs of the community. In turn, the involvement of local self-government, or Panchayati Raj Institutions, within the community, has also increased accountability within the health system. Through a variety of schemes and incentives, the NRHM has provided a substantial face-lift to the rural public health system in terms of infrastructure, human resources, access to care, and utilization of health services—improvements which have had a positive impact on health outcomes.

was launched in 2004 in an effort to integrate and coordinate activities that were hitherto running as parallel surveillance systems under different vertical disease programmes. The IDSP also incorporates risk factors for chronic non-communicable diseases, such as tobacco and alcohol use, and diet and physical activity, which were not covered under earlier programmes [27].

In 2008 the central government announced the addition of an urban analogue to this scheme, namely the National Urban Health Mission (NUHM). Urban Social Health Activists (USHAs), urban counterparts of the ASHAs, will be trained and recruited to promote urban health, particularly for homeless and street children, focusing on decreasing the levels of malnutrition and prevention of infectious disease through improved vaccination coverage. If the NUHM strengthens health systems for the urban population as envisaged, then, together with the NRHM, India will have taken a significant step towards its goal of universal primary healthcare for all, and the USHA (meaning 'dawn') may indeed provide a ray of hope to the urban poor.

These steps towards integration are landmarks in the development of the health system, and are indicative of a paradigm shift over the last 50 years in Indian health policy.

Public health education

Public health education in India has been limited in its scope and slow in its development. Even while the need for public health training was recognized by policy makers at the time of India's Independence, much emphasis was placed on the social reorientation of physicians through additional short-term training in public health, embedded within medical curricula. As a result, public health remained mostly confined to the medical fraternity and failed to develop into an interdisciplinary science. Even the long-term postgraduate programmes were labelled 'community medicine' and remained closeted in the restrictive medical paradigm.

The Sree Chitra Tirunal Institute for Medical Science and Technology in south India was one of the first to offer public health training programmes for non-medical graduates in the 1990s, but still produces only a small number of graduates each year [28]. The Public Health Foundation of India (PHFI) (Box 10.2) was recently launched in an attempt to infuse greater public health expertise into

Box 10.2 Public Health Foundation of India (PHFI)

The Public Health Foundation of India (PHFI) was launched in 2006 as a large-scale, sustainable response to growing concern over emerging public health challenges in India. It recognizes the fact that meeting the shortfall of health professionals is imperative to a sustained and holistic response to the public health concerns in the country [29].

The mandate of this not-for-profit organization, created through a public–private partnership, is to build and strengthen capacity for training, research, and policy development in public health. These goals are operationalized through the setting up of several institutes of education and training for public health programmes at the graduate and postgraduate level, the establishment of pathways for public health action that are truly multisectoral, and the advancement of a transdisciplinary research agenda which would inform policy and empower programmes. PHFI has engaged multiple stakeholders spanning national and international academia, central and state governments, civil society organizations, and industry leaders.

The PHFI is now at an advanced stage in establishing nine Institutes of Public Health in different regions of India, through partnerships with various state governments, and is developing a broader public health agenda through multisectoral action facilitated by interdisciplinary academic programmes and research.

For further information see: http://www.phfi.org

the health system and broaden the scope of the cross-cutting discipline of public health to extend beyond the health sector. Intiatives such as PHFI are attempting to establish synergistic links between these diverse disciplines and the health system to improve the design and delivery of health care through policy and systems-relevant research and training programmes in public health.

Overcoming barriers to progress

There are a number of barriers, both within and outside the health sector, which need to be overcome in order to improve the practice of public health in India. These arise from the different roles of central and state governments, the major role of the private sector, and, as everywhere, the shortfall in an adequate public health workforce.

Health has been defined as a state subject by the Indian constitution, i.e. it clearly assigns the duties of 'public health and sanitation, hospitals, and dispensaries' to state governments. The control of communicable diseases, drugs, medical education, and mental health are under the joint jurisdiction of the state and central government. Despite health being a deliverable responsibility of the states, state governments have played a small role in the decision-making process. Because of wide interstate differentials in the availability of financial resources for health, most health schemes have been centrally sponsored. Programme design has also taken place at the centre, leaving only the task of implementation to the state governments. Thus the centre has emerged as the dominant actor within the health sector. In heavily engaging itself with financing and design, it has slowly withdrawn from its former role of stewardship.

The liberalization of India's markets has produced a sharp rise in the provision of health services by the private sector. The growth of the private sector was welcomed and even encouraged by the government through the provision of grants and subsidies during its transition to an open market economy in the 1990s. Today, private providers are mainly located in urban and wealthy areas, where services fetch higher user fees. It is no surprise that out-of-pocket expenditure in India is one of the highest in the world. Estimates suggest that 32.5 million people fall below the national poverty line because of out-of-pocket payments in India each year [19].

While preventive and promotional health services still remain the primary responsibility of the public sector, over the years the private sector has expanded from its initial domain of tertiary care to include areas of secondary and primary care as well. Thus it is the dominant provider of health care in the country. Growth of secondary and tertiary hospitals in the public sector has not kept pace with the private sector. Despite the high cost attached to private health care, poor regulation of these facilities has raised concern over the quality of care delivered. There are several gaps in service in the less developed areas of the country, especially in the provision of secondary and tertiary care, where public infrastructure does not exist and the private sector has not delivered. According to the NCMH, about 25 per cent of people in Madhya Pradesh and 11 per cent in Uttar Pradesh could not access medical care because they were too far from any facility [17]. The private sector needs to be regulated and creatively involved to be complementary to, and not compete with, the public sector, and health systems need to be reconfigured to reflect India's vision of universal health care for all.

Despite the presence of over 165 medical colleges in the modern system of medicine and over 400 in the traditional Indian system throughout the country, there is a serious shortage of trained health-care providers, particularly in rural areas. Migration of doctors and nurses to other countries, their reluctance to work in rural areas, and their preference for the more lucrative private sector have resulted in shortages and maldistribution of human resources within the public health system. Several state governments have attempted to address this shortfall by task-shifting and task-sharing strategies. The burden of the ANM is now shared by the ASHA. While achieving the desirable skill-mix at health centres still remains a challenge, the presence of an ASHA within each village has significantly enhanced early medical attention and referral to a health facility, particularly benefiting areas where access to care is poor, and shortages of health personnel are substantial. However, rural health care is severly handicapped by a lack of doctors and nurses even as public health services overall are enfeebled by a lack of public health expertise.

Although financial allocations to the health sector are increasing and new national health programmes are being implemented to increase the outreach of health services, public health has not adequately engaged with policies which are traditionally considered to be outside the health sector. Policies related to agriculture, food processing, water resources, urban design, environment, trade, and education, which have a profound impact on the health of the population, are among those which need to become sensitive to and supportive of public health. Taxation and regulation are also measures which, when judiciously applied, can influence the determinants of health. Tobacco control is a public health imperative which requires such multisectoral action. India's response to the growing epidemic of non-communicable diseases has now begun to develop, commencing with comprehensive legislation for tobacco control (2003), and now extending to a new national programme on cardiovascular diseases, diabetes, and stroke (2008). This commitment must now extend to policies and actions outside the health sector. Public health in India must evolve to involve all of government in policy making for health and all of society in advancing health action.

Conclusion

As India gears up for accelerated economic growth in the twenty-first century, it faces a formidable array of public health challenges arising from a staggered health transition and accentuated by uneven development. Even as its health system is attempting to expand outreach and upscale quality, shortfalls in both human and financial resources are limiting the access of many sections of the population to affordable clinical care as well as to preventive and promotional public health services.

With a young demographic profile and an anticipated expansion of the population mainly in the 15–59 year age group over the next two decades, India needs to invest substantially in initiatives for strengthening public health so that its productive human resources can develop and deliver to full potential. The advocacy, by an increasingly assertive civil society, that health is an inalienable human right which entitles every citizen to health-enabling services across their lifespan has also placed public health more centrally in India's development discourse.

As a result, several new initiatives have been launched to increase health financing, improve health services, meet shortages in the health workforce, and infuse public health expertise into health policies and programmes. Even as these are evaluated for success, sustainability, and scalability, other efforts must be vigorously mounted to favourably influence the multiple determinants of health and bridge the gaping health inequalities that separate the many states and population groups.

Over the next decade, India's innovations in reinforcing the architecture of public health and its experiences in revitalizing its health services will be of interest to other low- and middle-income countries which face similar problems of health transition.

References

[1] Ministry of Health and Family Welfare, New Delhi: Government of India, November 2007.
[2] Bhat PN. Maternal mortality in India: an update. *Stud Fam Plann* 2002; **33**: 227–36.
[3] National Polio Surveillance Project (2008). *AFP Surveillance Bulletin*. New Delhi: Government of India, July 2008.
[4] Registrar General of India. *Sample Registration System Bulletin*. New Delhi: Government of India, 2007.
[5] Ministry of Health and Family Welfare. *National Health and Family Survey-III*. New Delhi: Government of India, 2006.

[6] Shukla A. Key public health challenges in India: a social medicine perspective. *Social Med* 2007; **2**: 1–7.

[7] UNSTATS. Available online at: http://mdgs.un.org/unsd/mdg/Default.aspx (accessed 20 May 2008)

[8] National Commission on Macroeconomics and Health. *Background Papers: Burden of Disease in India*. New Delhi: Government of India, 2005.

[9] Patel V, Chatterjie S, Chisholm D, *et al*. Chronic disease and injuries: the emerging priority public health agenda. *Lancet*; in press.

[10] Banerji D. *Landmarks in the Development of Health Services in the Countries of South Asia*. Delhi: Consul Press, 1997.

[11] Sharma VP. Re-emergence of malaria in India. *Indian J Med Res* 1996; **103**: 26–45.

[12] National Vector Borne Disease Control Programme, *Ministry of Health and Family Welfare*, New Delhi: Government of India, 2007.

[13] Central TB Division, Ministry of Health and Family Welfare. *TB India 2008- RNTCP Status Report 2008*. New Delhi: Government of India, 2008.

[14] WHO. *Global Burden of Disease Estimates, 2004*. Geneva: WHO, 2008.

[15] Steinbrook R. HIV in India: a downsized epidemic. *N Engl J Med* 2008; **358**: 107–9.

[16] *World Diabetes Foundation Annual Review 2007*. Available online at: www.worlddiabetesfoundation (accessed 20 December 2008).

[17] Ministry of Health and Family Welfare. *The Report of the National Commission on Macroeconomics and Health*. New Delhi: Government of India, 2005.

[18] Ministry of Health and Family Welfare. India's health system: The financing and delivery of health care services. In: *Report of the National Commission on Macroeconomics and Health*. New Delhi: Government of India, 2005.

[19] O'Donnell O, Doorslaer E, Rannan-Eliya R, *et al*. *Explaining the Incidence of Catastrophic Expenditures on Health Care: Comparative Evidence from Asia*. EQUITAP Project, Working Paper 2, Erasmus University, Rotterdam, the Netherlands 2005.

[20] Ministry of Health and Family Welfare. *National Rural Health Mission. Framework for Implementation, 2005–2012*. New Delhi: Government of India, 2005.

[21] Duggal R, Gangolli L. Introduction to review of healthcare in India. In: Gangolli L, Duggal R, Shukla A (eds). *Review of Healthcare in India*. Mumbai: Centre for Enquiry into Health and Allied Themes, 2005; pp. 3–4.

[22] Central Bureau of Health Information. *Human resources in health sector. National Health Profile 2007*. New Delhi: Government of India, 2007; pp. 136–7.

[23] WHO. *Not Many Here, Too Many There*. New Delhi: WHO, 2007

[24] Gangolli L, Gaitonde R. Programmes for control of communicable diseases. In: Gangolli L, Duggal R, Shukla A (eds). *Review of Healthcare in India*. Mumbai: Centre for Enquiry into Health and Allied Themes, 2005; pp 75–100.

[25] Kapil U, Pradhan R. Integrated Child Development Services scheme (ICDS) and its impact on nutritional status of children in India and recent initiatives. *Indian J Public Health* 1996; **43**: 21–5.

[26] Murlidharan R, Kaul V. Integrated early childhood development—the Indian experience. In: Eldering L, Leseman P, Paul P.M (eds). *Effective Early Education: Cross Cultural Perspectives*. London: Routledge, 1999; pp 297–304.

[27] Reddy KS, Shah B, Varghese C, Ramadoss A. Responding to the threat of chronic diseases in India. *Lancet* 2005; **366**: 1746–51.

[28] Beaglehole R, Bonita R. *Public Health at a Crossroads: Achievements and Prospects* (2nd edn). Cambridge: Cambridge University Press, 2004.

[29] Chen L. Philanthropic partnerships for public health in India? *Lancet* 2006; **367**: 1800–1.

Chapter 11

Public health in Australia and New Zealand

Peter Davis, Vivian Lin, and Robin Gauld

Introduction

Public health in Australia and New Zealand reflects a special set of historical and geographical circumstances reflected in some of the most favourable health outcomes in the world. The pattern reached its height in the 1950s and 1960s with cultural and social protection, political and economic stability, and relative insulation. Since then these conditions have been reshaped both by reforming governments [1] and by the pressures of globalization and regional transformation. In this chapter we review the unique historical experience of public health in these two countries, evaluate their more recent achievements, and assess their likely prospects in rapidly changing regional and global circumstances.

Societal context

Australia and New Zealand represent the furthest and final reach of the British colonial venture. Despite this common historical heritage, there are important differences between the two countries. These are to be seen in their political systems (Australia is federal, New Zealand is unitary), in levels of migration (high and varied for Australia, traditionally low and controlled in New Zealand), in size, in standard of living, and in economic and demographic growth (all more developed in Australia), and in focus of regional engagement (Australia towards Asia, New Zealand to the South Pacific). However, in most important respects the two countries have much in common.

Beyond these distinctive historical and societal features, both countries share many features relevant to public health with the rest of the developed world. For example, with affluence and the demographic transition have come ageing of their populations. Economic deregulation has been associated with the decline of protected industries and growing social inequality. Changes in the role of women and in home and family life have accompanied industrial restructuring and shifts in patterns and levels of workforce participation. Overlying these fundamental demographic, economic, and social changes are important ideological movements—individual rights, women, labour, indigenous peoples, the environment—and major shifts in perceptions of health and the role of the state. These cultural and ideological movements have much in common with the recent historical experience of other economically developed societies.

Health and policy context

Both Australia and New Zealand are at a stage of the epidemiological transition characteristic of other economically advanced societies. Both countries have well-developed welfare states and elaborate administrative and governance structures. Policy is also heavily influenced, and delivered, by a range of non-governmental bodies in the health field. Finally, both countries have undergone nearly a quarter of a century of structural reform and change in the health field, much of it oscillating between competing political tendencies and ideological perspectives [2].

Epidemiological transition

Australia and New Zealand follow the pattern of societies that advanced through the late stages of the epidemiological transition. Both have birth rates below replacement levels and substantial populations in the retirement years, both display a pattern of ill-health, including mental health problems, that has moved well beyond the communicable diseases, with relatively low levels of mortality, and both enjoy superior life expectancy [3] (Table 11.1).

Table 11.1 Demographic indicators for New Zealand and Australia

Demographic indicator	New Zealand[1]	Australia[2]
Total population (million)	4.18	20.3
Percentage population over 65 (%)	12.3	13.0
Total fertility rate	2.1	1.8
Infant mortality rate (deaths per 1000 live births)	5.1	5.0
Life expectancy at birth		
Males	77.9	78.5
Females	81.9	83.3

[1] Data for 2007 [4].
[2] Data for 2005 [5].

A feature of both societies are sub-populations which vary in their progress through the health transition and which differ markedly in health experience. Australian Aborigines still have high birth and death rates and high rates of communicable disease. New Zealand Maori have only recently passed through the transition, and some Pacific groups in New Zealand are still showing high birth rates. Furthermore, the favourable statistics on life expectancy (Table 11.1) are primarily those of the majority populations of European origin, particularly those in affluent circumstances. The indigenous population groups, together with other disadvantaged socio-economic and ethnic groups, fare much more poorly in health outcomes [6,7].

Welfare state tradition

Australia and New Zealand follow the tradition of the other English-speaking democracies in taxation and welfare state provision. While clearly committed to a comprehensive system of social protection and state involvement in health and education and a range of other fields, the levels of taxation and public funding in these countries do not match those of many European countries. The level of private funding for health care in Australia and New Zealand is substantial, but close to the OECD average. Overall funding as a percentage of GDP also registers close to where one might expect these countries to be, given their relative position of national wealth (Table 11.2).

Administrative and governance structures

While Australia and New Zealand follow the 'Westminster' tradition of parliamentary government, and share a similar party political structure, they diverge on key institutional features. New Zealand has a unitary system and a single-chamber parliament, and election is by proportional representation. There is

Table 11.2 Economic indicators for New Zealand and Australia

Economic indicator	New Zealand[1]	Australia[2]
GDP per capita (PPP in $US)[3]	26,200.0	33,300.0
Percentage of GDP on health (%)	8.4	9.8
Percentage of private health expenditure (%)	22.6	32.0
Percentage of health budget allocation for public health (%)	2.0	2.1

PPP, purchasing power parity.
[1] Data for 2005 [8].
[2] Data for 2004–05 [9,10].
[3] Data for 2006 [11].

Box 11.1 Maori health initiatives

New Zealand's earliest hospitals dated from the 1840s. These were intended primarily for use by indigenous people, but the rapidly increasing white settler population soon displaced Maori patients in most localities. From the 1850s central government subsidized general practitioners to treat Maori. From the 1890s until the late 1930s, when universal medical benefits were introduced under the first Labour government, approximately one-sixth of all GPs were engaged in this scheme. In 1920 the Department established a separate Division of Maori Hygiene, headed by a Maori doctor. This was disbanded in 1930 when responsibility for Maori health was returned to Medical Officers of Health [12].

Disparities between Maori and non-Maori health increasingly exercised the minds of politicians and policy-makers from the 1930s. Until the 1980s, Western medicine, together with improved economic and housing conditions, was seen as the solution. However, a growing commitment to Maori self-determination saw the introduction of 'by Maori for Maori' health services during the 1990s. There was also a revival of traditional healing, whose practitioners, the tohunga, had been outlawed in 1907. Today, there are about 200 Maori health services, many of which include traditional healers. Maori concepts of health which place equal importance on family, mental, spiritual, and physical health are also widely accepted and promoted within New Zealand health policy and across the health system.

also a historical treaty relationship with Maori, with its own associated strand of public health development (Box 11.1). Australia, in contrast, is a federation with a considerable dilution of central government power through the principle of subsidiarity (powers are exercised by the states, or as close as possible to the community, unless stipulated otherwise by the constitution). The Australian parliament has two chambers and is elected by a process that is closer to the traditional constituency system (at least for the lower house). There is no formal recognition of indigenous rights in the Australian constitutional system and Aboriginal Australians did not gain the right to vote until 1968.

Despite the difference in constitutional character, both countries have experienced similar challenges and trajectories in the delivery of health services, including public health. Thus, initially, public health functions were jealously defended at the local level, with central government relegated to a broad regulatory role. However, issues of funding and the threat of epidemics moved such responsibilities upwards, so that, by 1900 in New Zealand and by 1901 in Victoria, Australia, public health legislation, building on the 1848 Public Health Act in England, were passed establishing governmental agencies with responsibilities in the area. Upon Federation in 1901, the new Australian government had little involvement in public health issues, except quarantine (Quarantine Act 1908); the states maintained governance over public health, in accordance with the constitutional framework. In both countries central government responsibilities in health care only crystallized and grew rapidly in the second half of the twentieth century. Local government retained key powers in environmental health and regulation.

A turbulent period

The period since the early 1970s has been one of partisanship, ideological debate, and almost constant health system restructuring. Issues of public health have been a major theme and, to an important extent, a litmus test of wider philosophical trends. The 1970s saw a renewed commitment from left-of-centre governments in both countries to public investment in health, most strikingly with Medibank in Australia. The debate over the role of the state re-ignited in the late 1980s with the return of similar governments, while the 1990s saw a trend towards health restructuring stimulated by neo-liberal concepts [13]. This also coincided with a weakening of public health commitments at the political and bureaucratic level, with savage budget cuts across the health system in the Australian states and territories.

The debates of the 1970s resulted in greater campaigning and activism in public health, fuelled by broader social and ideological changes [14]. This was a challenge to the 'old public health' and brought in an active health promotion agenda. These gains were consolidated with a refreshing of national institutions in the 1980s. This was particularly evident in Australia [15]. Both countries initiated goals and targets, major screening programmes, and significant initiatives on HIV/AIDS and tobacco control. These advances were slowed, but not entirely reversed, in an environment in the 1990s that was ideologically and politically more hostile to public health. Indeed, the Australian National Public Health Partnership (NPHP), established in 1996 and replaced in 2006, was an initiative from public health officials to strengthen the system and to respond to the challenges from new public sector management [16,17].

New challenges

However, the 2006 replacement of the National Public Health Partnership (NPHP) with the Australian Health Protection Committee (AHPC) and the Australian Population Health Development Principal Committee (APHDPC) is again indicative of a priority change to greater focus on preparedness for possible pandemic and on targeted health issues. The Sydney Olympic Games in 2000, the threat of potential terrorism after the attacks on the USA in September 2001, and the 2003 outbreak of Sudden Acute Respiratory Syndrome (SARS), together with the more recent threat of possible human-to-human spread of avian influenza, all provided impetus for this shift. Health promotion receded to the background, other than disease prevention and early intervention aimed at reducing the incidence of avoidable chronic disease (e.g. through the Australian Better Health Initiative (ABHI)) [18]. Tackling problems of overweight and obesity in the general population is a particular area of priority in the goal of reducing chronic disease [19].

In contrast, in New Zealand there has been renewed commitment since 2000 to the 'new public health'—a focus on the social determinants of health in addition to traditional public health concerns. This is represented in health system restructuring and development of local 'district health boards' which plan and fund services in accordance with national population health goals. The aim of new 'primary health organizations' is to improve primary care access, reduce inequalities, and enhance population health (see Box 11.3 on p.235).

Public health infrastructure

In its origins, public health emerged in Australia and New Zealand strongly influenced by the British model. This early legal and legislative framework has had an enduring influence, but more important since has been the particular logistical and health challenges of both countries. As ever, the resourcing and administrative arrangements for the public health function have been controversial. Nevertheless, there are some notable achievements in the information base for public health decision-making, in workforce development, and in research and development activities. These areas are all fluid and under constant negotiation, but, despite setbacks and a lack of consistent and long-term strategic guidance and development, they suggest that there is a considerable vigour and creativity underpinning public health in Australia and New Zealand.

Legal framework

The origins of the legal framework for the public health function in both countries lie in the great legislative initiatives of late-nineteenth century Victorian Britain. While the early settlers assumed that they were escaping the worst excesses of industrial Europe, many of the conditions of urban squalor were replicated in the Antipodes. These circumstances, together with concerns about the potential for the spread of epidemic disease associated with large-scale migration, prompted early efforts to define the core public health function, establish the associated administrative structures, and secure the necessary funding. The 1918 influenza epidemic added urgency and impetus to the evolution of a public health administration. The special requirements of disadvantaged indigenous peoples and of providing coverage over large sparsely populated areas gave a distinct character to public health responsibilities and structures.

The role of the Medical Officer of Health was central to the early public health framework, and remains important to this day. As defined in the early legislation, the Medical Officer of Health had important statutory responsibilities for the control of communicable disease, particularly epidemics and outbreaks, and around this core function was established the broader range of health protection duties, generally also of a regulatory and enforcement character. To the early responsibilities in infectious disease control were added food safety and hygiene, venereal disease, aspects of living and environmental conditions (generally handled by local rather than central government), general monitoring and surveillance activities, and screening (e.g. tuberculosis).

Regulation

The agenda of the 'new public health' extended the legal and enforcement mandate of public health (e.g. tobacco control and alcohol licensing). However, it also complemented this traditional function with the educational and empowerment strategies of health promotion. The Ottawa Charter provided a complementary vision and regulatory strategy. Further, concerns with privacy, confidentiality, and non-discrimination (as in the case of HIV/AIDS) elaborated and complicated the once more straightforward legal basis for the public health function. Monitoring and surveillance no longer went uncontested. More 'positive' duties have also been added. The ability to conduct health impact assessment of public policy proposals in Tasmania, to develop municipal public health plans in Victoria and Queensland, and to fund health promotion activities through tobacco tax hypothecation (Box 11.2), have been some recent Australian achievements.

The New Zealand Public Health and Disability Services Act 2000 is explicitly designed to stimulate locally planned service innovations that improve population health. When passed, a new Public Health Bill, introduced in 2008, will provide for health impact assessments (albeit on a voluntary basis) and for a stronger local government role in promoting and protecting the public health of New Zealanders. Novel legal and ethical issues are also emerging with the new genetics. Thus in the case of genetically modified organisms, the appropriate balance between the precautionary principle, fundamental to the public health

Box 11.2 Health promotion foundations

In 1987, the Victorian parliament passed the Tobacco Act—the first act of its kind internationally—setting aside a portion of the tax on tobacco sales for health promotion activities [20]. The passage of the legislation was achieved with active lobbying by a broad coalition, led by the Anti-Cancer Council of Victoria, and underpinned by substantial health and economic research and public opinion surveys. The Act banned advertising of tobacco products at public events (with limited exemptions such as the Grand Prix) and, as a trade-off, the arts and sports sponsorship was 'bought out' by the Victorian Health Promotion Foundation. In doing so, the Foundation required art and sporting organizations to enter into part-nerships with health sector organizations to promote health messages. In addition, the Foundation funded community-based health promotion programmes and public health research.

Western Australia also passed similar legislation in 1990 and established an equivalent foundation for health promotion. In 1996, the tobacco industry was successful in having the Federal High Court declare the state taxation arrangements to be unconstitutional. As a consequence, the tax is now collected by the Commonwealth and transferred to the state treasuries, who then provide the foundations with their budgets.

ethos, and the growth- and development-oriented agendas of key economic and scientific interests has been in contention.

Legislation

Each jurisdiction in Australia (state, territory, and federal) has a plethora of legislation covering traditional public health issues of environmental health, infectious disease control, food safety, tobacco control, etc. Quarantine, national security, disease surveillance, and therapeutic goods are of particular focus at the Commonwealth level. Biosecurity and gene technology are areas with newly forming regulatory frameworks of relevance to public health. At the national level, focus is currently on extending and improving the disease surveillance system. The Australian government Gene Technology Act 2000 established a national scheme to regulate gene technology, providing a frame-work for coordination across all levels of government. The National Health Security Bill 2007, passed in October 2007, gives effect to Australia's treaty commitments under the revised International Health Regulations and also establishes a national regulatory scheme to minimize the security risk posed by security-sensitive biological agents.

In December 2003, the Australian and New Zealand Governments signed an agreement to establish a joint regulatory scheme for therapeutic products (medicines, medical devices, and complementary medicines) in both countries. Passage of legislation to enact the joint Australian and New Zealand Therapeutic Products Authority (ANZTPA) was suspended by the New Zealand government in July 2007 when it was determined that there was insufficient support for the bill. Opposition to the proposed legislation was largely on the grounds of the belief that it is inappropriate to regulate complementary medicines in the same manner as pharmaceutical products.

Administrative structures

The fortunes of public health have always been closely associated with the activities of the state. The legal and regulatory frameworks exemplify that relationship. However, with these powers and responsibilities have come potentially complicated administrative arrangements. In both Australia and New Zealand there has been a tension between centralism and localism. With the abolition of the provinces in New Zealand in 1867, public health became a central government function. But the exact deployment of public health services has oscillated between central government—the Department and then Ministry of Health—and various local and regional agencies as the New Zealand system has undergone a series of reorganizations. Added to this is the role of local government in delivering environmental and resource management services.

With its unitary and unicameral political system, there has never been any doubt about the national and uniform application of public health legislation in New Zealand. Certainly, the reforms of the 1990s seemed set to erect, for a country of little more than four million, a relatively complicated structure of advisory, purchasing, and delivery agencies running in parallel to personal health services that continues to this day, but the mandate was unitary and national [21]. In the case of Australia, however, jurisdiction at the level of the states has led not only to conflict with the Commonwealth but also to difficulties in ensuring national uniformity. For example, a nationally consistent list of notifiable diseases was achieved only in 2000. The replacement of the NPHP has led to the removal of intergovernmental coordination mechanisms in a number of areas, which is likely to slow down harmonization of programmes.

Financing and resource allocation

Just as the rise of public health has historically been associated with the growing role of the state in social stewardship, so the financial viability of the sector has been closely tied to the fortunes of government. In the early stages of development public health was reliant on the uncertain and variable support of local government. It was this inconstancy in financial support and the lack of adherence to fundamental public health precautions, particularly in times of epidemic threat, that forced central government in New Zealand, and state and federal authorities in Australia, to take on both financial and administrative responsibility for public health. To the basic role of disease control and related enforcement functions have been added other activities in the areas of prevention, such as maternal and child health services, school dental services, and services for indigenous peoples. Other related areas of expenditure that are sometimes considered to be in the broad realm of public health touch upon primary care, where immunization and other preventive activities receive special funding and administrative support.

In Australia and New Zealand the proportion of 'health vote' directed to core public health functions has rarely risen above 2 per cent (see Table 11.2). This figure is in line with that for other developed countries. This funding has come exclusively out of taxation. In addition, governments have supplemented general tax revenue support with funding from hypothecated sources (see Box 11.2). While this additional funding for health promotion was welcomed, it also allowed health authorities to 'cost shift' and move out of direct funding of these activities in some instances. For example, as part of budget cuts in 1991, the Health Department of Victoria shed its entire health promotion unit of about 90 staff, and the recurrent cost of a range of public health programmes was passed on to the Victorian Health Promotion Foundation during the 1993 budget cuts.

By the late 1990s, the arrangement whereby the Australian federal government provided funding to the states and territories for specific public health programmes (Specific-Purpose Payments (SPPs)) underwent reform as this arrangement was considered to encourage vertical programme development, thus limiting horizontal integration of public health services and messages across diverse setting and populations. Public Health Outcome Funding Agreements (PHOFAs) replaced the input-oriented SPPs. The new funding arrangement had the Commonwealth providing the states/territories with a pool of funds via one agreement to which the jurisdictions were accountable against a set of outcome indicators [22]. In late 2008, further new National Partnership Payments have been devised, to the Commonwealth funding with agreed national reforms.

In New Zealand the reforms of the 1990s affected the stability, mix, and rationale of funding for public health. The incorporation of central government regional public health services into the Area Health Boards of the late 1980s seemed to herald a historic realignment in which the public health agenda would take its rightful place alongside that of the personal health services in a set of fully regionalized health authorities. Instead, the period into the early 1990s was one of retrenchment. Core public health functions remained, but resources and personnel ebbed away with the pressure from clinical services and the unravelling of the infrastructure of public health nursing [23]. The funding of public health remained in reduced circumstances throughout the 1990s, despite an attempt to establish an independent advisory authority (the Public Health Commission) and the re-emergence (and de-integration) of regional public health services [24]. Since 2000 there has been something of a turnaround. With renewed commitment to public health, all government-funded health providers in New Zealand are expected to focus on preventive care, population health improvement, and community engagement. This has created new organizational changes (Box 11.3).

Box 11.3 Public health and primary health organizations

The New Zealand government's 2001 Primary Health Care Strategy has been the catalyst for creating some 81 primary health organizations (PHOs) covering 97 per cent of the population. Government requirements for PHO formation mean each has a multidisciplinary composition including GPs and other primary care providers. Each is governed by provider members and community representatives, is capitation funded, and must have an enrolled patient population. Key objectives for PHOs are to reduce health inequalities, improve primary care service access, involve the community in service planning and governance, and develop strategies to improve and promote population health. The government has provided substantial new funding to support PHOs, especially for programmes to promote health, reduce chronic disease, and improve primary care service access.

The advent of PHOs produces exciting new opportunities for public health. The increasing public health emphasis within primary care and, particularly, general practice settings, has led to alliances with public health services. It has focused general practice more strongly on determinants of health and meant a closer engagement of primary care with communities and other health-influencing sectors such as local government and welfare services. Data show that primary care access has increased, but it is not yet clear whether PHOs are improving health [25]. PHOs have added a new layer of organization within the New Zealand health system, and complicated the service delivery landscape. Nonetheless, numerous new initiatives and innovations have resulted, but there remains no national clearing-house, creating difficulty for those seeking best practice [26].

Controversies of the kind associated with the implementation of new pro-grammes (e.g. major screening initiatives [27]) have raised issues about the proper economic evaluation of public health when assessed alongside the demands for resources in personal health. With increasing concern from gov-ernments about 'value for money', the desirability for greater economic analy-ses (such as cost-effectiveness analysis) has been expressed. These tools have not been used extensively, partly because of the paucity of appropriate data, and partly because most decision-making is based around changes at the mar-gins. Programme-based marginal analysis (PBMA) has been one tool used, particularly in New South Wales and South Australia, because it better approx-imates administrative decision-making [28].

Economic analyses

In the late 1990s, the importance of economic analysis for informing health financing decisions became increasing apparent. The first study of health expenditure for Aboriginal Australians was undertaken in response to Conservative political arguments that far too much health funding was being spent on Aboriginal health. Deeble [29] demonstrated that, compared with people at a similar socio-economic level (i.e. comparable health need), per capita expenditure was low, especially in relation to payments for Medicare benefits and pharmaceutical benefits, and this meant less access to primary care. The Deeble Report laid the foundation for primary care reforms which are continuing.

Further work was commissioned on the financial and economic return on investment of selected public health programmes in Australia since the 1970s [30]. The Abelson Report in 2003 concluded that investment in public health programmes (reduction of tobacco consumption, HIV/AIDS prevention, immunization, and road safety programmes) resulted in net benefit. For instance, for every A\$1 of expenditure on public health programmes to reduce tobacco consumption, an estimated saving of A\$2 is made for government (through reduction of costs associated with smoking-related disease/prema-ture death and improved population health status). Despite interest in the report, the establishment of a mechanism for scaling up recurrent funding of health promotion and disease prevention strategies was too difficult in an environment unsympathetic to health promotion. However, building from the Abelson Report, and concerns about the ever-escalating costs of Medicare and pharmaceutical benefits, interest is still rising around 'purchasing preven-tion' with health policy studies looking further at prevention investment returns [31].

The New Zealand Ministry of Health has developed the use of data from burden of disease analyses and information on inequality to prioritize public health strategies [32]. The government pharmaceutical purchasing agency has applied cost–utility analyses to drug subsidy decisions, just as its Australian counterpart applies a stringent cost-effectiveness analysis. The application of systematic economic analyses of this kind remains limited, while public health authorities struggle with new approaches for financing and resource allocation.

Investment in intellectual and human capital

One of the key issues in the infrastructure for public health relates to the investment in what might be called the intellectual and human capital required for the performance of core public health functions. These relate to information base, research and development (R&D), and workforce development.

Surveillance systems

Australia and New Zealand have progressively enhanced their national collections of health data. For example, since the 1970s there has been a gradual but continuous process of aligning the collection of hospital morbidity data with national definitions and minimum datasets. However, it has been more difficult to forge population health data into a coherent system, and reliance is still placed on a range of mechanisms. These include notification (historically important in communicable disease control), registries (cancer being the best developed but still not adequate in New Zealand), and official, ad hoc, and regular surveys (at both federal and state level in Australia). In addition, surveys have been funded by non-government organizations such as the National Heart Foundation, and national public health strategies (e.g. HIV, drugs and tobacco) have invested in their own surveys.

This patchwork of data represents a significant commitment to an information base. However, the potential of such data for policy and programme development and evaluation is unfulfilled, and there are still major gaps, such as psychosocial factors, social and environmental determinants of health, public health activities (outputs and expenditures), and trend data on major risk factors [33]. A 2001 data collection and information systems stocktake provides some hope for improvement in New Zealand. It has provided the impetus for improving national collection standards, creating a series of population health datasets, and ensuring that information systems are compatible [34]. A subsequent update in 2005 reported limited progress.

Research and development

Establishing a sustainable and adequately funded framework for R&D in public health has been a long-standing issue in both countries. For example, the

Medical Research Council in New Zealand was established in 1937 with early initiatives in preventive medicine [35], yet biomedical research soon overwhelmingly dominated the Council's funding priorities. In 1990 the Council was renamed the Health Research Council and a statutorily recognized public health committee was established. This was modelled to an extent on an equivalent committee within the Australian counterpart, the National Health and Medical Research Council (NHMRC), which was initially set up in 1927. However, under different political circumstances in the mid-1990s, the NHMRC took the decision to abolish a distinct public health identity. In a subsequent review of health and medical research [36], the categories of research were redefined away from 'biomedical vs. clinical vs. public health', towards 'basic vs. priority-driven'. This review resulted in a doubling of government funding in health research in the 1999–2000 federal budget. A 2004 report to assess the outcome of the returns subsequent to the increased investment showed some successes in research productivity and quality and in the creation of new businesses [37]. By 2006, however, NHMRC shifted its research funding framework towards disease streams (such as cancer and cardiovascular).

A different approach was adopted with the development of the Cooperative Research Centre (CRC) for Aboriginal Health (building from the work of its 1997–2003 predecessor, the CRC for Aboriginal and Tropical Health). The introduction of end-user-driven research enables health research in the Aboriginal health sector to be cognisant of a broad indigenous research reform agenda, to ensure that research is directly relevant and provides benefits to Aboriginal people, and to be controlled by Aboriginal people. The CRC for Aboriginal Health mediates relationships between researchers, the Aboriginal health sector, and government agencies, and has facilitated ongoing projects around understanding the social determinants of Aboriginal health, prevention of chronic conditions, and strengthening the social and emotional well-being of Aboriginal families and communities.

Public health workforce

Public health workforce development has been a strong and continuing theme in both Australia and New Zealand. A crucial development was the emergence of postgraduate programmes in public health drawing on students from well outside traditional spheres. In Australia this expansion occurred in the late 1980s with the commitment of funds by government for the Public Health and Education Research Program (PHERP) within faculties of medicine, with a strong orientation towards epidemiology and public health research. This was followed by developments in non-medical institutions—health science faculties—with a strong orientation to health promotion and a foundation in the social sciences. In addition, in the 1990s some health authorities (New South Wales and Victoria) opted for stronger practice-based training programmes.

The blossoming of multiple approaches and programmes has accompanied debates about the nature of the public health workforce—whether it is a speciality, a credentialled profession, a dimension of the job of other workers, or just a set of competencies that can be deployed in many (particularly intersectoral) tasks. The recommendations from the 2005 PHERP review reflect the general trend in public health towards capacity development in specific areas of policy priority, i.e. obesity, biosecurity, and disaster response. However, it also focused on the need for public health education institutions to recruit indigenous Australian students; and for public health education to demonstrate quality, impact, and relevance, achieving core foundation competencies as sought by employers [38].

The strong public health emphasis in New Zealand's post-2000 health policies has created a demand for a spectrum of skills, from specialist epidemiologists and public health physicians through to experience in community development and health promotion. However, there remains a need to emulate the Australian practice-oriented training programmes.

Public health strategies

Public health activities in Australia and New Zealand have shown a vigour and creativity that reflects an ability to work outside the 'bureaucratic square' with groups in touch with community concerns, and to integrate these associations into sustained, strategically focused, and officially sanctioned and funded campaigns [39]. In both countries the three most commonly recognized achievements in the past two decades are HIV prevention and control, tobacco control, and reduction in motor vehicle crashes. A review of the Australian experience with these campaigns identified three factors critical to success in each case: strategic policy direction, technical capacity, and the availability of supportive structures [40]. In both Australia and New Zealand the HIV/AIDS epidemic has largely been contained (although after a downward trend in incidence between 1987 and 2000, incidence of HIV diagnosis is now on the rise in both countries [41,42]) and smoking rates have fallen dramatically (although there are still concerns about young people), as have road deaths. In each case the formula for success involved some combination of community engagement and mobilization, well-funded and targeted research, strategic regulatory change, and a climate of political support.

Reorienting the health system

Despite these successes, there remain areas of uncertainty in establishing and following through on key priorities. From the 1980s authorities in both countries sought to establish strategic priorities for action. In Australia this started with the report of the Better Health Commission [43], continued through the subsequent identification of official goals and targets [44], and culminated in the late-1990s with an attempt to declare a number of national health priorities and to link these targets through to monitored indicators. By 2006, the Council of Australian Governments, comprising the prime minister and first ministers, finally adopted the Australian Better Health Initiative, with A$500 million invested in chronic disease prevention and control. Following the change of government in November 2007, there has been further emphasis on prevention, with a Preventative Health Taskforce and a National Health and Hospital Reform Commission established in 2008. A national prevention and health promotion agency has been proposed by both groups.

New Zealand went through much the same cycle, with a strong performance orientation in the health reforms of the 1990s [45], extremely elaborate health [46] and disability [47] strategies, and a range of related strategies. Important recent strategies have been developed to deal with obesity and type 2 diabetes. These include the Healthy Eating, Healthy Action plan that aims to improve nutrition and physical activity [48]. In 2007, following the recommendations of a parliamentary select committee, the government announced a cross-sectoral ministerial committee to ensure a cohesive long-term approach to countering obesity and type 2 diabetes. The government's various strategies are notable for their emphasis on reducing health inequalities, improving the health of Maori and Pacific people, and promoting community participation in all aspects of service planning and delivery.

Priority setting

While entirely laudable as an attempt to introduce a more rational and systematic process into priority setting and monitoring for public health, there is a degree of ambivalence about the experience. Thus many interest groups and lobbies have sought to influence the process. In Australia, for example, by the mid-1990s there were over 30 national public health strategies, including official national health priorities (cardiovascular health, cancer control, injury prevention and control, mental health, diabetes mellitus, asthma, and arthritis and musculoskeletal conditions), which frequently competed for scarce resources rather than forging alliances for common action. In some instances politically effective lobbies (such as the rural sector in Australia) have forced themselves up the list of priorities. Furthermore, it is not always clear that this engagement with the mainstream of the health system has resulted in anything more than a co-option of the health improvement agenda rather than significant gains for public health.

The policy emphasis in Australia since 2000 on clustering conditions and risk factors, such as through the development of a national chronic disease prevention strategy [49], was a way of bringing resources, expertise, and interest groups into more effective working arrangements. The 2006 Australian Better Health Initiative, aimed at reducing the burden of chronic disease and improving workforce productivity, is now attempting to put greater focus on prevention across the health system through actions across four areas: prevention, early detection and early treatment, integration and continuity of prevention and care, and supporting self-management of chronic disease. While New Zealand's various strategies are widely supported for their public health objectives, there has been concern about 'over-strategization' and the related demands that this places on the various public health services, district health boards, and primary health organizations. In response, in 2007 the government issued a set of 10 focused 'targets' for the health sector [50].

Primary care

Primary care is one area in particular where ambivalence about public health's engagement with personal health services has come to the fore. In both Australia and New Zealand, governments have identified a role for GPs in delivering disease prevention and, to a more limited extent, health promotion services [51]. This has resulted from a combination of both a desire to fund primary care more substantially and a philosophical commitment to advance a more population-wide orientation in the organization and funding of general practice. Also, in practical terms, governments were seeking ways to deliver on immunization targets and to enhance screening and other programmes in a growing number of areas (now including smoking, nutrition, and physical activity in Australia).

The public health community has been divided over these initiatives. In debates at professional forums, some have applauded the expanded efforts and resources for primary care, while others have been alarmed that GPs are being well supported to undertake activities for which they are neither trained nor well placed to do, and in so doing potentially diverting resources out of public health (see Box 11.3).

Environmental and other challenges

Finally, there are areas where the public health agenda remains undeveloped. For example, there has been a tendency even in the area of communicable disease for funding to be 'crisis dependent'. Thus in 1988, a large outbreak of legionnaires' disease in Wollongong led to the investment of resources into area-based public health units all across New South Wales. In 1997, a series of food-borne disease outbreaks in Victoria led to the consolidation of the whole of government responsibility for food safety within the health portfolio.

In other areas, the public health response lags behind the requirement. In the late 1990s, public health interventions for mental illness began to receive attention in Australia with the development of a national strategy and action plan [52], which was further updated in 2006 with a focus on mental health promotion, prevention, and early intervention [53]. In 2000, a national initiative to raise awareness about issues associated with depression, anxiety, and related substance misuse disorders (*beyondblue*) was established, and in 2006 the Australian government committed A$1.9 billion over 5 years to improve access to mental health services and provide additional support to people with mental illness and their families and carers.

Despite the development of environmental protection authorities and the rise of the environmental movement, environmental health (as a field of public health practice and as a public health concern) largely disappeared from the public agenda and public consciousness until, in 1999, the Australian government adopted the National Environmental Health Strategy [54]. Today the Office of Health Protection provides project management for activities developed through the Environmental Health Committee (enHealth), although the agenda is largely driven by the federal government rather than in partnership with states and territories who have the main carriage of environmental health responsibilities. Hepatitis C, which until recently failed to receive much public support, is now the focus of a national strategy [55], but the funding remains limited despite its potential to affect large numbers of people.

Multicultural health promotion, despite the population mix, has also received little to no political and bureaucratic support, other than language services [56]. While the New Zealand government has been slow to update the 1956 Health Act, which governs the scope and activities of public health officials, it swiftly passed the Law Reform (Epidemic Preparedness) Act 2006 in response to the SARS outbreak and the threat of avian influenza. For a range of reasons—part technical, part political and ideological—the response in these areas has remained largely reactive, rather than one of pursuing a preventive strategy. That said, the new Public Health Bill, noted above, does embody a risk-assessment and management approach that is tied into government concerns about obesity and type 2 diabetes.

Conclusion

Public health in Australia and New Zealand presents a mixed picture. As expected for economically developed economies, they have favourable health profiles.

Yet significant inequalities and disadvantages are in evidence, particularly among the indigenous peoples, although, following a proactive policy programme, there are indications of a reduction in both counties [57]. Both countries have established public health systems with a clearly acknowledged mandate, strategic direction, and the requisite and full range of technical resources. Yet funding, professional identity, and ideological rationale remain contested and, at times, uncertain. There is considerable evidence of vigour, creativity, and engagement with the concerns of the community, but public health is also bureaucratically constrained and sometimes at odds with powerful constituencies, but decreasingly so in post-2000 New Zealand where population health is now at the forefront of much health policy. With the new Australian government elected in November 2007, prevention is expected to receive greater policy attention.

There are also a number of areas where public health needs to work outside established boundaries. Health inequalities, the health of indigenous peoples, most strikingly the Aborigines, the concerns of refugees and migrants, and mental health promotion all work at the margins of traditional categories of public health analysis and action. The interconnectedness of health issues is also something that the general approach to public health has yet to grapple with—for instance the campaign to combat overweight and obesity, which focuses its messages on the broad population, largely ignores health issues related to underweight and fad dieting.

There are also challenges of a more global nature—climate change, genetically modified organisms, emerging diseases, and the opportunities and dilemmas of the new health information technology, including e-health. Finally, the public health community has to consider its mandate. The 'new public health' has provided one source of regeneration and redefinition, but it has also created persistent divisions within the profession. There still remain lines of ambivalence, between technical and advocacy models, between enforcement and empowerment strategies, between professional and lay concepts of public health, and between state-sponsored and community-inspired agendas for action. Above all, the dynamic global environment and the growing density of regional relations supply a new set of challenges for a model of public health which, to date, has been closely tethered to the administrative and financial structures of the modern nation state.

Despite these challenges and uncertainties, public health policy has evolved from a history of medical dominance to an accommodation of interest group pluralism, while public health practice has similarly shifted from a rather singular professional approach to one acknowledging multiple perspectives. There are some signs that the next stage may well be one of more integrative practice and a greater emphasis on investment for health and preventive medicine, but much will depend on the cohesion of health policy and the profession, as well as the views of politicians and the communities they represent.

Acknowledgements

We are grateful to Derek Dow for preparing an earlier version of Box 11.1, and to Rachel Canaway for checking Australian sources.

References

[1] Castles F, Gerritsen R, Vowles J. *The Great Experiment. Labour Parties and Public Policy Transformation in Australia and New Zealand*. Auckland: Auckland University Press, 1996.

[2] Bloom A (ed). *Health Reform in Australia and New Zealand*. Melbourne: Oxford University Press, 2000.

[3] Davis P, Mathers C, Graham P. Health expectancy in Australia and New Zealand. In: Robine J-M, Jagger C, Mathers C, Crimmins E, Suzman R (eds). *Determining Health Expectancies*. Chichester: John Wiley, 2003; pp.391–408.

[4] Statistics New Zealand. *Population indicators*. Available online at: http://www.stats.govt.nz/tables/population-indicators.htm (accessed 31 July 2007).

[5] Australian Bureau of Statistics. Available online at: http://www.ato.gov.au (accessed 11 September 2007).

[6] Blakely T, Tobias M, Robson B. Ajwani S, Bonne M, Woodward A. Widening ethnic mortality disparities in New Zealand 1981–99. *Social Sci Med* 2005; 61: 2233–51.

[7] Anderson I, Crengle S, Kamaka M L, *et al*. Indigenous health in Australia, New Zealand, and the Pacific. *Lancet* 2006; 367: 1775–85.

[8] Organization for Economic Cooperation and Development. *OECD Health Data 2007*. Paris: OECD, 2007.

[9] Trewin D. *2007 Year Book Australia*. Canberra: Australian Bureau of Statistics, 2007.

[10] Australian Institute of Health and Welfare (AIHW). *National Public Health Expenditure Report 2004–05*. Canberra: AIHW, 2007.

[11] Central Intelligence Agency. *The World Factbook 2007*. Washington, DC: Central Intelligence Agency.

[12] Dow DA. *Maori Health and Government Policy 1840–1940*. Wellington: Victoria University Press, 1999.

[13] Ashton T. The health reforms: to market and back? In: Boston J, Dalziel P, St. John S (eds). *Redesigning the Welfare State: Problems, Policies, Prospects*. Auckland: Oxford University Press, 1999; pp. 134–53.

[14] Baum F. *The New Public Health* (3rd edn). Melbourne: Oxford University Press, 2008.

[15] Lin V, King C. Intergovernmental reforms in public health. In: Bloom A (ed.), *Health Reform in Australia and New Zealand*. Melbourne: Oxford University Press, 2000; pp. 251–63.

[16] Adams T, Lin V. Partnership in public health. *World Health Forum* 1998; 19: 246–52.

[17] Lin V, King C. Intergovernmental reforms in public health. In: Bloom A (ed). *Health Reform in Australia and New Zealand*. Melbourne: Oxford University Press, 2000; pp. 251–63.

[18] Australian Government Department of Health and Ageing (DoHA). *Australian Better Health Initiative: Promoting Good Health, Prevention and Early Intervention*. Available online at: www.health.gov.au/internet/wcms/publishing.nsf/Content/feb2006coag03.htm (accessed 2 October 2007).

[19] Lin V, Robinson P. Australian public health policy in 2003–2004. *Aust New Zealand Health Policy* 2005; **2**: 7.

[20] Galbally R. Placing prevention at the centre of health sector reform. In: Bloom A (ed.), *Health Reform in Australia and New Zealand*. Melbourne: Oxford University Press, 2000; pp. 264–76.

[21] Barnett P, Malcolm LA. To integrate or deintegrate? Fitting public health into New Zealand's reforming health system. *Eur J Public Health* 1998; **8**: 79–86.

[22] Lin V, King C. Intergovernmental reforms in public health. In: Bloom A (ed). *Health Reform in Australia and New Zealand*. Melbourne: Oxford University Press, 2000; pp. 251–63.

[23] Armstrong A, Bandaranayake D. *Public Health in New Zealand. Recent Changes and Future Prospects. Public Health Monograph Series*. Wellington: Department of Public Health, Wellington School of Medicine, University of Otago, 1995.

[24] Krieble TA. *The Rise and Fall of a Crown Entity: A Case Study of the Public Health Commission*. Wellington: Victoria University of Wellington, 1996.

[25] Health Services Research Centre. *Evaluation of the Implementation and Immediate Outcomes of the Primary Health Care Strategy*. Wellington: Health Services Research Centre, Victoria University of Wellington, 2005.

[26] Gauld R, Mays N. Reforming primary care: are New Zealand's new primary health organisations fit for purpose?. *BMJ* 2006; **333**: 1216–18.

[27] Ministry of Health. *Investigation into Cervical Screening in the Tairawhiti Region, Health Funding Authority: Final Report*. Wellington: Ministry of Health, 2001.

[28] Deeble J. *Resource Allocation in Public Health: An Economic Approach*. Melbourne: National Public Health Partnership, 1999.

[29] Deeble, J. *Expenditures on Health Services for Aboriginal and Torres Strait Islander People*. Canberra: Commonwealth Department of Health and Family Services and Australian Institute of Health and Welfare, 1998.

[30] Abelson P, Taylor R, Butler J, *et al. Returns on Investment in Public Health: An Epidemiological and Economic Analysis*. Canberra: Commonwealth Department of Health and Ageing, 2003.

[31] Wilcox S. Purchasing prevention: making every cent count. Background Paper, National Health Policy. Roundtable, Melbourne, Australian Institute of Health Policy Studies, 8 August 2006.

[32] Ministry of Health. Evidence-based health objectives for the New Zealand Health Strategy. *Public Health Intelligence Occasional Bulletin 2*. Wellington: Ministry of Health, 2001.

[33] National Public Health Partnership. *National Public Health Information Development Plan*. Melbourne: National Public Health Partnership, 1999.

[34] WAVE (Working to Add Value to E-information) Advisory Group. *From Strategy to Reality: The WAVE Project*. Wellington: Ministry of Health, 2001.

[35] Dow DA. *Safeguarding the Public Health. A History of the New Zealand Department of Health*. Wellington: Victoria University Press, 1995.

[36] Health and Medical Research Strategic Review Committee. *The Virtuous Cycle. Working Together for Health and Medical Research*. Canberra: Department.of Health and Aged Care, 1999.

[37] *Sustaining the Virtuous Cycle for a Healthy, Competitive Australia. Investment Review of Health and Medical Research. Final Report, December 2004 (The Grant Report)*. Canberra: Commonwealth of Australia, 2004.

[38] Durham G, Plant A. *PHERP: The Public Health Education and Research Program— Review 2005, Strengthening Workforce Capacity for Public Health*. Canberra: Commonwealth of Australia, 2005.

[39] National Public Health Partnership. *Key Achievements in Public Health*. Melbourne: National Public Health Partnership, 1998.

[40] National Health and Medical Research Council. *Health Australia Review*. Canberra: Health Advancement Standing Committee, 1997.

[41] New Zealand Ministry of Health. HIV and AIDS information. *AIDS New Zealand*. 2007; 59 *Issue 59*: 1–4. ISSN 1170 2656.

[42] National Centre in HIV Epidemiology and Clinical Research (NCHECR). *HIV/AIDS, Viral Hepatitis and Sexually Transmissible Infections in Australia—2006 Annual Surveillance Report*. NCHECR, The University of New South Wales, Sydney and the Australian Institute of Health and Welfare, Canberra, 2006.

[43] Commonwealth Department of Health. *Report of the Better Health Commission*. Canberra: Australian Government Printers, 1985.

[44] Australian Health Ministers Advisory Council. *Health for All Australians: Report of the Health Goals and Targets Committee*. Canberra: Australian Government Printers, 1988.

[45] Ministry of Health. *Progress on Health Outcomes Targets (Te Haere Whamua Ki Nga Whainga Hua Mo Te Hauora)*. Wellington: Ministry of Health, 1996.

[46] Ministry of Health. *The New Zealand Health Strategy*. Wellington: Ministry of Health, 2000.

[47] Ministry of Health. *The New Zealand Disability Strategy: Making a World of Difference*. Wellington: Ministry of Health, 2001.

[48] Ministry of Health. *Healthy Eating, Health Action (Oranga Kai—Oranga Pamau): A Strategic Framework*. Wellington: Ministry of Health, 2003.

[49] National Health Priority Action Council (NHPAC). *National Chronic Disease Strategy*. Canberra: Australian Government Department of Health and Ageing, 2006.

[50] Minister of Health. *Health Targets: Moving Towards Healthier Futures 2007/08*. Wellington: Ministry of Health, 2007.

[51] General Practice/Population Health Joint Action Group. *Consultation Paper: General Practice and Population Health*. Canberra: Department of Health and Aged Care, 2001.

[52] Australian Health Ministers Advisory Council. *National Mental Health Promotion and Prevention Action Plan*. Canberra: Commonwealth Department of Health and Aged Care, 1999.

[53] Council of Australian Governments (COAG). *National Action Plan on Mental Health 2006–2011*. Available online at: www.coag.gov.au/meetins/140706/index.htm#related (accessed 2 October 2007).

[54] National Public Health Partnership, EnHealth Council, and Commonwealth Department of Health and Aged Care. *National Environmental Health Strategy*. Canberra: Commonwealth Department of Health and Aged Care, 1999.

[55] *National Hepatitis C Strategy 2005–2008*. Canberra: Commonwealth of Australia, 2005.

[56] Liamputtong P, Lin V, Bagley P. Ethnic communities and health reforms. In: Gardner H, Liamputtong P (eds). *Health, Social Policy, and Communities*. Melbourne: Oxford University Press, 2002.

[57] Thomas D, Condon J, Anderson I, *et al.* Long-term trends in indigenous deaths from chronic diseases in the Northern Territory: a foot on the brake, a foot on the accelerator. *Med J Aust* 2006; **185**: 145–9.

Chapter 12

Ethical issues

Daniel Wikler and Richard Cash

Introduction

Ethical dilemmas arise at almost every turn in the practice of global public health. For example:

- Practitioners who would save lives through public health measures must decide which lives to save.

- Interventions usually protect health, but because they sometimes carry risks, the claims of people who might be harmed must be heard.

- Practitioners who intervene and those who are affected may have different preferences and values.

- Public health programmes sometimes require compromises with values such as privacy and liberty.

- Public health requires research involving human subjects, but there is an incomplete consensus on the social contract between subjects, scientists, sponsors, and society.

- The pursuit of global public health takes place in an unjust world, demanding that its practitioners judge when and to what extent to compromise their ideals and standards in order to remain effective.

- Practitioners of public health must sometimes choose between the objectives and interests of the communities they serve, the donors and sponsors, and themselves.

In this chapter we survey a few of these ethical quandaries as a stimulus to consideration of ethical dimensions of global public health. After some general remarks on ethics, we take up: ethical issues encountered in global public health practice, ethical dimensions of health resource allocation, and ethical issues in research involving human subjects. Our goal is to identify ethical issues that bear further reflection. We leave the task of proposing standards and solutions to others [1–3].

A proposed Public Health Code of Ethics, written by a working group of the Public Health Leadership Society, is posted on the website of the American Public Health Association at http://www.apha.org/programs/education/proge-duethicalguidelines.htm/(accessed on 16th February 2009).

Responsibilities and values

Ethical issues are those involving actions and policies that are right or wrong, fair or unfair, just or unjust. There is no consensus on methods for resolving ethical dilemmas and controversies [4]. Nevertheless, we cannot escape ethical dilemmas. When confronted, our responsibility is to reason our way through them, identify the best options (or the least bad ones), and to act according to our best judgement.

In view of the importance of health, the burden of disease, and the numbers of individuals involved, few fields of professional activity face ethical choices as potentially momentous as those encountered in public health. A decision to emphasize prevention of HIV infection over treatment of AIDS in the poorest countries, for example, might represent the most efficient use of available resources to keep the population healthy. But it also means that people suffering from AIDS will have fewer health care resources, although their lives might have been prolonged longer with better treatment. As is typically the case in global health, the ethical dilemma must be faced by societies, not merely by individual health workers. Indeed, there are multiple agents involved, both individual and collective, including patients, doctors, families, organizations, professions, and nations. In addition to having conflicting interests, and answering to different constituencies whose interests may conflict, these agents may not accept the same sets of moral rules.

Whose responsibility?

Only the cooperative effort of individuals, local and national agencies, the private sector, and donors and governments can protect global public health. All agree on this general proposition, but not on the actual assignment of responsibility to the respective agents. For example:

◆ Although many pharmaceutical firms have donated drugs to low- and middle-income countries, high prices continue to impede access to essential medicines. In many cases, the marginal cost of producing the drugs is low; moreover, since few people in low- and middle-income countries can afford them, the high cost of these drugs brings little profit. By ordinary moral calculations, the case for providing these drugs in the poorest countries at cost, or even free, is overwhelming [5]. However, as publicly owned for-profit enterprises, the primary responsibility of the drug manufacturers is to stockholders.

+ All who suffer from disease deserve the sympathy of others. But individuals can reduce their risk of getting many illnesses, including diabetes, cancer, and cardiovascular disease, if they take elementary precautions. Do those who become ill because they have made imprudent choices have a strong claim on their fellow citizens' resources? The WHO was faulted for placing tobacco control high on its agenda, on the grounds that whether to smoke is a matter of individual choice [6,7], just as, in many countries, tobacco companies have successfully defended themselves in court by emphasizing the responsibility of the individual smoker [8]. The notions of culpability and fault play central roles in legal thinking. Do they have any place in global health policy?

+ Sponsors of health research in developing countries offer benefits to the host community that go beyond any treatment offered in the course of the investigation. In the past sponsors had no obligations to host communities beyond the standard protections offered to the participants themselves. But ethics advisory agencies have urged that sponsors of research be required to demonstrate that any treatments proved effective by research in developing countries be useful to and accessible by those who live there [9,10].

In these and other cases, the outcomes turn not only on economics and politics, but also reflect ethical judgements. Refusing to aid countries that do not provide for their own citizens punishes individuals for the failings of their governments. Addiction to tobacco generally occurs before the age of majority [11], and this counts strongly against the claim that tobacco control is not a legitimate public health function. Requiring sponsors of research sited in developing countries to become donors to health systems could make research on tropical diseases unaffordable. These considerations point to the substantive ethical debates needed in assigning responsibility.

Whose values?

Whose values should guide those who face ethical dilemmas in the course of public health work? Deference to the values of the community may enhance acceptance and compliance with public health advice. But public health workers can sometimes benefit communities by insisting on compliance with non-traditional norms and values: discouraging female circumcision, endorsing condoms and male circumcision to prevent the spread of sexually-transmitted diseases, and refusing to abide by cultural norms that accord inferior status or stigma to women, sex workers, homosexuals, and lower castes.

Except when the subject is reproduction or sex, fundamental moral beliefs tend to be universal. Every culture champions the honest, the selfless, and the brave, and disdains those who are corrupt, insensitive, selfish, or untrustworthy. Where opinions differ, disagreements within borders are often as great as those across them. What sometimes presents itself as a difference in moral beliefs may, on analysis, simply reflect different beliefs about scientific facts. These differences may be difficult to bridge, but they do not require a choice between one moral outlook and another [12].

International treaties, including human rights conventions, that have been ratified by the government of the host community can serve as a common point of reference in the case of inter-cultural ethical differences, as can codes or guidelines of reputable professional societies or international organizations. The latter are sometimes devised specifically to protect the practitioner's freedom to act according to conscience in the face of pressure. An example is the proposed convention on 'dual loyalties' for health professionals, drafted by Physicians for Human Rights, designed to reinforce the dedication of health workers to the well-being of their patients regardless of the demands of state security agencies or employers [13].

Ethical issues in public health practice

As in clinical medicine, the ethics of public health practice are based on the fundamental principle of professional dedication to the best interests of the clients. However, the ethics of public health are distinctive in many ways.

- ◆ Public health takes into consideration the interests of the group or society as a whole, even when this may conflict with the best interests of some individuals. At the same time, individual rights must be respected [14].

- ◆ Interventions on a public scale, such as fluoridation of the water supply, do not always permit individual informed consent.

- ◆ With public health interventions, particularly those that are preventive, it may be difficult or impossible to identify those who will benefit, or those who have benefited. Thus, individuals may not be able to weigh benefit against cost, risk, and other burdens.

- ◆ In some public health interventions, particularly during catastrophes, disasters, and epidemics, health authorities may invoke the power of the state, even including the use of force.

- ◆ In the case of global public health, the potential reach across national, cultural, and economic boundaries adds further moral complexity.

- ◆ Since research and monitoring may have serious unintended and harmful consequences, they should be built into public health interventions (See Box 12.1).

Individuals and groups

The dilemma of choosing between individual and group interests in public health practice is most clearly at stake in the case of infectious disease epidemics.

Box 12.1 Unintended consequences of public health interventions: arsenic in tube wells [15–17]

For 25 years there has been a major effort to improve rural standards of water and hygiene in Bangladesh. The installation of tube wells has been the most important element of the programme with over 95 per cent of the population now relying on groundwater from tube wells for drinking. Control of cholera and other water-borne enteric diseases was the stated purpose of increasing the availability of tube wells, although these wells were not routinely tested for microbial counts, heavy metals content, or toxic chemicals. In 1985, a physician in West Bengal, India, began noticing patients with clinical signs of arsenic intoxication. (High levels of arsenic ingestion are associated with skin pigmentation and increased rates of a variety of cancers.) A check of tube wells revealed arsenic levels that were many times the recommended levels. As these areas bordered Bangladesh, authorities were informed but neither the government nor international donors, who had contributed significantly to tube-well construction, took serious action. A national programme has identified areas of high arsenic concentrations in tube-well water; a quarter of the population, or about 30 million people, are drinking water with significantly high levels of arsenic. Possible strategies to lower arsenic intake from water include treating water at the pump, in-home treatment of water, community-level water treatment, sealing wells with high arsenic content and returning to the use of treated surface water or collected rainwater, and sinking deeper wells below the water table with high arsenic content. Many of these interventions are too costly, require continuing maintenance, or may be culturally unacceptable. Government and some NGOs have mounted programmes to reduce arsenic levels locally; however, there has been no effective national programme to reduce tube-well arsenic levels. On a sub-national level, some NGOs have been promoting sinking of deeper wells to mitigate the problem.

When public health authorities place limitations on travel, commerce, and other activities of daily life, some individuals may suffer losses that exceed any protective benefits. But the ethical issue arises in ordinary times. Reporting requirements for sexually transmitted diseases may benefit the general population, but weigh heavily on the individual. Vaccination, while very safe, can impose risks that a child's parents might prefer to avoid if neighbouring children agree are immunized. In this case, it is in the best interest of each child to be the single individual who is not vaccinated, but if more than a few parents try to secure this advantage for their children, the potential loss of herd immunity may threaten their children as well as the others. In addition, society might have to carry the financial burden should any of the non-immunized children become ill and require expensive treatment.

Public health practitioners in the past sought to minimize these conflicts by reducing risks to individuals as much as possible, consistent with the public health goal. For example, safer vaccinations reduce the risk to children, and protection of confidentiality minimizes the social harm caused by contact tracing in sexually transmitted diseases. But where the conflicts were unavoidable, the ethical norms of public health practitioners, unlike those of individual physicians, often accepted the claims of the group. These priorities contributed to the success of public health over the past century in reducing mortality and morbidity; but mass sterilization programmes, carried out in the name of public health, were also reflections of these priorities. The involvement of the state's power necessitates continuous ethical reflection on goals and on the means chosen to accomplish them.

The range of possible accommodations between individual and group interest is illustrated in differing approaches to HIV/AIDS. For example, Cuba's early success in limiting the impact of sexually transmitted HIV/AIDS was due in part to a decision to subject individuals at risk to testing and to segregate those infected with the disease from the general population [18,19]. However, UNAIDS and other major international agencies have placed human rights at the centre of their strategy [20]. This may reflect strategy as well as principle. The prospect of containing the spread of infectious disease by emphasizing human rights may be particular to HIV/AIDS, which is spread through actions performed in private, such as unsafe sex and illicit drug use, and hence generally beyond the reach of the state. They argued that only by assuring the individuals that their interests would be protected could they be recruited to join in a public health effort by modifying their behaviour. But not all agree that expedience and ethics coincide for HIV/AIDS, and some have expressed concern at the idea that a rights-based approach partially absolves government of a complete commitment to an aggressive public health strategy [21].

Individual perceptions of risk

The emphasis on prevention that partially distinguishes public health from clinical medicine gives rise to further ethical difficulties. Population health may be the highest priority for public health practitioners, who concern themselves with aggregates and thus assign high priority to interventions that promise significant reductions in morbidity or premature mortality for society as a whole at modest cost, risk, or inconvenience. However, individuals are not primarily concerned with aggregates.

The difference in perspectives is apparent in the case of interventions that offer slight reductions in risk for large numbers of people. Standard medical practice for risk factors is to identify those at highest risk and to assist them in reducing their personal risk to normal levels. But when the distribution of risk follows the normal bell-shaped curve, interventions that reduced the risk of those at normal or near-normal levels might have a larger aggregate impact, even if the risk reduction is modest [22]. The reason is that there are many more people in the latter category than in the high-risk category.

In the case of hypertension, for example, the medical approach identifies patients with very high blood pressure and offers suggestions for behaviour changes and, if necessary, drugs. The benefits to the individual—avoidance of premature death or serious disability—may easily outweigh any costs or burdens. A population-level approach might seek to reduce risks for those at normal or near-normal levels—a much larger group—by seeking 10 per cent reductions in the salt levels of processed food or food served in restaurants. In this case some of these individuals might question the value or desirability of the intervention, especially when not chosen by them, since the likelihood of personal benefit is very small. It will be of no direct interest to these individuals that there are many others similarly situated and that the sum of these small reductions in risk could represent a significant improvement in health at the population level.

This difference in perspective also plays a role in the relative priority placed on 'identified' and 'statistical' lives. For example, a community may fail to allocate sufficient funds to put caps on unused wells, but if a child falls into one, no expense will be spared for the rescue. From the population-level perspective, this cannot be justified. But the wrongness of failing to save an identified individual at peril is more apparent to many than that preventing this eventuality, whose ('statistical') identity does not become known. The rescue, whether of a child from a well or a patient needing expensive surgery, addresses the needs of 'identified' lives that attract the sympathy of all [23–25]. The arguable result is a persistent misallocation of resources away from preventive public health in the direction of curative clinical services [23–26].

Individuals vary in their perception of risk, and may be reluctant to accept the need for sacrificing liberties or changing lifestyles as the public health practitioner recommends [27]. In the case of less well-educated populations in poor countries, the gap in knowledge and perception may be much wider. The potential exists for distrust, or conversely for excessive trust (at the expense of meaningful deliberation) [28,29]. Public health practitioners may find allies in political authorities that claim to speak for their fellow-citizens and can order compliance, thus increasing acceptance but possibly at the expense of norms of self-determination. Public support for preventive measures that impose burdens of cost and loss of liberty is less certain when those who benefit and those who pay the price are not the same individuals. This is an issue inherent in public health prevention, in which the lives saved are 'statistical'—no-one can know which individuals would have been afflicted had the prevention not have occurred.

Issues in health promotion

Attempts in all countries to change health-related behaviour on a mass scale face numerous ethical problems, whether the chosen means are communication, incentives, coercion, or some combination. Although taxes on cigarettes are known to be an effective instrument in reducing the toll taken by tobacco [30,31], the individual's own calculation of the relative gain and loss may be different from that of the public health practitioner. Residents of the American state of Nevada, who have some of the least healthy living habits in the country, may look across the state line at their pious clean-living neighbours in Utah and decide that, on the whole, they prefer the lifestyle they already enjoy (although, statistically speaking, they will not enjoy it for as long) [32]. But in wealthy countries most smokers, even young people, wish that they could quit [33]. Recent work in behavioural economics defends the view that taxes and other curbs on smoking and other self-destructive addictive behaviour can be understood as a benefit to those who are targeted [34].

Libertarians reject such interventions on principle as paternalistic, regardless of their potential health benefit [35,36]. But the relation of the government to the individual in health promotion is more subtle than the spectre of the paternalistic 'nanny state' might suggest. Further research in behavioural economics has identified methods that guide individuals to more self-protective choices without withdrawing any options, such as removing high-calorie desserts from easy reach in the cafeteria line [37,38]. More generally, a 'stewardship' model of health promotion seeks to enable people to make healthy choices and to act on them, removing constraints on good choices and incentives for risk-taking without restricting liberty [39].

'First, do no harm' and the obligation to serve

Primum non nocere ('First, do no harm') is a venerable principle of medical ethics. Is this tenable in public health? It is of course an important goal. But the price of obedience in some cases would be to refrain from interventions that offer protection from death or serious harm in order to protect some people from lesser harms. For example, fortifying flour sold in food stores with folic acid reduces neural tube defects among newborns, but at the same time may mask the symptoms of vitamin deficiency in older people that would have prompted them to seek medical attention [40].

Similarly, while physicians have a general obligation to assist patients in need, doing so can create a role conflict in public health. Basic epidemiological data are lacking in most poor countries, hampering the development of effective public health strategies. Public health workers who collect these data must make ethical choices between their primary mission and the inevitable demands for better personal health care. Provision of services would take time away from data collection and could render the data unrepresentative, undermining the rationale for stationing observers in the first place.

In some cases reasonable compromises may be very difficult to achieve. The WHO has been concerned over the possibility that disease may be spread by vaccination and other public health interventions because of improper re-use of needles and inadequate sterilization of syringes. Observation of injection practices is indispensable if the authorities are to know whether the intervention does more good than harm. But what should the observer do if he/she sees that an individual is about to receive an unsafe injection? Intervening so that it does not take place would probably skew the data; indeed, intervention might result in the observer's being asked to leave at once. To stand by and say nothing would seem unconscionable to many, and could damage the good name of the health agency. WHO elected to intervene in all such cases.

Ethical dimensions of resource allocation

Public health interventions benefit some and not others. Choosing who will benefit requires ethics as much as it does economics and science. Attention to the ethics of public health resource allocation, particularly in international contexts, has only recently been undertaken [41–43]. The starting point for resource allocation in global public health is cost-effectiveness—maximizing health benefits per unit of cost. Conceptualizing, measuring, and calculating cost-effectiveness, and allocation strategies based on cost-effectiveness allocation, is complex and involves numerous ethical judgements [44,45]. The ethical nature of some of these choices may not be evident. But ethics can play a role even in measuring costs. The overall economic loss to a society when a productive or wealthy person becomes ill may be greater than when illness befalls a poor person, but we may decide to exclude these differences in cost so as to avoid counting the health and life of one person as being more valuable than those of another [46]. Measuring health gains also involves a series of value-laden assumptions and decisions. For example, we must decide whether health benefits are worth less if they occur in the future than if they occur soon. Similarly, we must assign a value to prevention of disabilities and to measures to relieve them. Disabled people typically regard their disabilities as less burdensome than others do. If we adopt their assessments, then measures to prevent disability will count as less cost-effective (because the benefit will count less), but efforts to extend the lives of the disabled may count as more so (because the lives extended will be counted as healthier). If we adopt the valuations of the non-disabled, these results are reversed. These uncertainties require choices among values rather than further measurement or calculation [45].

A maximizing strategy based on measures of cost-effectiveness makes resources go as far as possible, but the resulting allocation might conflict with ordinary notions of fairness [47]. People who are already well off may get the most benefit from a given health resource. For example, professionals who have access to health care and who can and do comply with physician advice may show more benefit in a hypertension treatment programme than poor unemployed men even though the latter have higher rates of hypertension [48]. It follows that 'more health', in terms of total reduction in hypertension, could be realized if the well-to-do population were treated in place of the needier one. But to steer scarce resources away from the poor because their deprivation limits the benefit that they can realize seems to punish them twice over. Existing inequalities in health status would be exacerbated if the resources went to the better off.

Similarly, maximizing strategies face potential conflicts with norms of universality and inclusiveness. Consider a region in which 80 per cent of the population live on the plain and the remainder in inaccessible highland villages. A vaccination campaign with limited funds has just enough money to vaccinate the 80 per cent, but given the much higher cost of vaccinating the mountain-dwellers, they would be left out. Suppose that a donor provides the funds necessary to vaccinate the remaining 20 per cent. This would achieve inclusiveness and offer equal treatment. But a maximizing health resource allocator might choose instead to vaccinate the same 80 per cent who live in the plain for a second disease if, as is highly likely, the result would be a greater gain in mortality and morbidity.

Allocators must also decide between targeting inequalities and attending to absolute deprivation. Some Latin American countries are among the world's most economically unequal, but people in the lower social strata in these nations tend to be better off than their counterparts in sub-Saharan Africa [49]. Should the objective be to reduce inequality, or to raise the level of the worst-off as high as possible? In poor countries where meagre health budgets are spent largely on a handful of tertiary care hospitals, following a rule of maximization is practically the same strategy as narrowing inequalities. And measures that help the worst-off tend to decrease inequalities.

Ethics and research involving human subjects

During the decades that followed the Second World War, scientists throughout the world came to accept the need for commonly accepted standards of conduct for scientists and prior ethical review of experiments involving human subjects. A trial of physicians who conducted medical experiments under the Nazi regime was held in Nuremberg, and upon their conviction the court offered a code of conduct that remains the basis for ethical evaluation of research. The World Medical Association, a group created to restore the good name of the medical profession after the horrors of the war years, issued its Declaration of Helsinki in 1964. Revised five times subsequently, the Declaration expanded the scope of the Nuremberg Code and is the most widely cited standard of conduct today. A set of guidelines published in 1993 by the Council of International Organizations of Medical Sciences (CIOMS), a non-governmental organization established by WHO and UNESCO, has served as an elaboration of the Declaration of Helsinki [50]. The CIOMS guidelines are also periodically revised.

These international standards, and the process of prior ethical review to which research is now subjected, have served both scientists and the public well. Although originally resisted by many scientists as a bureaucratic intrusion on their work, these review committees are more often seen as a key element in the social contract under which scientists are authorized to recruit ordinary citizens for their experiments. The public, in turn, is given an assurance that they will not be asked to participate in an experiment unless it has been carefully examined by a group of scientists and laymen, with attention paid to both the frankness of the scientists' disclosure of risks and benefits, and the adoption of any protection needed for the participants.

But not all is well in this field. Even in the richest countries, review committees are overwhelmed by their workload and short of staff, resulting at times in long delays before approving projects. The expansion of the scope of the committee's deliberations, including not only new fields such as population genetics, but also novel aspects of all research, such as conflict of interest, stretches the committees' expertise and adds to expense and delay. Numerous reviews of the system of ethical scrutiny that have been conducted by agencies of the US government have portrayed a system undergoing stress; and the American system is widely regarded as the world's best-developed and certainly its most lavishly funded.

The system of ethical review of research involving human subjects works best for the kinds of studies it was intended to oversee: conventional medical research projects funded and carried out in the same high-income country in which the review takes place. The Declaration of Helsinki, created to prevent any recurrence of the abuses of the Nazi era, is designed to ensure that no minority will be deprived of the protections given to fellow-citizens enrolled in medical research.

For this very reason, however, the existing systems of ethical review, including both the committees and the international guidelines, have faced difficulties in connection with global public health. This often involves sponsors and scientists from a wealthy country working in a poor one, usually in collaboration with nationals of the latter. Following established procedures, collaborative research is to be reviewed at all the institutions of the several participants, and must be approved by all of them. But review committees in many poor countries have been few in number until very recently. Resources, such as staff support and even photocopying, have been hard to come by. Research in epidemiology and other sciences specific to public health presents further challenges, since the issues require expertise that is often lacking. The building of capacity for ethical review in developing countries is a high priority and must be supported and funded by national and international organizations.

However, the most significant ethical problems in global public health research involve substance rather than process. In international health research involving developing countries, the disparities are between nations; and the treatment given to participants in the research is often superior to that available to their fellow-citizens. Nevertheless, a number of international collaborative trials have been subjected to vociferous ethical criticism. In the critics' view, the basic question is whether scientists are using a single standard of ethical conduct [51–53]. If they are, according to this view, any experiment they would perform in a poor country must be one that would be permitted in their home countries. The studies that were most strongly criticized did not meet that standard. Whether this is an appropriate standard is another matter entirely. As many observers have pointed out, it would seem to rule out any attempt to gauge the efficacy and safety of a new inexpensive affordable treatment if a better therapy were on the market, regardless of its cost (Box 12.2).

There are other areas of controversy in international collaborative public health research. Conflicts of interest between researchers and institutions are a growing problem [54]. Host nations are beginning to insist on some kind of broader community benefit if their citizens are to be used as experimental material. Concern is also growing that methods of informing potential subjects and obtaining their uncoerced informed consent are inadequate and insufficiently monitored.

Box 12.2 Testing a vaccine: a hypothetical case

A US-based company developed a vaccine against HIV-1 that appeared promising in animal studies. Phase I trials demonstrated that the vaccine was safe and produced significant antibody levels in most volunteers. The company now wants to begin phase II trials and decided to carry out the study in a large city of a South East Asian country where previous surveillance had identified a cohort of intravenous drug users (IUDs) with a high rate of conversion to HIV-1 (of the same strain to which the vaccine had been developed). The company agreed to cover the cost of the study and further agreed to give the vaccine free of charge to the IDU population of the city and at cost to the country for 5 years, if it proved effective. The study was to be a randomized double-blind prospective study with one group receiving the vaccine and the other tetanus toxoid. All potential participants were to be tested for HIV-1 prior to being enrolled in the study. If they were HIV+, they were referred to one of the municipal hospitals where HIV+ patients were treated by the standard method recommended by the Ministry of Health. This meant that all infections were treated, but that control patients were not given anti-retroviral therapy. The Municipal Corporation would provide lifetime care. The proposal was reviewed by the ethical review boards of the company and the Ministry of Health and approved. An AIDS activist group strongly objected to the fact that the study did not provide state-of-the-art care for those who became HIV+ during the study. They argued that the study would not have been approved in the USA and that the only reason it was being conducted in this South East Asian country was because of the reduced cost. The company countered that the use of state-of-the-art therapy would in itself be unethical because the treatment regime would not be sustainable and only a small group would have access to this therapy. By offering the best care available in the world, the study would be giving an unfair inducement to the participants. The Ministry of Health agreed with the company.

This study raises several ethical questions. Is the study unethical because participants are not being offered the best care available in the world if they become HIV+? Should the vaccine be tested if it is presently unaffordable to the country? If the developer of the vaccine had been a small local Thai company, would the use of 'best available treatment' compared with 'standard local therapy' be viewed differently?

Resources for ethics

The profession of public health lags far behind clinical medicine and biotechnology in focusing attention on ethical issues. While courses in ethics are now standard in medical schools, they have been rare in schools of public health [55]. Texts are only now beginning to appear [2,3,56,57]. Nevertheless, the trend towards explicit consideration of ethical issues in public health education and institutions is unmistakable. In many countries, the advent of national bioethics commissions and governmental bioethics agencies provides a public forum for deliberation on these issues [58]. The WHO has created a Department of Ethics, Equity, Trade and Human Rights. A global professional society, the International Association of Bioethics, holds world congresses biannually which offer forums for discussion of ethical issues in public health, with particular emphasis on developing countries.

The role of ethics in global public health

For many practitioners of global public health, 'ethics' is perceived as a watchdog or regulator. It lurks in the ethical review boards to which scientists must submit proposals for research involving human subjects. It may present itself in conflict-of-interest requirements and investigations. Viewed in a favourable light, these review boards keep global health research and practice ethical, avoiding ethical blunders, intentional or otherwise.

Understood as a check on behaviour, the actions of ethical committees and the like are not inevitably a force for good. Watchdog agencies can stumble, degenerate into bureaucracies, or even run amok. The chief executive of a major global health foundation labelled ethics as 'a major threat to global health' [59]. He had in mind decisions by ethical review committees that unjustifiably (in his view) threatened important research initiatives. One need not look far to find adverse consequences of the misapplication of familiar ethical principles. A case in point was the reluctance of governments in some developing countries to approve a vaccine for rotavirus that had been withdrawn from the American market for safety reasons. The ethical principle relied upon in these discussions was the equal value of children's lives, regardless of nationality—if the vaccine was not safe enough for American children, it could not be safe enough for children in low- and middle-income countries [60]. But this ethical perspective did not take into account the vastly greater threat posed by rotavirus to the health of children in these countries, which was far greater than any risks posed by the vaccine [61]. The price paid by this ethical mis-step may have been hundreds of thousands of children's lives [62,63] as the development of a new vaccine has taken over 10 years.

More positively, ethics can be viewed less as a check on illegitimate behaviour than as a problem-solving activity in which nearly everyone in global health must play a part. Personal virtues, such as honesty and sincerity, do not in themselves offer consistent solutions to moral dilemmas in global health that rise because of conflicts among legitimate goals. Along with epidemiology and other disciplines, ethics can contribute to the development of optimal global health policy and practice.

References

[1] Kass NE. An ethics framework for public health. *Am Public Health* 2001; **91**: 1776–82.

[2] Holland S. *Public Health Ethics*. Cambridge: Polity Press, 2007.

[3] Bayer R, Gostin L, Jennings B, Steinbock B. *Public Health Ethics: Theory, Policy, and Practice*. Oxford: Oxford University Press, 2006

[4] Roberts MJ, Reich MR. Ethical analysis in public health. *Lancet* 2002; **359**: 1055–9.

[5] Thomas A. *Street Price: A Global Approach to Drug Pricing for Developing Countries*. London: VSO, 2001.

[6] Scruton R. *WHO, What and Why?: Transnational Government, Legitimacy and the World Health Organization*. London: Institute of Economic Affairs, 2000.

[7] Scruton R. Tobacco and freedom. *Wall Street Journal* (European edn), 7 January 2000.

[8] Brandt A. *The Cigarette Century: The Rise, Fall, and Deadly Persistence of the Product that Defined America*. New York: Basic Books, 2007.

[9] National Bioethics Advisory Commission (USA). *Ethical and Policy Issues in International Research: Clinical Trials in Developing Countries*. Bethesda, MD: National Bioethics Advisory Commission, 2001.

[10] London AJ, Kimmelman J. Justice in translation: from bench to bedside in the developing world. *Lancet* 2008; **372**: 82–5.

[11] Warren CW, Riley L, Asma S, *et al*. Tobacco use by youth: a surveillance report from the Global Youth Tobacco Survey project. *Bull WHO* 2000; **78**: 868–76.

[12] Macklin R. *Against Relativism: Cultural Diversity and the Search for Ethical Universals in Medicine*. Oxford University Press, 1999.

[13] International Dual Loyalty Working Group (Physicians For Human Rights and School of Public Health and Primary Care). *Dual Loyalty and Human Rights In Health Professional Practice: Proposed Guidelines & Institutional Mechanisms*. Cape Town: School of Public Health and Primary Care, 2002.

[14] Callahan D, Jennings B. Ethics and public health: forging a strong relationship. *Am J Public Health* 2002; **92**: 160–76.

[15] Smith AH, Lingas EO, Rahman M. Contamination of drinking-water by arsenic in Bangladesh: a public health emergency. *Bull WHO* 2000; **78**: 1093–1103.

[16] *Combating a Deadly Menace: Early Experience with a Community-Based Arsenic Mitigation Project in Bangladesh, Research Monograph Series No. 16*. Dhaka: BRAC Research and Evaluation Division, August 2000.

[17] Chowdhury AMR. Arsenic crisis in Bangladesh. *Sci Am* 2004; **291**: 87–91.

[18] Hanson H, Groce N. Human immunodeficiency virus and quarantine in Cuba. *JAMA* 2003; **290**: 2875.

[19] Bayer R, Healton C. Controlling AIDS in Cuba. the logic of quarantine. *N Engl J Med* 1989; **320**: 1022–4.

[20] Mann JM. Medicine and public health, ethics, and human rights. *Hastings Center Rep* 1997; **29**: 6–13.

[21] Burr C. The AIDS exception: privacy vs. public health. In: Beauchamp DE, Steinbock B (eds). *New Ethics for the Public's Health*. Oxford: Oxford University Press, 1999; pp. 211–24.

[22] Rose G. *The Strategy of Preventive Medicine*. Oxford: Oxford University Press, 1993.

[23] Eddy DM. The individual vs. society: is there a conflict? *JAMA* 1991; **265**: 1446, 1449–50.

[24] Eddy DM. The individual vs. society: resolving the conflict. *JAMA* 1991; **265**: 2399–401, 2405–6.

[25] Emanuel EJ. Patient v. population: resolving the ethical dilemmas posed by treating patients as members of populations. In: Danis M, Clancy C, Churchill LR (eds). *Ethical Dimensions of Health Policy*. Oxford University Press; 2002; pp. 227–45.

[26] McKie J, Richardson J. The rule of rescue. *Soc Sci Med* 2003; **56**: 2407–19.

[27] Fitzpatrick M. *The Tyranny of Health: Doctors and the Regulation of Lifestyle*. London: Routledge, 2001.

[28] Leichter, HM. *Free to be Foolish. Politics and Health Promotion in the United States and Great Britain*. Princeton: Princeton University Press, 1991.

[29] Callahan D (ed.) *Promoting Healthy Behavior. How Much Freedom? Whose Responsibility?* Washington, DC: Georgetown University Press, 2001.

[30] Guindon GE, Tobin S, Yach D. Trends and affordability of cigarette prices: ample room for tax increases and related health gains. *Tob Control* 2002; **11**: 35–43.

[31] Groosman M, Chaloupka FJ. Cigarette taxes: the straw to break the camel's back. *Public Health Rep* 1997; **112**: 290–7.

[32] United Health Foundation. *America's Health: United Health Foundation State Health Rankings 2001 Edition*. Available online at http://www.unitedhealthfoundation.org/rankings2001/rankings.html (accessed 30 March 2002).

[33] Perry RF, Saper CB, Kessler DA. Nicotine addiction in young people. *N Engl J Med* 1995; **333**: 1225–6.

[34] Gruber J Mullainathan S. *Do Cigarette Taxes Make Smokers Happier?* Working Paper 8872, National Bureau of Economic Research, Cambridge, MA, 2002.

[35] Sullum J *For Your Own Good: The Anti-Smoking Crusade and the Tyranny of Public Health*. New York: Free Press, 1998.

[36] Wikler D. Personal and social responsibility for health. In: Anand S, Peter F, Amartya Sen A (eds). *Public Health, Ethics, and Equity*. Oxford: Oxford University Press, 2005; pp. 107–31.

[37] Thaler R, Sunstein C. *Nudge: Improving Decisions About Health, Wealth, and Happiness*. New Haven, CT: Yale University Press, 2008.

[38] Loewenstein G, Brennan T, Volpp K. Asymmetric paternalism to improve health behaviors. *JAMA* 2007; **298**: 2415–17.

[39] Nuffield Council on Bioethics. *Public Health: Ethical Issues*. London: Nuffield Council on Bioethics, 2007.

[40] Tucker KL, Mahnken B, Wilson PW, et al. Folic acid fortification of the food supply. potential benefits and risks for the elderly population. *JAMA* 1996; **276**: 1879–85.

[41] Battin M, Rhodes R, Silvers A. *Health Care and Social*. New York: Oxford University Press, in press.

[42] Wikler D, Marchand S. Macroallocation of health care resources. In: Singer P, Kuhse H *Companion to Bioethics*. Oxford: Blackwell, 1998.

[43] Wikler D, Murray C (eds). *Fairness and Goodness: Ethical Issues In Health Resource Allocation*. Geneva: WHO, in press.

[44] Menzel P, Gold M, Nord E, *et al*. Toward a broader view of values in cost-effectiveness analysis of health. *Hastings Center Rep* 1999; **29**: 7–15.

[45] Wikler D, Brock D, Marchand S, TanTorres T. Quantitative methods for priority-setting in health: ethical issues. In: Ashcroft R, Dawson H, Draper H, McMillan JR (eds). *Principles of Health Care Ethics* (2nd edn). Chichester: John Wiley, 2007; pp. 563–8.

[46] Murray C. Rethinking DALYs. In: Murray C, Lopez A (eds). *The Global Burden of Disease*. Cambridge, MA: WHO/Harvard University Press, 1996.

[47] Nord E. *Cost–Value Analysis in Health Care: Making Sense out of QALYs*. Cambridge: Cambridge University Press, 1999.

[48] Stason WB, Weinstein MC. Public-health rounds at the Harvard School of Public Health. Allocation of resources to manage hypertension. *N Engl J Med* 1977; **296**: 732–9.

[49] Gwatkin DR. Health inequalities and the health of the poor: What do we know? What can we do?. *Bull WHO* 2000; **78**: 3–18.

[50] Bankowski Z *International Ethical Guidelines for Biomedical Research Involving Human Subjects*. Geneva: Council for International Organizations of Medical Sciences, 1993.

[51] Angell M. Ethical imperialism? Ethics in international collaborative clinical research. *N Engl J Med* 1988; **319**: 1081–3.

[52] Angell M. The ethics of clinical research in the Third World. *N Engl J Med* 1997; **337**: 847–9.

[53] Lurie P, Wolfe SE. Unethical trials of interventions to reduce perinatal transmission of the human immunodeficiency virus in developing countries. *N Engl J Med* 1997; **337**: 853–6.

[54] Lo B, Wolf LE, Berkeley A. Conflict of interest policies for investigators in clinical trials. *N Engl J Med* 2000; **343**: 1616–20.

[55] Coughlin SS, Katz VVH, Mattison DR. Ethics instruction at schools of public health in the United States. *Am J Public Health* 2000; **90**: 768–70.

[56] Beauchamp DE, Steinbock B (eds). *New Ethics for the Public's Health*. Oxford: Oxford University Press; 1999.

[57] Coughlin SS, Beauchamp TL (eds). *Ethics and Epidemiology*. New York: Oxford University Press, 1998.

[58] Bulger RE, Bobby EM, Fineberg HV (eds). *Society's Choices: Social and Ethical Decisionmaking in Biomedicine*. Washington, DC: National Academy Press, 1995.

[59] Anonymous. Private communication (identity withheld to protect the executive's career).

[60] Mulholland EK. Global control of rotavirus disease. *Adv Exp Med Biol* 2004; **549**: 161–8.

[61] Bresee JS, El Arifeen S, Azim T, *et al*. Safety and immunogenicity of tetravalent rhesus-based rotavirus vaccine in Bangladesh. 2001 *Pediatr Infect Dis J* **20**: 1136–43.

[62] Milstien J, Cash R, Wecker J, Wikler D. Development of priority vaccines for disease-endemic countries: risk and benefit. *Health Aff (Millwood)* 2005; **24**: 718–28.

[63] Coffin SE, Nelson RM. Optimizing risks and benefits: the case of rotavirus vaccine. In: Kodish E (ed). *Ethics and Research with Children: A Case-based Approach*. Oxford University Press, 2005; 46–62.

Chapter 13

Putting the public into public health: towards a more people-centred approach

Sarah Macfarlane and Alec Irwin

Introduction

The public health challenges described in this book may at first generate a sense of disempowerment. Many of the global and national determinants of health may seem to be largely beyond people's control (see Chapter 1). However, there is evidence that, by linking their strengths and skills, public health professionals and communities confronting health challenges can get a grip on these problems and begin to solve them. Where this is happening, new modes of collaborative action are emerging that expand the traditional boundaries of public health.

Taking the global perspective makes it necessary to broaden responsibility for public health beyond a single professional model and to seek out a more coordinated response from multiple players (Chapters 1 and 2). The predominantly epidemiological skills of public health practitioners are no longer sufficient. We argue that the public, as members of communities or as employees of multidisciplinary public health organizations, should drive the public health agenda. Public health practitioners, policy-makers, and researchers should be trained to form partnerships with communities in the formulation of public health priorities, programmes, and values. To meet the expectations of its 'global' qualifier, public health must reflect the opinions and contributions of the global community that it serves.

The evolution of public health

The term 'public health' is used in a variety of ways, for example as a condition, an activity, a discipline, a profession, an infrastructure, a philosophy, or even a movement (Chapter 1). The term is given attributes and responsibilities, presented with huge challenges, and then judged. Yet it is not clear where the ownership of public health lies. Common to most definitions of public health as a discipline, is a sense of the public interest: 'the art and science of preventing disease, promoting health, and prolonging life through the organised efforts of society' [1]. The mission of public health was seen as 'fulfilling society's interests in assuring conditions in which people can be healthy' [2]. But when 'public health fails', who exactly fails? When 'public health succeeds', who exactly succeeds? When public health is 'at the crossroads', who exactly chooses the direction?

The modern concept of public health originated about 200 years ago in Europe and the USA when fear of morbidity and mortality from infectious diseases stimulated scientists, social workers, statisticians, religious leaders, philanthropists, and governments to search for ways to protect the public's health. It was quickly understood that disease outbreaks were associated with poverty and poor sanitary conditions. Later, as the germ theory matured, medical interventions became significant. In the early twentieth century, just as Flexner led the overhaul of American medical schools, John D. Rockefeller supported the establishment of schools of public health around the world. From then on, there has been a debate about the nature of the so-called schism introduced between public health and medicine [3]. Today, traditional public health practitioners claim 'global health' as public health without recognizing that its emergence provides the opportunity to heal the schism by broadening the players and disciplines involved.

Public health action itself has been marked by persistent internal tensions between a reliance on technological solutions implemented by highly trained experts, and more inclusive models of health action, rooted in the concept of health as a social process and incorporating the right of communities to participate in shaping their own health. The quantitative and technological face of public health has generally been the most prominent, particularly in the period since the Second World War. Public health processes and achievements have been primarily couched in a scientific language through which health problems are described and assessed and solutions are explored and evaluated. With the aim of preventing death, disease, and disability, populations are studied and interventions determined on the basis of epidemiological evidence, in terms, for example, of 'disability adjusted life years' (Chapter 2). Mass public education campaigns are designed, implemented, and evaluated by technical experts. Human issues of suffering and distress, and the potential for happiness, health, and well-being, are summarized in terms such as 'risk factors', 'social capital', 'social determinants', and 'equity', which may appear abstract and remote from the lived experience of the communities most directly concerned.

However, in addition to its scientific requirements and focus on narrowly defined disease conditions, public health can use other epistemologies, such as those of a more qualitative nature, and also investigate issues of quality of life, well-being, good health, and social justice in a more inclusive participatory manner.

Health for All

A significant expression of this approach was the Health for All movement which gained prominence in the 1970s, emphasizing the concept of primary health care. The manifesto of Health for All was the 1978 Declaration of Alma Ata, in which primary health care was described as 'essential health care ... made universally acceptable to individuals and families in the community through their full participation' and practised so as to nurture the 'self-reliance and self-determination' of communities [4]. In addition, primary health care as set forth at Alma Ata incorporated critical analysis of the social and economic roots of health and sickness, including the health impact of global economic inequalities and development policies.

The architects of the Alma Ata vision drew lessons from the community-based health programmes that had developed over the preceding two decades in Bangladesh, China, Guatemala, India, Nicaragua, the Philippines, Tanzania, and many other countries [5]. Across their geographical diversity, these community-based programmes shared common traits, such as: reduced reliance on advanced technology and highly specialized medical personnel, a holistic model of health with strong attention to social and environmental determinants, and a fundamental commitment to community participation and empowerment in health action. China's rural health workers (figuratively referred to as 'barefoot doctors') are the most famous examples of this approach [6]. In some regions, particularly Latin America, community-based programmes have been linked to vigorous social medicine movements. These movements sought to connect health action among disadvantaged communities to broader efforts for political change and social justice, in many cases inspired by Marxist analyses [7].

The Health for All campaign launched at Alma Ata failed to achieve many of its ambitious objectives, for reasons that are still debated. In the 1980s and 1990s, trends in the global economy weakened the capacity of countries to act on health. During this period, many developing countries slashed their health and social sector budgets under economic 'structural adjustment programmes' imposed by the World Bank and International Monetary Fund. As the effects of such programmes were felt, economic and health gaps between rich and poor widened, and the vision of equitable health progress faded [8].

Despite this mixed historical picture, the approach to health action shaped in community-based health programmes and formalized at Alma Ata constitutes an enduring legacy for public health. Indeed, to mark the thirtieth anniversary of Alma Ata, the WHO is devoting its annual report to primary health care. WHO Director-General Margaret Chan has argued that the global community 'will not be able to reach the health-related Millennium Development Goals unless we return to the values, principles, and approaches of primary health care' [9].

Ottawa Charter for Health

The Alma Ata vision has remained a rallying point for 'people-centred' approaches to public health which question top-down technocratic models. The health promotion movement is one such questioning voice. In 1986 the Ottawa Charter for Health Promotion, subtitled the New Public Health, redefined the concept of health promotion. The Charter defined health as being 'created by caring for oneself and others, by being able to take decisions and have control over one's life circumstances, and by ensuring that the society one lives in creates conditions that allow the attainment of health by all its members' [10]. The Charter provided five action streams—a checklist for what needs to be done to promote health at a societal and local level:

- build healthy public policy
- create supportive environments
- strengthen community action
- develop personal skills
- reorient health services to a health promotion perspective.

The term 'health promotion' was added to that of 'health protection' as a core activity for public health. Some governments now define public health as health protection plus health promotion [11]. The term 'health protection' refers to the more regulatory, centralized, and reactive aspect of public health; 'health promotion' is more self-determined, community-based, and developmental—'the process of enabling people to exert control over the determinants of health and thereby improve their health' [10]. The characteristics of 'people-centred' approaches are contrasted with the more conventional epidemiological approach to public health in Table 13.1.

Bangkok Charter for Health Promotion

The 2005 Bangkok Charter for Health Promotion emphasized the importance of supporting the 'rights, resources and opportunities' for communities and civil society to undertake health promotion, and pointed out the need for capacity building in this regard [12]. Tang et al. [13] demonstrated how technical

Table 13.1 Contrasting approaches to public health

	Orthodox	People-centred
Groups of interest	Populations, at-risk groups	Aggregations (communities, cultures, etc.)
Aims	Containing and lowering premature death, disease, and disability	Enhancing health, well-being, and quality of life
Values	Social justice, equity, human rights, social issues, prevention of suffering, science	Empowerment, self-determination, community, culture, diversity, equity, enhancement of quality of life
Means of knowledge building	Epidemiology, evidence-based, rigorous study designs	Participatory, qualitative, quasi-experimental, evaluative
Conceptual drivers	Risk, disease, prevention, 'medical model', determinants of disease	Strengths, health and well-being, promotion, people, empowerment, community, 'social model', determinants of health
Means of intervention	Policy, large top-down population interventions, regulation, media, education and early treatment	Community development, self-determined and participatory action, information and resourcing, action based on wishes
Professional approach	Planning, policy development, expert-driven decisions and priorities, intersectoral collaboration among services, reactive	Facilitation of people-driven priorities, partnerships, enabling community control, resource-getting, proactive
Overall feel	Cool, committed, scientific, measured	Passionate, enthusiastic, intuitive, active

assistance can be provided to health workers to build such capacity during a project to improve disease prevention in China funded by the World Bank. Raeburn *et al.* [14] reviewed approaches to capacity building and concluded that 'action centred on empowered and capable communities, in synergistic collaboration with other key players, may be the most powerful instrument available for the future of health promotion in a globalized world'.

A People's Charter for Health

In December 2000, about 1500 participants from international organizations and civil society groups came together at the People's Health Assembly in Dhaka, Bangladesh, in order to return the goals of Alma Ata to the development agenda [15]. A People's Charter for Health was prepared as a call for action to treat health as a human right, tackle the broader determinants of health, develop a people-centred health sector, and ensure people's participation for a healthy world [16]:

> Equity, ecologically-sustainable development and peace are at the heart of our vision of a better world—a world in which a healthy life for all is a reality; a world that respects, appreciates and celebrates all life and diversity; a world that enables the flowering of people's talents and abilities to enrich each other; a world in which people's voices guide the decisions that shape our lives . . .

The People's Health Movement (PHM) is now a well established global advocacy group with regional focal points and a strong grassroots base in many countries (Box 13.1).

Individual and collective responsibility

As individuals and members of communities, we each have responsibility for our own health, our children's health, and other people's health through commonly

---

Box 13.1 The People's Health Movement (PHM)

The PHM owes its genesis to many health networks and activists concerned by the growing inequities in health over the last 25 years. The PHM calls for a revitalization of the principles of the Alma Ata Declaration which promised Health for All by the year 2000 and complete revision of international and domestic policy that has been shown to impact negatively on health status and systems.

The People's Charter for Health includes the following objectives:

- To promote the Health for All goal through an equitable, participatory, and inter-sectoral movement and as a Rights Issue.

- To encourage government and other health agencies to ensure universal access to quality health care, education, and social services according to people's needs and not people's ability to pay.

- To promote the participation of people and people's organizations in the formulation, implementation, and evaluation of all health and social policies and programmes.

- To promote health along with equity and sustainable development as top priorities in local, national, and international policy-making.

- To encourage people to develop their own solutions to local health problems.

- To hold accountable local authorities, national governments, international organizations, and corporations.

accepted or legally enforced behaviour. As members of populations, we expect to be protected by our governments and by international agencies. In order to maintain the public's health, international, national, and local public health infrastructures have been created, and public health professionals have been appointed to work for our common good. But there is evidence that this process is not working fairly, for example the tremendous burden of disease in poor populations and the increasing inequalities between population groups. A commonly promoted solution is for international and national systems to measure and monitor inequalities, and to search for solutions. But, until there is better communication between the public and their appointed servants, the public health practitioners, progress in reducing inequalities will be painfully slow.

The pivotal role of community control

The Ottawa Charter championed a people-centred approach to public health when it defined health promotion as 'the process of enabling people to increase control over, and to improve, their health' [10]. The people dimension implies a bottom-up grass-roots perspective—the view of the ordinary person in the context of his/her everyday life, culture, and community. This dimension may be contrasted with the traditional academic, political, bureaucratic, or structural dimension, where analyses of determinants and risk are the dominant discourse, and the view is remote from the subjective realities of ordinary people. The control aspect is closely allied to the concept of 'empowerment', which is the crucial political and psychological dimension for a more people-centred approach to public health.

Empowerment

'Empowerment' designates transformative processes of social participation whereby previously marginalized and excluded communities gain voice in the key decisions that affect their well-being [17]. Such processes signify the concrete redistribution of political power and control over resources among social groups. This essentially political concept of empowerment emerged in the 1960s and 1970s through the work of Brazilian educator Paolo Freire, the international women's movement, and the liberation struggles of ethnic minority groups in many countries, including indigenous groups in Latin America and African Americans in the USA.

However, it is important to observe the different way in which the concept of 'empowerment' has been used recently by some global development institutions. During the 1990s, notions of social participation and empowerment were increasingly appropriated by mainstream development agencies, including the World Bank. Whereas the original use of these terms within progressive social movements had defined empowerment primarily in political terms, the development mainstream has now subtly recast community empowerment as a *substitute* for political change and the redistribution of resources. Community empowerment came to function as a code word for the shrinking of the public sector and the offloading of responsibilities from central governments to local actors—often without a corresponding transfer of resources, capacities, and tools. This has led some critics to suggest that the use of the term 'empowerment' allows major development organizations to 'say they are tackling injustice without having to back any political or structural change' [18].

'Empowerment' remains a multidimensional and contested concept—vital for guiding people-centred health action, but vulnerable to interpretations that can greatly weaken its relevance. The main criterion for assessing whether health and other public policies are truly empowering communities is the notion of increased control highlighted by the Ottawa Charter. Empowerment signifies the expansion by marginalized and dominated communities of their effective control over the political and economic processes that affect their well-being.

Power and control issues shape people's health through many different mechanisms. Differences in people's ability to control the key social processes in which they are involved (e.g. their work activities and relationships) are seen by some researchers as the principal 'cause' of the relation between health status and the social gradient—the further down the social scale, the less the power and control one has as a member of society, and the poorer one's health [19]. The Wilkinson hypothesis on inequality and poor health can be accounted for in these terms [20], i.e. the greater the gap in oppotunities poor people perceive in society, the greater their sense of disempowerment, the higher their levels of stress, and hence the poorer the health and well-being.

Public health action includes many examples of communities mobilizing to assert greater control over aspects of their collective well-being and thereby propelling changes in social power dynamics and public policy. Some of the strongest recent cases have emerged from the HIV/AIDS fight. South Africa's Treatment Action Campaign (TAC), formed in 1998, is a popular movement demanding access to lifesaving anti-retroviral therapy for the country's poor and marginalized people living with HIV (Box 13.2).

Enablement

The **enabling** dimension is important for defining the nature of the relationship between those holding the power and resources and the general population. If communities are to be enabled to have more control over their health and its determinants, then the resources—financial, knowledge, expertise,

Box 13.2 Treatment Action Campaign—successful community action

At the time of the creation of the Treatment Action Campaign (TAC), the dominant view in global public health was that, although combination anti-retroviral therapy was rapidly turning HIV/AIDS from a death sentence into a manageable chronic illness for people in high-income countries, its provision in low-income settings, particularly Africa, was not 'cost-effective'. This exclusion of the poor from access to life-saving treatment created a situation that TAC's members diagnosed as a form of global health apartheid. (Not coincidentally, many of the group's leaders had forged their organizing skills as activists in South Africa's anti-apartheid struggle). Through community education and mobilization, mass marches and demonstrations, legal action, and media campaigns, TAC energized a powerful people-driven response. The group successfully challenged the pricing and intellectual property policies of international pharmaceutical companies which were fighting to maintain inflated prices for anti-retroviral medications in the South African market. TAC also successfully used the court system to sue the South African government of Thabo Mbeki over its failure to tackle HIV/AIDS. TAC's legal action and mass campaigns were instrumental in accelerating the roll-out of programmes to prevent mother-to-child transmission of HIV and expand access to anti-retroviral treatment in the public sector. In the process, TAC became a force to be reckoned with on the South African national political scene and a powerful voice in global public health. The group constitutes one of recent history's most compelling examples of effective social movement-building [21].

facilities—need to be made available to them. Given the relative fragility of community processes in the face of other societal pressures, there must also be policy and legislative structures in place to protect community development. This is especially true in the early phases of community development when networks, organizational structures, resources, and capacities are being built to enable people to work together effectively.

A classic example of a community development study in Modello and Homestead Gardens in Florida, USA, shows what can be achieved in work facilitated by a professional [22]. These areas were low-income housing projects, with high rates of crime, drug abuse, teenage pregnancy, child abuse, and violence. Processes included relationship-building in the community,

Box 13.3 A case study from Venezuela

Barrio Adentro was created in 2003 under the government of President Hugo Chavez as part of an ambitious national agenda to combat social exclusion and poverty. The programme aimed to expand health service coverage among Venezuela's poorest citizens by answering the long-standing (and long unmet) demand of low-income communities for quality health services in their local neighbourhoods. Just as importantly, Barrio Adentro's planners were committed to seeing that services were delivered in a way that strengthened neighbourhood capacities and social networks, and enabled local people to exercise ownership. The programme worked by rapidly constructing a large number of comprehensive diagnostic centres and other facilities in poor and previously under-served neighbourhoods. These facilities were staffed with skilled health personnel (originally including a substantial contingent of Cuban physicians), and the new facilities and resources were placed under the oversight of local health committees which comprised ordinary citizens—including many low-income people previously denied a voice in decisions related to their health.

parenting classes, leadership identification and training, building a strong parent–teacher association that went on to organize many community activities, a tenants' council, community-initiated residential treatment programmes, job training, and tutoring programmes. Community morale visibly improved in a short time, and within 2 years there were major reductions in most negative social and health indicators, including a 60 per cent drop in child abuse, a 65 per cent reduction in drug trafficking, a 50 per cent reduction in reported parent and child drug abuse, an 80 per cent reduction in serious delinquency referrals, and a major reduction in teenage pregnancy.

An impressive recent example of how government public health action can respond to community demands and enable pro-active community processes related to health comes from the Barrio Adentro (Into the Neighbourhood) programme in Venezuela (Box 13.3). In addition to rapid gains in coverage for key health interventions, Barrio Adentro has had a dramatic enabling effect on communities' organizing capacities and confidence that they can tackle their own problems. As one member of a local health committee puts it [23]:

> It used to be that here they made all the decisions for us. We were like puppets. But that's not true any more. Now we are an organized health committee, which has had to pioneer everything. We are the ones who figured out how to organize housing construction, the ones who sit on the land tenure committees … We are going to be our own advocates in solving our problems.

The connection to the primary health care model formulated at Alma Ata is explicit. Indeed, Mirta Roses, Director of the Pan American Health Organization, calls Barrio Adentro 'primary health care in its essential form'. She describes the programme as the cutting edge of a historical process through which Latin American communities have 'struggled to improve their level of health through social justice and the building of a newly empowered citizenry' [24].

Evaluation of public health interventions

There is no clearer demonstration of a public health success than the control of an outbreak of cholera, measles, or typhoid, just as there is no clearer demonstration of failure than the outbreak of cholera, measles, or typhoid. Epidemics can result in the downfall of politicians, the resignation of professionals, and the death of many people. It is little wonder that public health interventions that can demonstrate reduction in disease incidence are highly sought after.

The conventional procedures for evaluating public health interventions are based on rigorous study design and quantifiable outcome measures in intervention and control populations. Results are reported in terms of reduction in disease rates, increase in uptake of services, or changed behaviour between the groups. Success is demonstrated by the existence of a statistically significant difference in outcome measure between the groups. It is difficult and usually not desirable to apply such procedures to interventions that emanate from within the community, and this is where the debate about evaluation begins.

Advocates of the people-centred approach point out that intervention studies designed from the top down are not flexible or participatory enough to formulate and implement the solutions that are most agreeable to communities and that their evaluations do not necessarily reflect community values of effectiveness. On the other hand, advocates of the epidemiological approach point out that evaluations of community-driven interventions are usually so subjective that there is no way of knowing if they can or should ever be brought to scale.

Methods of evaluating community development projects include a variety of quasi-experimental naturalistic designs, demonstration projects with goal-attainment measures set by communities, and participatory action research. There have been some attempts to build systems of evaluation that serve traditional and 'new' (people-centred) public health approaches [25]. For example, health impact assessment attempts to assess the way in which policies and interventions affect people's health using a mixture of information-gathering techniques [26]. In Eastern Nova Scotia, Canada, The People Assessing Their Health (PATH) project has developed community health impact tools tailored to the special needs of individual communities [27].

Little formal evaluated research on people-centred approaches, or even on community development programmes as they relate to public health, is available in the mainstream academic literature. There are substantial numbers of informal unpublished evaluation reports. Reviews of injury prevention projects indicate that success is often not high for community-based programmes where there is little actual community participation, but the opposite may be true where there is significant and meaningful community participation [28]. A quasi-experimental study in New Zealand involving over 4000 people in an urban locality using a multicultural approach with a high degree of community and local government involvement demonstrated significant reductions in child hospitalization rates, a significantly higher awareness of injury prevention safety messages, higher rates of seatbelt use, and better fencing of home swimming pools [29].

On the other hand, the Department of Nursing Education of the University of the Witwatersrand evaluated the community participation component of the Muldersdrift Health and Development Programme [30].Using standard criteria they observed that although community participation had increased, there had been little shift in control over decision-making and the allocation of resources. They concluded that a people-centred approach had not been achieved, and that power over planning and resources should remain in the hands of the partners if community participation was to remain progressive and sustained.

For many years, Health Canada (a federal department) has funded rural and urban communities across Canada to undertake their own community health projects, often with consultation from regional experts, but under the control of the community. These projects are selected from a formal application process and have to meet a number of criteria, one of which is that they be evaluated. In this way, these projects meet the requirement of 'community control'.

The way forward

The current global context presents public health with an array of emerging challenges—but also significant new opportunities to build people-centred approaches in public health action. Processes such as economic globalization, environmental degradation and climate change, the proliferation of armed conflict in some parts of the world, fluctuations in the availability of basic commodities, and widening economic and health gaps between the world's 'haves' and 'have-nots' make new demands on public health practice. Flexibility to adapt to changing contexts and anticipate new challenges is a crucial attribute of public health leadership in this new era.

At the same time, while contexts evolve and shift, certain core principles of people-centred health action provide sustained orientation. Public health work that genuinely seeks to include 'the public' aims to promote equity and social justice. Equity in health means the elimination of those health differences among population groups that are systematically produced by social conditions—avoidable or correctable and unfair [31].

Achieving equity

Throughout the history of the discipline, the most insightful public health leaders have understood that public health's concern with the well-being of socially disadvantaged groups necessarily implies their active engagement in efforts to achieve a more equitable distribution of health-enabling conditions. Improving the health of disadvantaged groups requires analysing and tackling the social and economic inequities that determine people's chances for health. This does not mean that public health adopts a uniform political ideology. Public health practitioners can and do defend very different views on the specific types of economic and social policy change that will most rapidly generate conditions for greater health equity in contemporary societies. Indeed, pursuing and refining this collective debate on the population health effects of different public policy models is one of the most important challenges—and one of the great opportunities—that lie ahead for the next phase of public health's development. Analysing with greater precision the health consequences of policies conceived to stimulate economic growth and/or ensure a more equitable distribution of the benefits of economic and technological progress stands among the discipline's most urgent tasks. Some of public health's most creative current research is engaged with this problem [32,33].

What is clear is that public health cannot be indifferent to the way in which societies distribute resources, prestige, and power among their members. By its very nature, public health is deeply engaged with these fundamental questions of social cohesion, social exclusion, and the underlying dynamics of political economy. That is why the question of a 'people-centred', participatory mode of action is so central to public health—more so than to many other scientific and scholarly disciplines [34]. Because public health efforts to achieve greater health equity are about changing the way society works, those efforts must include the participation of the people who make up society—especially those who face systematic discrimination and marginalization.

Honouring participation

This is true for ethical and human rights reasons, because it is right for people to have a voice in the processes (including public health action) that shape important aspects of their lives. Independent of moral and human rights justifications, however, it can also be argued that participation has a pragmatic value: enabling community participation in public health efforts may increase the likelihood that these efforts will be successful, on long-term outcomes measures because people are likely to lend greater and more lasting support to processes in which they have participated and feel invested. The practical value of participation remains for the moment too weakly researched and evaluated in the public health literature, although numerous suggestive examples exist (including those cited in this chapter). Pursuing and deepening research in this area constitutes another important task for public health in the years ahead.

Future research will broaden and systematize our understanding of what makes participatory processes succeed or fail, and it will draw the lessons for how public health professionals, technical experts in other fields, and members of affected communities can best collaborate to achieve health gains. Contributing to this 'people-centred' evolution defines a new agenda for public health education.

Conclusion

It is vital not to equate a people-centred approach with a purely emotive attitude and a denigration of science. Working with communities does not mean jettisoning public health's intellectual rigor and its quantitative tools. On the contrary, the most effective community-based health advocates, for example those associated with the Treatment Action Campaign and the Barrio Adentro programme, show an unwavering commitment to clear science and clear outcomes. The epidemiologists, statisticians, physicians, nurses, and programme managers who work for Barrio Adentro are not asked to forget their specialized training. They are asked to put that training at the service of the community—and in turn to let the community's concerns and experience inform the questions science asks and answers.

Poor and vulnerable communities do not have the leisure to indulge in ineffective solutions. Communities and public health practitioners have a common interest in getting rapidly to what works. And part of what works is people working together. This shared commitment is the basis of a people-centred approach.

References

[1] Acheson D. *Independent Inquiry into Inequalities in Health*. London: Stationery Office, 1998.

[2] Institute of Medicine, Committee for the Study of the Future of Public Health. *The Future of Public Health*. Washington, DC: National Academy Press, 1988.

[3] White KL. *Healing the Schism. Epidemiology, Medicine, and the Public's Health.* New York: Springer, 1991.

[4] WHO–UNICEF. *Primary Health Care. A Joint Report by the Director General of the World Health Organization and the Executive Director of the United Nations Children's Fund.* New York: WHO, 1978.

[5] Newell KW (ed). *Health by the People.* Geneva: WHO, 1975.

[6] Werner D, Sanders D. *Questioning the Solution: the Politics of Primary Health Care and Child Survival.* Palo Alto, CA: Health-Wrights, 1997.

[7] Tajer D. Latin American social medicine: roots, development during the 1990s and current challenges. *Am J Public Health* 2003; **93**: 2023–7.

[8] Kim JY, Millen J, Irwin A, Gershman J (eds). *Dying for Growth: Global Inequalities and the Health of the Poor.* Monroe, ME: Common Courage Press, 2000.

[9] Chan M. The contribution of primary health care to the Millennium Development Goals. *International Conference on Health for Development, Buenos Aires, Argentina, 16 August 2007.* Available online at: http://www.who.int/dg/speeches/2007/20070816_argentina/en/(accessed 31 August 2008).

[10] WHO. *The Ottawa Charter for Health Promotion.* Ottawa: WHO/Canadian Public Health Association/Health Canada, 1986.

[11] New Zealand Ministry of Health. *Preparing the New Zealand Strategic and Action Plan for Public Health. Discussion Document for Consultation.* Wellington: Ministry of Health, 2001.

[12] WHO. *The Bangkok Charter for Health Promotion in a Globalized World.* Geneva: WHO, 2005.

[13] Tang K., Nutbeam D, Kong L, Wang R, Yan J. Building capacity for health promotion—a case study from China. *Health Promot Int* 2005; **20**: 285–95.

[14] Raeburn J, Akerman M, Chuengsatiansup K, Mejia F, Oladepo O. Community capacity building and health promotion in a globalized world. *Health Promot Int* 2007; **21** (Suppl 1): 84–90.

[15] Chowdhury Z, Rowson M. The people's health assembly. *BMJ* 2000; **321**: 1361–2.

[16] PHA. *People's Charter for Health.* Dhaka, Bangladesh: PHA Secretariat. Available online at: http://www.pha2000.org

[17] Secretariat of the Commission on Social Determinants of Health. *A Conceptual Framework for Action on the Social Determinants of Health.* Geneva: WHO, 2007. Available online at: http://www.who.int/social_determinants/resources/csdh_framework_action_05_07.pdf (accessed 30 July 2008).

[18] Fiedrich M, Jellema A, Haq N, Nalwoga J, Nessa F. *Literacy, Gender and Social Agency: Adventures in Empowerment. Research Report for ActionAid UK by DFID, 2003.* Cited in: Luttrell C, Quiroz S, Scrutton C, Bird K. Understanding and operationalising empowerment. Available online at: www.poverty-wellbeing.net/document.php?itemID=1547&langID=1 (accessed 30 July 2008).

[19] Marmot M. Achieving health equity: from root causes to fair outcomes. *Lancet* 2007; **370**: 1153–63.

[20] Wilkinson R, Pickett K. *The Spirit Level.* London: Allen Lane, 2009.

[21] Friedman S, Mottiar S, Pickett K. The Spirit Level. London: Allen Lane. *2009 A Moral to the Tale: The Treatment Action Campaign and the Politics of HIV/AIDS.* Discussion paper, University of KwaZulu-Natal, Program on 'Globalisation, Marginalisation,

and New Social Movements in Post-Apartheid South Africa.' Durban: University of KwaZulu-Natal, 2004. Available online at: http://www.nu.ac.za/ccs/files/Friedman%20Mottier%20TAC%20Research%20Report%20Short.pdf (accessed 30 July 2008).

[22] Mills R. *Substance Abuse, Dropout and Delinquency Prevention: The Modello/Homestead Gardens Public Housing Early Intervention Project*. Coconut Grove, FL: RC Mills, 1990.

[23] Pan American Health Organization. *Mission Barrio Adentro: The Right to Health and Social Inclusion in Venezuela*. Caracas: Pan American Health Organization, 2006; pp. 36–7.

[24] Pan American Health Organization. *Mission Barrio Adentro: The Right to Health and Social Inclusion in Venezuela*. Caracas: Pan American Health Organization, 2006; pp. i-ii.

[25] Nutbeam D. Evaluating health promotion: progress, problems and solutions. *Health Promot Int* 1998; **13**: 27–44.

[26] WHO. *Informal WHO Consultative Meeting: Health Impact Assessment in Development Policy and Planning, Cartagena, Colombia, 28 May 2001*. Geneva: WHO, 2002.

[27] People Assessing Their Health Project. http://www.path-ways.ns.ca/flash/index.html (accessed 23 May 2002).

[28] Klassen T, Mackay M, Moher D, Walker A, Jones A. Community-based prevention interventions. *Future Child* 2000; **10**: 83–93.

[29] Coggan C, Patterson P, Brewin M, Hooper R, Robinson E. Evaluation of the Waitakere Community Injury Prevention Project. *Inj Prev* 2000; **6**: 130–4.

[30] Barker M, Klopper H. Community participation in primary health care projects of the Muldersdrift Health and Development Programme. *Curationis* 2007; **30**: 36–47.

[31] Whitehead M, Dahlgren G. *Levelling Up: A Discussion Paper on Concepts and Principles for Tackling Social Inequities In Health*. Copenhagen: WHO Regional Office for Europe, 2006.

[32] Chung H, Muntaner C. Political and welfare state determinants of infant and child health indicators: an analysis of wealthy countries. *Soc Sci Med* 2006; **63**: 829–42.

[33] WHO. *Knowledge Networks of the WHO Commission on Social Determinants of Health*. Available online at: http://www.who.int/social_determinants/knowledge_networks/final_reports/en/index.html (accessed 30 July 2008).

[34] Raeburn J, Rootman I. *People-Centred Health Promotion*. Chichester: Wiley. 1998.

Chapter 14

Strengthening public health for the new era

Robert Beaglehole and Ruth Bonita

In this chapter we summarize the state of global public health and suggest the way forward for improving the practice of global public health. We begin by reviewing the main themes from the earlier chapters: the daunting context, the weakness of the public health infrastructure and workforce, the challenges presented by the broad scope of public health, and the ongoing renaissance of public health. We describe our vision for public health and outline the steps required to achieve this vision. We emphasize the need to strengthen public health training, especially at the postgraduate level, and the ability of public health practitioners to carry out their multiple activities, especially at the country level. Although the focus is on low- and middle-income countries, strengthening public health training and practice is required in all countries. We are optimistic that we are entering an era in which the public health perspective will become more central to the health and development agendas [1].

The state of global public health

The daunting global context

The first general theme of earlier chapters is that, despite impressive health gains in almost all countries over the last few decades, the challenges facing public health practitioners remain great, and are often more difficult to address than in the past (Chapters 1 and 2). The unfinished agenda of the control of communicable diseases, for example HIV/AIDS, malaria, and tuberculosis, is now compounded by the emergence of new pandemics, notably chronic (non-communicable) diseases, the effects of violence, global environmental changes, and the increasing recognition of the importance of the underlying determinants of health.

It is encouraging that some (mostly wealthy) countries have the essentially preventable epidemic of HIV/AIDS more or less under control. These successes have been achieved at great cost and are primarily due to preventive campaigns (including facilities for injecting drug users), the availability of effective and relatively affordable drugs, de-stigmatization, and the presence of an appropriate health service infrastructure. However, in several countries in Africa the HIV/AIDS epidemic is affecting large segments of the population and overwhelming already stretched health services. A strong economic case can be made for giving more attention to the prevention of HIV/AIDS and especially to discouraging multiple sexual partners [2]. Cheap anti-retroviral drugs are not yet available for the majority of patients, despite donations and recent reductions in prices, and the health service infrastructure in most countries is not adequate to cope with the escalating case load. Fortunately, some low- and middle-income countries, for example Malawi [3] and Thailand [4], have demonstrated that good progress in controlling the epidemic is possible, but this requires strong and sustained political leadership together with new resources and strengthened primary health care infrastructure [5]. The need for strong leadership for public health more generally is one we return to later.

In addition to the continuing communicable disease burden, there is a rapidly growing global burden of chronic diseases and mental health problems (Chapter 2). The burden is largely a consequence of the ageing of populations because of falling infant and child mortality rates and lower fertility [6]. Public health programmes have contributed to these favourable trends, although many other factors have been important, most notably female education and empowerment [7]. Urbanization and the globalization of risks are contributing to the chronic disease pandemic [8]. Unfortunately, the information base for estimates of future trends in chronic diseases and mental health problems, and their immediate and underlying causes, is still far from complete despite recent methodological developments (Chapter 2).

In addition, there are newly recognized public health problems such as those related to economic globalization and its impact on wealth creation and distribution [9], the effects of violence in all its manifestations, especially against women and children [10], global environmental changes, and threats to the sustainability of human well-being and health [11]. The globalization of the marketing and promotional techniques now being used to such great effect by transnational corporations, such as the tobacco [12] and food and beverage industries [13], are contributing to the growing burden of chronic diseases. As discussed in Chapter 1, these larger challenges present particular problems for public health scientists; the usual study designs are not helpful in assessing the potential future risks to health from, for example, global warming. New methods and new partnerships with scientists in fields outside the health arena are essential for developing credible projections of likely health effects of these global changes. Even when these projections appear robust, it is difficult to ensure the support of policy-makers to implement the necessary changes because of the powerful interest groups involved.

The public health implications of global environmental changes illustrate the difficulties facing public health practitioners. Although the overwhelming majority of environmental scientists are pessimistic about the state of the world [14], a few assert that all is well and that general environmental conditions are improving [15]. Unfortunately, the prosperity of growing economies in recent decades has not created new wealth; it depended on drawing upon ecological 'capital'. The world has been operating in ecological deficit for decades, extracting resources without restoring the ecological capital balance. This exploitation of natural resources in the interests of economic growth cannot continue indefinitely.

The prognosis for the future well-being of the Earth and the health of its human inhabitants is grim (Chapter 1). The Kyoto Accord on global warming highlighted the problems faced by public health practitioners when dealing with global issues. The USA, a major contributor to the global problem, declined to take part in the treaty which addressed the projected impact of global warming, preferring to protect national economic growth, even though this sustained growth will further exacerbate the environmental problem and its public health consequences. It remains to be seen how seriously the post-Kyoto discussions address global climate changes, especially given the recent global financial turmoil.

The general issue, and one which extends beyond the domain of public health, is the sustainability of human society; the over-consumption of natural resources by people in wealthy countries severely constrains the ability of poor populations to improve their standard of living (Chapter 1) [16]. Given the low likelihood of technical solutions to global environmental issues, the only long-term solution is for wealthy populations to reduce the extravagant nature of their standard of living and the over-consumption of natural resources on which it is based. We urgently need to move towards sustainable global patterns of living, rather than those based on excessive consumption by a minority.

The public health workforce

The public health workforce contributes to the organization, delivery, and evaluation of health services directed towards both individuals and populations. All countries have a public health workforce using a variety of organizational structures [17]. An effective public health workforce is essential for the task of improving health system performance, especially in low- and middle-income countries. It is also central to the process of building intersectoral activities to ensure that the underlying determinants of population health status are addressed [18].

The public health workforce is characterized by its diversity and complexity; it includes people from a wide range of occupational backgrounds who are involved in protecting, promoting, and/or restoring the collective health of whole or specific populations (as distinct from activities directed to the care of individuals) [19]. In a few countries, notably the USA, it is also involved in ensuring patient care for poor populations.

The second major theme from the earlier chapters is that in all countries and regions described in this book, the public health workforce is not in a position to respond appropriately to the old, let alone the new, challenges (Chapters 7 and 8). With very few exceptions, governments have neglected public health workforce development and the public health infrastructure in general [20]. For too long workforce issues were left to be solved by the market. There needs to be greater attention to workforce development and retention, including the public health workforce, in the context of a much greater international mobility of health workers [21].

In all countries the proportion of the health budget allocated to public health activities is less than 5 per cent, and usually of the order of 1–2 per cent. This deplorable state of affairs is found in wealthy countries, such as the USA where the public health system has been seriously under-funded for more than 30 years [22], and to an even greater extent in poor countries. Workforce issues are complex and include size, composition, balance between medical and other health science graduates, training methods and skills acquisition, and migration. Secure career pathways and appropriate remuneration packages are of great importance in all countries. In addition, training programmes require evaluation and the performance of the workforce requires assessment. Building the public health workforce is a long-term undertaking and will require a substantial commitment of new resources from both recipient countries and donor agencies.

The scope of public health

The third theme is the need to clarify the scope of public health practice. All would agree that public health extends well outside the health sector, yet we are hampered by insufficient experience of effective intersectoral action and a lack of preparation for confronting the new challenges. The development and implementation of comprehensive tobacco control policies in many countries provides one positive example. The World Bank [23] has played an important role in developing the evidence base for essential economic policies for effective tobacco control, especially in low- and middle-income countries, and philanthropic foundations are also getting involved [24]. The WHO Framework Convention on Tobacco Control is the first public health treaty initiated by the Organization and has ramifications well beyond the health sector [25].

The renaissance of public health

The fourth theme from earlier chapters offers some cause for optimism. There are grounds for suggesting that a renaissance of public health is underway [1]. In Sweden (Chapter 4), and to a lesser extent in the UK (Chapter 3) and in Australia and New Zealand (Chapter 11), there is political support for public health and an expressed determination to confront health inequalities. However, translating this rhetoric into effective programmes is much more difficult and serious progress is yet to be achieved. Sweden offers a positive example based on cross-party political support (Chapter 4).

Fortunately, there are effective interventions against the few diseases which account for most of the excess premature mortality in poor populations [26]. It is increasingly recognized that achieving high coverage of these interventions requires not only new financial resources, but also a well-functioning health system. The public health infrastructure is a key component of health systems. In the effort to support the delivery of vertical disease control programmes, this infrastructure has been neglected and marginalized. However, there are examples of innovative approaches to public health training [27] that may herald the strengthening of the public health workforce in low- and middle-income countries (Chapters 8 and 10).

From a global perspective, health improvement is increasingly on the development agenda. This new focus on health is due in large part to the efforts of WHO and its effective advocacy for health improvement as a key component of economic and social development in poor countries [28]. This advocacy has contributed to the development of the Global Fund to Fight AIDS, Tuberculosis, and Malaria [29], the Report of the Commission on Macroeconomics and Health [30], and the Report of the Commission on the Social Determinants of Health [18]. It seems that momentum is being maintained and increased resources are becoming available (at least for infectious diseases and maternal and child health), including from the USA [31].

A vision for public health

There are at least five interrelated general features which would characterize a reinvigorated practice of public health.

- Public health practitioners will lead the response to immediate health crises, for example HIV/AIDS, and to emerging problems such as the health impact of global environmental change and the pandemic of chronic diseases.

- Public health practitioners will lead the ongoing health sector reforms which, in turn, will be driven by the need to improve population health and health equity, rather than by the need to contain costs.
- Public health practitioners will be promoting and leading intersectoral actions for health improvement and health equity.
- Public health research, training, and practice will be a high priority in all health services and there will be adequate resources for public health practitioners to tackle a broad agenda. Public health research will clarify the ways diverse policies affect the health of the public. Public health practice will underpin timely and policy relevant information and surveillance systems for both communicable and chronic diseases and will be informed by global and regional perspectives.
- The values of public health will be explicit, and mutually reinforcing interactions will be established between practitioners, clinicians, and the communities they serve.

Achieving this vision

Broadening the scope of public health

A critical step in the reinvigoration of public health practice is for the workforce, in all its diversity, to affirm its professional commitment to a broad view of its mission, including the values of equity and ecological sustainability [32]. A useful beginning to this process would be to include such issues in all public health training programmes and to shift the focus of public health practice to overall population health improvement. Reducing social and economic deprivation has the potential to reduce the readily preventable burden of disease, both communicable and chronic, especially among disadvantaged groups. Public health scientists and practitioners can contribute to this goal by clarifying the links between social and economic factors and health status [18], identifying cost-effective approaches to overall health improvement [26], and being advocates for appropriate policies [33].

The deplorable health conditions of the poorest countries are now receiving increased attention, as are the major health inequalities in wealthy countries [18]. Achieving the goal of halving the number of people living in absolute poverty by the year 2015, the main Millennium Development Goal adopted at the Millennium Summit of the United Nations in September 2000, would do more to reduce health inequalities and improve global health status than any other measure. Although considerable progress has been made in China, this goal will not be reached in sub-Saharan Africa, given the still limited international financial commitments to sustainable development [34]. The achievement of this and other broad health goals will require major new resources. These, in turn, depend on the strong global political leadership which has been demonstrated around more specific infectious disease goals [29]. In the face of pressing disease treatment priorities and the desire for short-term results, most of the resources have so far been directed towards treatment programmes for the three specific diseases for which the Global Fund was established. Fortunately, there is now a growing emphasis on supporting health systems infrastructures [35].

The Report of the Commission on Macroeconomics and Health, published by the WHO in 2001, made a strong case for improving the health of the poor on economic grounds as well as, of course, on direct humanitarian grounds [30]. For example, the Commission suggested that endemic malaria is responsible for at least a 1 per cent per year lower growth rate than would be the case in the absence of the disease; these lower growth rates compound and, over time, have a major effect on national wealth creation. The Commission was forthright in its condemnation of the neglect of international health development by wealthy countries. It argued for large new contributions from the international donor community to support low-income and a few middle-income countries to improve the health status of their populations. While low- and middle-income countries themselves need to contribute to this endeavour, because of their fragile economies and debt burdens, much of the initial resources for health improvement will have to come from wealthy countries. Substantial new resources for health development have been made available by wealthy countries, development agencies, and foundations over the last decade [36], although there are questions about its allocation [37]. It is still a challenge for many poor countries to build the necessary political will to increase their budgetary commitments to health services and ensure effective governance for health. The WHO Commission on the Social Determinants of Health provides an important complementary approach to health development [18]. The importance of foreign policy to health development is only now realized and needs further support, especially in difficult financial times [38].

Strengthening the practice of public health

The core public health activities are monitoring population health status and its determinants, prevention and control of disease, injury, and disability, health promotion, and protection of the environment [39]. As we have seen in earlier chapters, few of the core public health functions are carried out to a high standard even in wealthy countries. The effect of the increased attention to essential public health functions, especially in Canada and Latin America

(Chapters 6 and 7), is yet to be assessed, especially among disadvantaged populations.

There are several reasons for the poor performance of public health practice. The recent ideological ascendancy of neoliberalism has narrowed the focus of public health; responsibility for health is increasingly located at the personal level as national authorities attempt to reduce their costs [40]. However, the determinants of health, and the most powerful means of health improvement, are increasingly located at the global and regional levels [18]. Since most public health work lies outside the conventional market framework and remains the responsibility of governments, its 'public good' nature must be stressed. The concept of global public goods for health is gaining acceptance, and this might assist the improvement of public health practice [41].

WHO is promoting the concept of stewardship of the health system whereby governments have a duty to provide overall leadership for the health system in terms of vision, priorities, and regulatory climate, irrespective of whether the funding for the system comes in full or in part from government sources [35].

The lack of an effective response to health inequalities highlights the current lack of leadership provided by most governments. Reducing health inequalities requires action on the underlying structural determinants of social and economic deprivation [42]. This approach is notably absent from government agendas, and public health efforts are mostly targeted at the health effects of exclusion [43]. These programmes are acceptable politically but they are not sufficient. Serious intersectoral action is required, as recently advocated by the Commission on the Social Determinants of Health [18]. Unfortunately, public health practitioners are not skilled in this type of work; it should be taught and researched in all academic public health programmes.

Reinvigorating public health teaching and research

Public health training has a long history, primarily in Europe and in North and Latin America [44,45]. The Rockefeller Foundation was instrumental in establishing many of the most prestigious schools of public health in the early decades of the last century [46]. More recently, WHO, UNICEF, and other international organizations have made major contributions to the training of health personnel in low- and middle-income countries. However, most of this effort has focused on the training of junior health personnel rather than on public health workers with a relevant postgraduate degree [47–50]. The International Clinical Epidemiology Network (INCLEN), initiated by the Rockefeller Foundation in the mid-1980s, focused over a 20-year period on providing epidemiological skills for physicians, but failed to address the needs for a modern public health workforce in a resource constrained setting [51].

From the perspective of low- and middle-income countries, traditional approaches to public health training have several limitations [52]:

- the emphasis on epidemiology and biostatistics and the relative neglect of other public health sciences;
- the isolation from ministries of health, other health providers, local communities, and other relevant scientific disciplines;
- the emphasis on institution-based teaching and the lack of direct field experience;
- the lack of public health practitioners in the field as role models;
- the consideration of public health as a medical speciality;
- the high cost of the training programmes in North America and Europe.

There is a need to reconnect public health education and research with public health practice. All too often academics, divorced from the communities they serve, have concentrated on research issues of questionable relevance to overall population health improvement and the reduction of health inequalities [53]. It is time to move beyond the exquisite refinement of causal associations and the search for new risk factors, for example for cardiovascular disease, and to focus more on understanding why whole populations are at risk of specific disease constellations [54]. There is also a need to support the broad scope of public health teaching and to resist the temptation to allow molecular epidemiology, clinical epidemiology, and health services management to dominate training and research programmes. An innovative project began in 1992 with the launch of the Public Health Schools Without Walls (PHSWOW) initiative in Africa (Box 14.1), later expanding to Asia. The programme was driven by the energy and initiative of the Rockefeller Foundation; CDC field-based training experience in epidemiology was also of conceptual importance to the new programme [55,56]. The guiding principle of the initiative was that public health training should be provided through a combination of rigorous academic and supervised practical experience, with a focus on the capacity to pursue rather than memorize knowledge [52].

Public health leadership

Strong political and professional leadership is essential to capitalize on the potential for the reinvigoration of public health practice. At the international level there is some cause for optimism. The WHO is highly regarded as a UN inter-governmental agency and has led several recent important global health initiatives: reinvigorating the response to HIV/AIDS and other infectious diseases, revising the International Health Regulations, and successfully ensuring the widespread acceptance of the Framework Convention on Tobacco Control.

Box 14.1 Public Health Schools Without Walls

The PHSWOW programme, and others like it (Chapter 10), aimed to train graduates competent to respond to practical health problems and to manage health services, especially at the district level. To achieve this goal, the ministry of health plays a significant role in these programmes. A feature of the PHSWOW curricula is the substantial period of supervised field training, up to 75 per cent of the course. During this time trainees are expected to acquire and demonstrate competence in key areas, including the ability to investigate important local health problems, design, manage, and evaluate health programmes, assess and control environmental hazards, and communicate effectively with colleagues, individuals, communities, and policy-makers.

An evaluation of the programme concluded that, despite the lack of clear initial goals and milestones for evaluation, the PHSWOW achievements could provide one foundation on which to build public health capacity in developing countries [57]. This programme has led to sustained advances in public health training in both Africa and Asia.

WHO has now embarked on an ambitious, and long overdue, effort to strengthen health systems based on a renewed emphasis on primary health care [58].

Until recently, WHO was the only global public health agency. The situation is now vastly more complicated, with WHO only one of more than a hundred global health agencies. Over the last three decades the World Bank has become a major actor, and not always a positive influence. Other key players are UNAIDS, UNICEF, the UN Population Fund, governmental agencies (USAID, SIDA, CIDA, JAICA, and DIFID), funds (Global Fund to Fight HIV/AIDS, Tuberculosis and Malaria, GAVI), foundations (Bill and Melinda Gates, Open Society Institute working with national Soros Foundations, Instituto Carso de la Salud, Doris Duke, Bloomberg Philanthropies) and a host of other organizations and NGOs, public and private, most of whom have very focused priorities.

The strengthening of global leadership will lead to stronger leadership of public health practice at the regional, national, and local levels. An educational focus on public health leadership in low-and middle-income countries is also required to ensure the development of the next generation of leaders who will place public health firmly on their country's agenda.

Modern electronic communication technology can build and support leadership and networks; creative technical and financial innovations are required to overcome the 'digital divide', especially in sub-Saharan Africa and South Asia [59]. Training centres in developed countries could contribute to distance learning programmes based on the full range of modern technology to support the goals of the training programmes in developing countries. The People's Open Access Education Initiative (People's-uni) is helping to build public health capacity using Internet-based e-learning, which has the potential to deliver high-quality learning resources any time and anywhere; although Internet access is by no means universal, it is improving quickly [60].

In many countries, academic public health specialists have the independence and autonomy to play a major public health leadership role. Closer ties between academic public health researchers and public health practitioners at the national level will also increase the value of this research. The credibility of public health professionals will be strengthened by closer partnerships with communities, their representatives, and other agencies working at the local level [61]. Full community participation in public health activities is the key to more responsive and effective programmes (Chapter 13). However, moving from the traditional top-down approach to health-improvement strategies to a more inclusive model will be difficult for most public health practitioners, and this emphasizes the importance of a new approach to public health educational programmes.

Responding to globalization

Public health practitioners can no longer ignore the impact of globalization on the determinants of population health status at the national level [62]. The key issue is the impact of the liberalization of trade rules on poverty, especially in poor countries. Increasing the developing world's share of global trade would do more to lift people out of poverty than increased aid spending [63]. Can the WTO Multilateral Trade Agreements be interpreted in a way that shifts the balance from protecting the economies of wealthy countries to promoting development where it is most needed [64,65]? Can the huge European Union and US subsidies for agriculture be reduced as part of the stalled Doha round of negotiations in favour of easier access for products from developing countries, without imposing new conditions [66]? These issues have major health implications for poor countries but are only now getting on to the public health agenda.

Comprehensive research and action agendas are required on the globalization and health interface. For example, what are the public health implications of the WTO Multilateral Trade Agreements [67]? What are the health impacts of the global marketing of energy-dense food products, alcohol, and tobacco? What will be the major health effects of global environmental changes?

The tools available for understanding the process and effects of globalization on population health status are still rudimentary, although environmental health scientists are leading the way. This research agenda provides an exciting opportunity for public health practitioners to take the initiative and position themselves at the forefront of civil society's response to globalization. Until now, the response has been lead by civil society groups who have, for example, made progress by increasing access to affordable drugs which had been constrained by the WTO agreement on intellectual property rights (TRIPS). The response from the pubic health community to most globalization and health issues has been, at best, muted [28].

The challenge for the international public health research community is to establish a mechanism for facilitating research that extends beyond national boundaries, perhaps through a new style of cooperative research—the public health equivalent of the Human Genome Project. The WHO is in an ideal position to lead this collaborative research agenda. It could usefully establish a globalization and health research database and associated website that would include relevant datasets from a range of disciplines and a registry of ongoing and completed research projects. An important research question, and one that the WHO is uniquely qualified to address, is the need to use more comprehensive surveillance data for the full range of diseases at a regional level and to collect new data unconstrained by national boundaries. The research endeavour, as with any another public health problem, is only the first step; it must go hand in hand with the appropriate public health response. The incorporation of the results of this research into education and learning programmes will ensure that the next generation of public health professionals is better equipped to address these emerging global issues.

Both scientists and policy-makers face unfamiliar and difficult challenges in addressing these broad public health issues. It is important to continue to identify, quantify, and reduce the risks to health that result from specific, often localized, social, behavioural, and environmental factors. It is also important to be increasingly alert to the influences on population health which arise from today's larger-scale social and economic processes and global environmental disturbances. Research within this framework will enhance the capacity to manage social and natural environments in ways that support and sustain population health.

Conclusion

The ultimate goal for public health practitioners is to ensure that the public health perspective is integrated into all health, social, and economic policies and programmes. Ideally, all public policy should have an explicit commitment to overall health improvement, health equity, and the sustainability of human societies. These goals are a long way from being realized, in part because this vision is not shared and the public health workforce is not yet equipped for these tasks.

As earlier chapters have emphasized, the challenges facing public health practitioners are huge. However, a reasonably optimistic future for public health can be predicted: several innovative public health training activities are underway, health is now high up the international development agenda, and major new funds for health improvement have been established [1]. The vision for public health outlined in this book is both necessary and achievable. Hopefully, as the reinvigoration of public health practice gathers pace, the public health perspective will become more central to the development process.

References

[1] Beaglehole R, Bonita R. Global public health: a scorecard. *Lancet* 2008; **372**; 1988–96.

[2] Horton R, Das P. Putting prevention at the forefront of HIV/AIDS. *Lancet* 2008; **372**: 421–2.

[3] Jahn S, Floyd S, Crampin AC, et al. Population-level effect of HIV on adult mortality and early evidence of reversal after introduction of antiretroviral therapy in Malawi. *Lancet* 2008; **371**: 1603–11.

[4] Clark S, Spencer S. Thailand glimpses success. *Lancet* 2004; **364**: 319–20.

[5] Beaglehole R, Epping-Jordan J, Chopra M, et al. Improving the management of chronic disease in low- and middle- income countries: a priority for primary health care. *Lancet* 2008; **372**: 940–9.

[6] Abegunde DO, Mathers CD, Adam T, Ortegon M, Strong K. The global burden and costs of chronic diseases. *Lancet* 2007: **370**: 1929–38.

[7] Caldwell JC. Routes to low mortality in poor countries. *Popul Dev Rev* 1986; **12**: 171–220.

[8] Stuckler D. Population causes and consequences of leading chronic diseases: a comparative analysis of prevailing explanations. *Millbank Q* 2008; **86**: 273–326.

[9] Kawachi I, Wamala S (eds). *Globalization and Health*. Oxford University Press, 2007.

[10] Ellsberg M, Jansen HAFM, Heise L, *et al.* Intimate partner violence and women's physical and mental health in the WHO multi-country study on women's health and domestic violence: an observational study. *Lancet* 2008; **371**; 1165–72.

[11] McMichael AJ, Woodruff RE, Hales S. Climate change and human health: present and future risks. *Lancet* 2006; **367**; 859–69.

[12] Frieden T, Bloomberg M. How to prevent 100 million deaths from tobacco. *Lancet* 2007; **369**: 1758–61.

[13] Anonymous. Curbing the obesity epidemic (editorial). *Lancet* 2006; **367**: 1549.

[14] Intergovernmental Panel on Climate Change (WGI). *Climate Change, 2007: The Science of Climate Change: Contribution of Working Group I to the Second Assessment Report of the Intergovernmental Panel on Climate Change*. Cambridge University Press, 2007.

[15] Lomborg B. *The Sceptical Environmentalist*. Cambridge: Cambridge University Press, 2001.

[16] McMichael AJ, Friel S, Nyong A, Corvalan C. Global environmental change and health: impacts, inequalities, and the health sector. *BMJ* 2008: **336**; 191–4.

[17] Porter D (ed.) *The History of Public Health and the Modern State*. Amsterdam: Rodopi, 1994.

[18] Commission on Social Determinants of Health. Closing the Gap in a Generation: Health Equity through Action on The Social Determinants of Health. *Final Report of the Commission on Social Determinants of Health*. Geneva: WHO, 2008.

[19] Rotem A et al. *The Public Health Workforce Education and Training Study: Overview of Findings*. Canberra: Australian Government Publishing Service, 1995.

[20] Beaglehole R, Dal Poz MR. Public health workforce: challenges and policy issues. *Hum Resour Health* 2003; **1**: 4.

[21] Omaswa F. Human resources for global health: time for action is now. *Lancet* 2008; **371**: 625–6.

[22] Nelson R. USA faces severe shortage of public-health workers. *Lancet Infect Dis* 2008; **8**: 281.

[23] World Bank. *Curbing the Epidemic*. Washington, DC: World Bank, 2000.

[24] WHO. *WHO Report on the Global Tobacco Epidemic, 2008: The MPOWER Package*. Geneva: WHO, 2008.

[25] Bettcher D DeLand K, Schlundt J, *et al*. International public health instruments. In: Detels R et al. (eds). Oxford: *Oxford Textbook of Public Health* (5th edn). Oxford University Press, 2009.

[26] Jamison DT, Breman JG, Measham AR, *et al*. (eds). *Disease Control Priorities in Developing Countries* (2nd edn). Washington, DC: World Bank and Oxford University Press, 2006.

[27] Sadana R, Petrakova A. Shaping public health education around the world to address health challenges in the coming decades. *Bull WHO* 2007; **85**: 902.

[28] Bonita R, Irwin A, Beaglehole R. Promoting public health in the twenty-first century: the role of the World Health Organization. In: Kawachi I, Wamala S (eds). *Globalization and Health*. Oxford University Press, 2007.

[29] Feachem RGA, Sabot OJ. An examination of the Global Fund at 5 years. *Lancet* 2006; **368**: 537–540.

[30] WHO. *Report of the Commission on Macroeconomics and Health. Macroeconomics and Health: Investing in Health for Development*. Geneva: WHO, 2001

[31] Bristol N. US Senate passes new PEPFAR bill. *Lancet* 2008; **372**: 277–8.

[32] Stuckler D, McKee M. Five metaphors about global-health policy. *Lancet* 2008; **372**: 95–7.

[33] Chapman S. *Public Health Advocacy and Tobacco Control: Making Smoking History*. Oxford: Blackwell, 2007.

[34] World Bank. New data show 1.4 billion live on less tha US$1.25 a day, but progress against poverty remains strong. Press Release, 26 August 2008. Available online at: http://web.worldbank.org/WBSITE/EXTERNAL/NEWS/0 (accessed 10 September 2008).

[35] WHO. *Everybody's Business. Strengthening Health Systems To Improve Health Outcomes. WHO's Framework for Action*. Available online at: http://www.wpro.who.int/NR/rdonlyres/5BA80B95-DC1F-4427-8E8B-0D9B1E9AF776/0/EB.pdf (accessed 15 May 2008).

[36] Kates J, Morrison JS, Lief E. Global health funding: a glass half full? *Lancet* 2006; **368**: 187–8.

[37] Sridar D, Batniji R. Misfinancing global health: a case for transparency in disbursements and decision making. *Lancet* 2008; **372**: 1185–91.

[38] Ministers of Foreign Affairs of Brazil, France, Indonesia, Norway, Senegal, South Africa, and Thailand. Oslo Ministerial Declaration—global health: a pressing foreign policy issue of our time. *Lancet* 2007; **369**: 1373–8.

[39] Bettcher DW, Sapirie SA, Goon EHT. Essential public health functions. *World Health Stat Q* 1998; **51**: 44–54.

[40] Beaglehole R, Bonita R. *Public Health at the Crossroads: Achievements and Prospects* (2nd edn). Cambridge: Cambridge University Press, 2002.

[41] Smith R, Beaglehole R, Drager N (eds). *Global Public Goods for Health*. Oxford: Oxford University Press, 2003.

[42] Kawachi I, Wamala S. Poverty and inequality in a globalizing world. In: Kawachi I, Wamala S (eds). *Globalization and Health*. Oxford: Oxford University Press, 2007.

[43] McKinlay JB, Marceau LD. A tale of 3 tails. *Am J Public Health*. 1999; **89**: 295–8.

[44] Fee E, Acheson R (eds). *A History of Education in Public Health: Health that Mocks the Doctors' Rules*. Oxford: Oxford University Press, 1991.

[45] Pan American Health Organization. Development of Public Health Education: Challenges for the 21st Century. *Nineteenth Conference of the Latin American and Caribbean Association of Public Health Education (ALAESP)*, Havana, 2–4 July 2000.

[46] Brown ER. *Rockefeller Medicine Men*. Berkeley, CA: University of California Press, 1980.

[47] WHO. *Health Manpower Requirements for the Achievement of Health for All by Year 2000. WHO Technical Report Series 717*. Geneva: WHO, 1985.

[48] WHO. *Regulatory Mechanisms for Nursing Training and Practice Meeting Primary Health Needs. WHO Technical Report Series 738*. Geneva: WHO, 1986.

[49] WHO. *Strengthening the Performance of Community Health Workers in Primary Health Care. WHO Technical Report Series 780*. Geneva: WHO, 1989.

[50] WHO. *Management of Human Resources for Health. WHO Technical Report Series 783*. Geneva: WHO, 1989.

[51] White KL. *Healing the Schism. Epidemiology, Medicine, and the Public's Health*. New York: Springer, 1991.

[52] Bertrand WE. *Public Health Schools Without Walls: New Directions for Public Health Resourcing(draft)*. New York: Rockefeller Foundation, March 1999.

[53] Pearce N. Traditional epidemiology, modern epidemiology, and public health. *Am J Pub Health* 1996; **86**: 678–83.

[54] Beaglehole R, Magnus P. The search for new risk factors for coronary heart disease: occupational therapy for epidemiologists. *Int J Epidemiol* 2002; **31**: 1117–21, 1134–5.

[55] Music SI, Schultz MG. Field epidemiology training programs: new international health resources. *JAMA* 1990; **263**: 3309–11.

[56] Goodman RA, Buchler JW, Koplan JP. The epidemiological field investigation. Science and judgement in public health practice. *Am J Epidemiol* 1990; 132: 9–16.

[57] Rockefeller Foundation. *Report to the Rockefeller Foundation. Enhancing Public Health in Developing Countries*. New York: Rockefeller Foundation, 2001.

[58] WHO. *Now More Than Ever. The World Health Report, 2008*. Geneva: WHO, 2008.

[59] Chandrasekhar CP, Ghosh J. Information and communication technologies and health in low income countries: the potential and the constraints. *Bull WHO* 2001; **79**: 850–5.

[60] http://peoples-uni.org (accessed 28 October, 2008).

[61] Raeburn J, Rootman I. *People-Centred Health Promotion*. Chichester: John Wiley, 1997.

[62] Erikson SL. Getting political: fighting for global health. *Lancet* 2008; **371**: 1229–30.

[63] Drager N, Fidler D. Foreign policy, trade, and health: at the cutting edge of global health diplomacy. *Bull WHO* 2007; **85**: 162.

[64] Bloche MG, Jungman ER. Health policy and the World Trade Organization. In: Kawachi I, Wamala S (eds). *Globalization and Health*. Oxford: Oxford University Press, 2007.

[65] Pollock AM, Price D. Market forces in public health. *Lancet* 2002; **359**: 1363–4.

[66] Lang T, Lobstein T, Robertson A, Baumhofer E. Building a healthy CAP. *Eurohealth* 2001; **7**: 34–40.

[67] Ransom K, Beaglehole R, Correa C, et al. The public health implications of the WTO multilateral trade agreements. In: Lee K, Buse K, Fustkian S (eds). *Crossing Boundaries: Health Policy in a Globalising World*. Cambridge: Cambridge University Press, 2002.

Index

Lightning Source UK Ltd.
Milton Keynes UK
UKOW04f1809151013